AF691114

Neuropsychiatric Disorders

Koho Miyoshi • Yasushi Morimura
Kiyoshi Maeda
Editors

Neuropsychiatric Disorders

Springer

Editors
Koho Miyoshi, M.D., Ph.D.
Director
Jinmeikai Research Institute for Mental Health
53-20 Kabutoyama-cho, Nishinomiya
Hyogo 662-0001, Japan

The former Professor
Department of Neuropsychiatry
Kyoto University Graduate School of Medicine
Kyoto, Japan

Yasushi Morimura, M.D, Ph.D.
Chief Executive Officer
Jinmeikai Foundation and Hospital
53-20 Kabutoyama-cho, Nishinomiya
Hyogo 662-0001, Japan

Ohmura Hospital
200 Kitayama-Ohmura, Miki
Hyogo 673-0404, Japan

Kiyoshi Maeda, M.D., Ph.D.
Professor
Department of Occupational Therapy
Kobe Gakuin University School of Rehabilitation
518 Ikawadani-cho, Nishi-ku
Kobe 651-2180, Japan

ISBN 978-4-431-53870-7 e-ISBN 978-4-431-53871-4
DOI 10.1007/978-4-431-53871-4
Springer Tokyo Dordrecht Heidelberg London New York

Library of Congress Control Number: 2010924621

© Springer 2010
This work is subject to copyright. All rights are reserved, whether the whole or part of the material is concerned, specifically the rights of translation, reprinting, reuse of illustrations, recitation, broadcasting, reproduction on microfilm or in any other way, and storage in data banks.
The use of general descriptive names, registered names, trademarks, etc. in this publication does not imply, even in the absence of a specific statement, that such names are exempt from the relevant protective laws and regulations and therefore free for general use.
Product liability: The publishers cannot guarantee the accuracy of any information about dosage and application contained in this book. In every individual case the user must check such information by consulting the relevant literature.

Printed on acid-free paper

Springer is part of Springer Science+Business Media (www.springer.com)

Preface

Neuropsychiatry is an integrating neuroscience of neurology and psychiatry that aims to investigate the psychiatric symptoms of neurological disorders as well as the neurobiological bases of psychiatric disorders, including organic mental disorders and endogenous psychoses. Additionally, neuropsychiatry aims to prevent or reduce the suffering of individuals with the psychiatric symptoms of cerebral disorders. The International Organization of Neuropsychiatry (ION), the forerunner of the current association, was established in Seville in 1996 and was reorganized as the International Neuropsychiatric Association (INA) in Toronto in 1998. Since then, it has continued to provide a forum for exchanging knowledge acquired by scientific activities in the field to accomplish the purposes of the association. Toward that end, international congresses have been held every 2 years in cities around the world: Seville (1996), Toronto (1998), Kyoto (2000), Buenos Aires (2002), Athens (2004), Sydney (2006), and Cancun (2008). In addition to the international congresses, regional congresses of neuropsychiatry have been organized regularly in Europe and Latin America. All the meetings have been successful and fruitful in stimulating progress in neuropsychiatry. As one of the results of the meetings, the monograph *Contemporary Neuropsychiatry* was published by Springer Japan in 2001.

This present monograph consists of papers from the Kobe Conference of the International Neuropsychiatric Association, which was held by the International Neuropsychiatric Association in collaboration with the Jinmeikai Foundation and the Japan Neuropsychiatric Association in Kobe, September 12–13, 2009. The meeting was originally planned to be a semi-closed workshop for the publication of this monograph in neuropsychiatry. Because the meeting was organized to be held between two international congresses of neuropsychiatry – the 7th INA Congress in Cancun (2008) and the 8th INA Congress in Chennai (2011) – it was planned so as to concentrate on rather limited areas of neuropsychiatry, namely, the clinical aspects of neuropsychiatric disorders.

As the editors, we are confident that this publication will stimulate further progress and research in neuropsychiatry in all parts of the world. We express our heartfelt gratitude for the contributions by all the authors who attended the meeting and submitted papers. We are very pleased to have received their excellent work in neuropsychiatry for this publication. We express our special appreciation to Dr. Perminder Sachdev, who allowed us to publish "The Core Curriculum of Neuropsychiatry," which originally appeared on the website of the International Neuropsychiatric Association in 2004, for standardizing the guidelines of training in neuropsychiatry.

We would like to acknowledge the support for the Kobe Conference of the International Neuropsychiatric Association by the Jinmeikai Foundation, Ohmura Hospital, the Federation of Pharmaceutical Manufacturers Association of Japan, the Osaka Pharmaceutical Manufacturers Association, Kaiseikai (Japan Psychiatric Association for Partnership), the Kobe Convention and Visitors Association, the Tsutomu-Nakauchi Foundation, Japan Eisai Pharmaceutical Company, Japan Pfizer Pharmaceutical Company, Japan Janssen Pharmaceutical Company, and Japan Eli Lilly Pharmaceutical Company.

Koho Miyoshi, M.D., Ph.D.
Yasushi Morimura, M.D., Ph.D.
Kiyoshi Maeda, M.D., Ph.D.
Editors

Contents

Contributors

Emmeline Agars
Brain and Ageing Program, School of Psychiatry, University of New South Wales, Sydney, NSW, Australia

David B. Arciniegas
Brain Injury Rehabilitation Unit, HealthONE Spalding Rehabilitation Hospital, Aurora, CO, USA;
Department of Psychiatry, University of Colorado School of Medicine, Aurora, CO, USA

Simone Brockman
School of Psychiatry and Clinical Neurosciences, University of Western Australia, Perth, WA, Australia;
Fremantle Hospital, Fremantle, WA, Australia

Luis Ignacio Brusco
Alzheimer Center, School of Medicine, Buenos Aires University, Buenos Aires, Argentina

Robertas Bunevičius
Institute of Psychophysiology and Rehabilitation, Kaunas University of Medicine, Palanga, Lithuania

Anthony S. David
Department of Psychiatry, Section of Cognitive Neuropsychiatry, Institute of Psychiatry, King's College London, London, UK

Masaaki Fukutake
Department of Psychiatry, Kobe University School of Medicine, Kobe, Japan

Eduardo Gastelumendi
Peruvian Psychiatric Society; Peruvian Psychoanalytic Society, Lima, Perú

Moises Gaviria
Department of Psychiatry, University of Illinois at Chicago, Chicago, IL, USA;
Advocate Christ Medical Center, Oak Lawn, IL, USA

James Gilleen
Department of Psychiatry, Section of Cognitive Neuropsychiatry, Institute of Psychiatry, King's College London, London, UK

Kathryn Greenwood
Department of Psychiatry, Section of Cognitive Neuropsychiatry, Institute of Psychiatry, King's College London, London, UK

Takashi Haraguchi
Department of Neurology, South Okayama Medical Center, Okayama, Japan

Ryota Hashimoto
Department of Psychiatry, Osaka University Medical School, Suita, Japan

Akira Homma
Department of Psychiatry, Center for Dementia Care Research and Training in Tokyo, Tokyo Metropolitan Institute of Gerontology, Tokyo, Japan

Hideki Ishizu
Zikei Hospital, Okayama, Japan

Michael D. Kopelman
Institute of Psychiatry, King's College London, London, UK;
Academic Unit of Neuropsychiatry, Adamson Centre, London, UK

Kenji Kosaka
Yokohama Houyuu Hospital, Yokohama, Japan

Takashi Kudo
Department of Psychiatry, Osaka University Medical School, Suita, Japan

Shigetoshi Kuroda
Zikei Hospital, Okayama, Japan;
Department of Neuropsychiatry, Okayama University Graduate School of Medicine, Dentistry and Pharmaceutical Sciences, Okayama, Japan

Kiyoshi Maeda
Department of Occupational Therapy, Kobe Gakuin University School of Rehabilitation, Kobe, Japan

Ian Grant McKeith
Wolfson Research Centre, Institute for Ageing and Health, Newcastle University, Campus for Ageing and Vitality, Newcastle upon Tyne, UK

Yoshio Mitsuyama
Psychogeriatric Center of Daigo Hospital, Miyazaki, Japan

Koho Miyoshi
Jinmeikai Research Institute for Mental Health, Nishinomiya, Hyogo, Japan;
The former Professor, Department of Neuropsychiatry, Kyoto University Graduate School of Medicine, Kyoto, Japan

Takashi Morihara
Department of Psychiatry, Osaka University Medical School, Suita, Japan

Yasushi Morimura
Jinmeikai Foundation and Hospital, Nishinomiya, Japan

Yoshio Morita
Department of Neuropsychiatry, Hyogo College of Medicine, Nishinomiya, Japan

Marco Mula
Division of Neurology, Maggiore Hospital, Amedeo Avogadro University, Novara, Italy

Naoki Nishiguchi
Department of Neuropsychiatry, Kinki University School of Medicine, Osakasayama, Japan

Yoshitaka Ohigashi
International Center, Graduate School of Human and Environmental Studies, Kyoto University, Kyoto, Japan

Masayasu Okochi
Department of Psychiatry, Osaka University Medical School, Suita, Japan

Spyridon Papapetropoulos
Department of Neurology, Miller School of Medicine, University of Miami, Miami, FL, USA;
Biogen Idec, Cambridge, MA, USA

Arthur J. Prange, Jr.
Department of Psychiatry, University of North Carolina at Chapel Hill, NC, USA

Perminder Sachdev
School of Psychiatry, University of New South Wales, Sydney, NSW, Australia;
Neuropsychiatric Institute, Prince of Wales Hospital, Euroa Centre, Randwick, NSW, Australia

Blake K. Scanlon
Department of Neurology, Miller School of Medicine, University of Miami, Miami, FL, USA;
Department of Psychology, University of Miami, Coral Gables, FL, USA

Osamu Shirakawa
Department of Neuropsychiatry, Kinki University School of Medicine, Osakasayama, Japan

Ingmar Skoog
Neuropsychiatric Epidemiology Unite, Department of Psychiatry,
Institute of Neuroscience and Physiology, Sahlgrenska Academy at Göteborg University, Göteborg, Sweden

Sergio E. Starkstein
School of Psychiatry and Clinical Neurosciences, University of Western Australia, WA, Australia
Fremantle Hospital, Fremantle, WA, Australia

Shinji Tagami
Department of Psychiatry, Osaka University Medical School, Suita, Japan

Masatoshi Takeda
Department of Psychiatry, Osaka University Medical School, Suita, Japan

Yasuyuki Tanabe
Department of Neurology, South Okayama Medical Center, Okayama, Japan

Toshihisa Tanaka
Department of Psychiatry, Osaka University Medical School, Suita, Japan

Seishi Terada
Department of Neuropsychiatry, Okayama University Graduate School of Medicine, Dentistry and Pharmaceutical Sciences, Okayama, Japan

Michael Trimble
Department of Neuropsychiatry, Institute of Neurology, London, UK

Julian Trollor
Brain and Ageing Program, School of Psychiatry, University of New South Wales, Sydney, NSW, Australia;
Department of Developmental Disability Neuropsychiatry, School of Psychiatry, University of New South Wales, Sydney, NSW, Australia

Rhonda DePaul Verzal
Director of Neuropsychiatry, Advocate Christ Medical Center, University of Illinois at Chicago, Chicago, IL, USA

Makiko Yamada
Molecular Imaging Center, National Institute of Radiological Sciences, Chiba, Japan

Osamu Yokota
Department of Neuropsychiatry, Okayama University Graduate School of Medicine, Dentistry and Pharmaceutical Sciences, Okayama, Japan

Part I
Introduction

Clinical Manifestations of Neuropsychiatric Disorders

Koho Miyoshi and Yasushi Morimura

Abstract Cerebral disorders commonly cause psychiatric symptoms. It is recommended to call psychiatric symptoms or syndromes that are caused by organic cerebral disorders "neuropsychiatric symptoms" or "neuropsychiatric syndromes." And, in this context, cerebral disorders, which cause psychiatric symptoms, are called neuropsychiatric disorders. The main characteristics of neuropsychiatric symptoms are (1) concurrent occurrence of the various psychiatric symptoms, (2) cognitive impairment as a core symptom, (3) the possibility of early cerebral symptoms, and (4) occasional resemblance to endogenous psychiatric disorders. The characteristics of neuropsychiatric symptoms, namely, anxiety, neurotic complaint, apathy, mood disorder, hallucinations, delusions, behavioral and personality changes, delirium, and cognitive impairment (dementia), are discussed briefly.

Keywords Cognitive impairment • Dementia • Neuropsychiatric disorders • Neuropsychiatry • Organic psychosis

Introduction

Almost all brain disorders may cause psychiatric symptoms [1]. Psychiatric symptoms caused by organic brain disorders could be called "neuropsychiatric" symptoms. Psychiatric manifestations caused by organic brain disease have been traditionally called organic mental disorders. In DSM-IV-TR, however, the term "organic psychosis" is not applied to the psychosis caused by organic cerebral disorders. Because the "organic" or neurobiological bases of psychoses, including

K. Miyoshi (✉) and Y. Morimura
Jinmeikai Research Institute for Mental Health,
Nishinomiya, Hyogo, Japan
e-mail: RX102704@nifty.com

K. Miyoshi et al. (eds.), *Neuropsychiatric Disorders*,
DOI 10.1007/978-4-431-53871-4_1, © Springer 2010

endogenous psychiatric disorders, have been revealed by recent investigations, it would be recommended not to use the poorly defined term “organic” to avoid implying that mental disorders other than “organic” mental disorders do not have a neurobiological component. Alternatively, the use of the term “neuropsychiatric symptoms” would be recommended to indicate psychiatric symptoms caused by organic cerebral disorders. In this context, organic cerebral disorders or neurological disorders that cause psychiatric symptoms could be called “neuropsychiatric disorders.”

Neuropsychiatric disorder commonly occurs in elderly patients and occasionally mimics endogenous psychoses. Therefore, the organic factors should be carefully evaluated in diagnostic procedures in patients with psychiatric symptoms among the elderly. The clinical manifestations and characteristics of neuropsychiatric symptoms, especially in elderly patients, are briefly discussed in this chapter.

Neuropsychiatric Symptoms and Neuropsychiatric Disorders

Neuropsychiatric symptoms could be defined as psychiatric manifestations of cerebral (neuropsychiatric) disorders. Cerebral disorders cause various psychiatric symptoms.

Some of these symptoms occasionally mimic the psychiatric manifestation of endogenous psychiatric disorders. In ICD-10 [2], psychiatric symptoms caused by organic cerebral disorders are classified as organic (including symptomatic) mental disorders. The psychiatric symptoms described in this classification are as follows: dementia in Alzheimer’s disease, vascular dementia, dementia in other diseases classified elsewhere, unspecific dementia, organic amnestic syndrome, not induced by alcohol and other psychoactive substances, other mental disorders caused by brain damage and dysfunction and by physical illness, including organic hallucinosis, organic catatonic disorder, organic delusional disorder, organic mood disorder, organic anxiety disorder, organic dissociative disorder, organic emotionally labile disorder, mild cognitive disorder, other specific mental disorders, and personality and behavioral disorders resulting from brain disease, damage, and dysfunction.

In the core curriculum of the International Neuropsychiatric Association, neuropsychiatric symptoms and syndromes are also classified as follows: cognitive disorders (dementias and predementia syndromes, nondementing cognitive disorders), seizure disorders, movement disorders, traumatic brain injury, secondary psychiatric disorders (psychosis, depression, mania and anxiety disorders secondary to “organic” brain disease), substance-induced psychiatric disorders, attentional disorders, and sleep disorders.

The core curriculum of the American Neuropsychiatric Association also defines the major neuropsychiatric syndromes as delirium, the dementias, and the major primary psychiatric disorders, including those of learning and communication, and motor skill disorders. Also, neuropsychiatric disorders are defined as neurological disorders with cognitive, emotional, behavioral features; neurodegenerative disorders (dementias), movement disorders, stroke, epilepsy, multiple sclerosis, traumatic brain injury, infections, neuroendocrine disorders, metabolic disorders, intoxication, etc. [3].

The term "neuropsychiatric disorders" should be applied to brain diseases that cause psychiatric symptoms. Therefore, organic cerebral disorders, including neurodegenerative diseases (Alzheimer's disease, frontotemporal lobar degeneration, progressive supranuclear palsy, corticobasal degeneration, Huntington's disease, and Lewy body disease), Creutzfeldt–Jakob disease, cerebrovascular disorders, subdural hematoma, encephalitis, traumatic brain injury, brain tumor, metabolic encephalopathy, intoxication, and normal pressure hydrocephalus, could be called neuropsychiatric disorders.

Characteristics of Clinical Manifestations of Neuropsychiatric Disorders

Multiple Neuropsychiatric Symptoms Occur Simultaneously

Brain diseases commonly cause neurological, neuropsychological, and psychiatric symptoms concurrently in the course of illness (Fig. 1). Therefore, clinical manifestations of the cerebral disorders usually are composed of these three components. Neurological symptoms, such as motor and sensory disturbances, are commonly encountered in neurological disorders. Neuropsychological symptoms, such as aphasia, apraxia, and agnosia, caused by the circumscribed lesion of the cerebrum, commonly occur in cerebral disorders. Also, diffuse lesions of the cerebrum usually cause neuropsychiatric symptoms such as cognitive impairment, mood disorder,

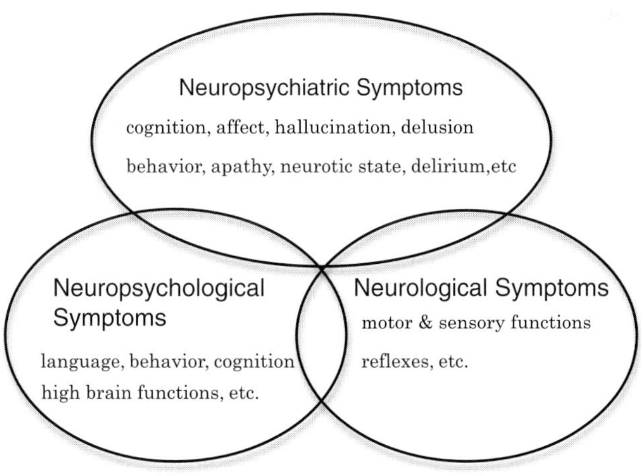

Fig. 1 Structures of the clinical manifestations of cerebral disorders

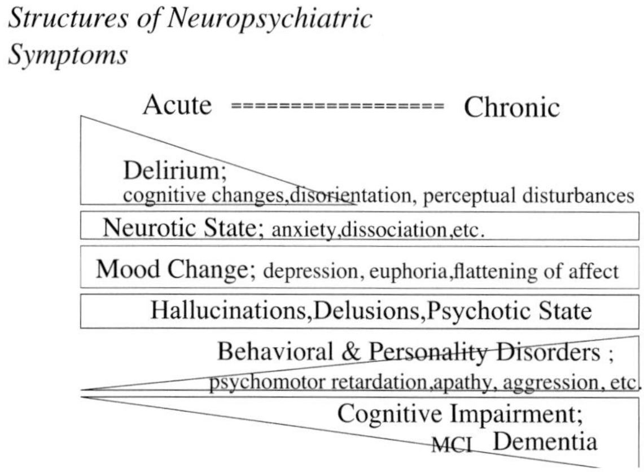

Fig. 2 Structures of the neuropsychiatric symptoms of cerebral disorders

apathy, hallucination, delusion, and behavioral disorders. These three components form complex clinical manifestations of neuropsychiatric disorders.

Multiple neuropsychiatric symptoms, such as cognitive impairment, disturbance of consciousness, anxiety, mood disorders, hallucination, delusion, behavioral change, and apathy, commonly occur concurrently in the course of cerebral disorders (Fig. 2). The psychiatric symptoms are usually accompanied by other psychiatric symptoms. Namely, depression, neurotic states, behavioral changes, apathy, and cognitive impairment occur simultaneously in Alzheimer's disease, and mood change, apathy, visual hallucination, and cognitive impairment are encountered concurrently in patients with Parkinson's disease. Any of the neuropsychiatric symptoms rarely occur independently in the course of illness. Clinical manifestations of neuropsychiatric disorders usually consist of the multiple components of psychiatric symptoms.

Probable and Possible Symptoms of Neuropsychiatric Disorders

Cognitive impairment is a core symptom of neuropsychiatric disorders. Almost all neuropsychiatric symptoms are intermingled with impairment of cognition, if evaluated carefully. If distinct cognitive impairment is evaluated in psychiatric patients, it could be a sign indicating the symptoms might be caused by cerebral disease.

Disturbance of consciousness, on the other hand, could be a clue for diagnosis of cerebral disorders, if the possibility of physical illness can be ruled out. In the diagnostic procedure, these two symptoms, namely, cognitive impairment and disturbance of consciousness, indicate that the psychiatric symptoms are probably caused by brain disease. Therefore, these symptoms could be called "probable" neuropsychiatric symptoms (Fig. 3).

Probable and Possible Neuropsychiatric Symptoms

1. Probable Neuropsychiatric Symptoms
–Cognitive impairment
–Disturbance of consciousness

2. Possible Neuropsychiatric Symptoms
–Neurotic complaints, anxiety
–Mood changes
–Psychotic States: Hallucination & delusion
–Behavioral and personality changes

Fig. 3 Probable and possible neuropsychiatric symptoms

On the other hand, psychiatric symptoms such as neurotic complaints, mood changes, hallucination, delusion, and behavioral and personality changes could possibly be caused by cerebral disorders. Therefore, these symptoms could be called "possible" neuropsychiatric symptoms (Fig. 3).

Neuropsychiatric Symptoms Could Be the Earliest Symptoms in Cerebral Disorders

Mild neuropsychiatric symptoms, such as anxiety, depression, apathy, and personality changes, occasionally precede dementia in cerebral disorders (Fig. 4). Mild psychiatric symptoms could be the earliest manifestations of the neuropsychiatric disorders. Occasionally these symptoms are composed of vague somatic complaints. Patients with neuropsychiatric disorders commonly complain of subjective work difficulties, forgetting the location of objects, decreased functioning in demanding employment settings, and difficulty in traveling to new locations in the early stage of their illness. Hypochondria, anxiety, irritability, dysphoria, dysthymia, depressive mood, agitation, euphoria, hypomanic mood, flattening of affects, sleep disorder, apathy, and psychomotor retardation may occur, preceding dementia, in the initial stage of brain disease.

Mild Neuropsychiatric Symptoms, precede Dementia

1) Neurotic Symptoms: Headache, vertigo, dizziness, fatigueability, listlessness, pain, weakness, hypochondria, anxiety, irritability,

2) Mood Disoders: dysphoria, dysthymia, depressive mood, agitation, euphoria, hypomanic mood, flattening of affect, sleep disorders,

3) Behaviors: apathy, psychomotor retardation, subjective work difficulties,

4) Cognitive Impairment: forgetting location of objects, decreased functioning in demanding employment settings, and difficulty in traveling to new locations.

Fig. 4 Mild neuropsychiatric symptoms that precede dementia

Cognitive impairment preceding dementia is called mild cognitive impairment (MCI) [4]. It is reported that MCI is commonly accompanied by neuropsychiatric symptoms such as depression, dysphoria, apathy, irritability, anxiety, agitation, aberrant motor behavior, and parkinsonian-like signs. Neuropsychiatric symptoms in the MCI stage could be the predictors of conversion to dementia [5].

Neuropsychiatric Symptoms Are Not Pathognomonic to a Certain Cerebral Disorder

Psychiatric symptoms are nonspecific to certain neurological diseases. Therefore, it usually is not possible to indicate what kind of disease causes the psychiatric symptoms in the patients. Almost all neuropsychiatric symptoms may occur in any of the cerebral disorders. For example, depressive mood and agitation occasionally occur in Alzheimer's disease, cerebrovascular disorders, and Parkinson's disease. Neurotic symptoms are commonly encountered in patients with Alzheimer's disease, traumatic brain injury, and seizure disorders, which means that no type of neuropsychiatric symptom is pathognomonic to a specific cerebral disorder.

Neuropsychiatric Symptoms May Mimic Endogenous Psychoses

Cerebral disorders may mimic endogenous psychoses. Paranoid-hallucinatory state and mood disorders could be caused by cerebral diseases. Visual hallucination, especially, commonly occurs in cerebral disorders. Delusions of persecution and infidelity are occasionally seen in patients with organic brain disorders. Less frequently, delusional misidentification occurs in neuropsychiatric disorders. Therefore, endogenous psychosis should be diagnosed carefully by excluding the possibility of cerebral disorders.

The neurobiological basis of the endogenous psychoses, such as schizophrenia and mood disorder, is still unknown. However, the pathophysiology of the endogenous psychoses could be revealed by neurobiological investigations of neuropsychiatric disorders in the future.

Neuropsychiatric Symptoms and Syndromes

Various neuropsychiatric symptoms and syndromes, such as anxiety, neurotic complaints, apathy, mood disorder, hallucination, delusion, behavioral change, personality alteration, and delirium, occur in patients with cerebral disorders and cause dementia in the advanced stages of illness (Fig. 5).

Diseases	MCI Type	Disturbance of Cognitive Functions	Mood Disorders	Volition	Neurotic State	Other Non-cognitive Symptoms	Other Neuropsychiatric Symptoms
Vascular Cognitive Impairment	Multiple or Nonmemory Domains MCI	Executive Function	Depression Emotional Incontinence	Apathy	Somatic complaints Anxiety	Personality Change	Delirium Neurological Signs
Alzheimer's Disease	Amnestic MCI	Memory	Depression Depressive Pseudo-dementia	Apathy	Somatic complaints Anxiety	Personality Change Delusion	
Frontotemporal Dementia	Nonmemory Domains MCI	Language Executive Function	Depression Hyperthymia	Apathy		Personality Change	
Parkinson's Disease	Nonmemory Domains MCI	Subcortical Dementia PDD (DLB)	Depression	Apathy Brady-phrenia	Somatic Complaints Anxiety		Parkinsonism
Dementia with Lewy Bodies	Memory Domains MCI	Memory or Nonmemory	Depression	Apathy		Visual Hallucination, Delusion	Delirium, Parkinsonism
Progressive Supranulear Palsy	Nonmemory Domains MCI	Subcortical Dementia	Depression	Apathy		Personality Change	Nuchal Rigidity Stiffness

Fig. 5 Neuropsychiatric symptoms in cerebral disorders

Anxiety and Neurotic Complaints

Anxiety commonly occurs in the initial stage of a neuropsychiatric disorder [6, 7]. However, it usually becomes less obvious as the progress of cognitive decline continues. Anxiety, intermingled with depressive mood or dysphoria, is one of the most common neuropsychiatric symptoms in Alzheimer's disease and vascular dementia. Somatic distress, such as headache, vertigo, dizziness, fatigability, listlessness, and feeling of weakness are occasional complaints. Excessive anxiety is usually accompanied by restlessness, irritability, muscle tension, fears, and respiratory symptoms of anxiety.

Apathy

Apathy, a syndrome of decreased initiation and motivation, is a common neuropsychiatric symptom in demented patients. The prevalence of apathy is reported to be almost 65% of patients with dementia and 70% in Alzheimer's disease patients. Although there is some overlap between apathy and depression, these two conditions are independent in the course of illness [8]. Apathy is significantly associated with more severe cognitive deficit and has been reported to reflect the interaction between cholinergic deficiency and neuropathological changes in the frontal brain regions. Increased apathy is associated with poor quality of life.

Mood Disorder

The prevalence of depression in cerebral diseases is strikingly high, particularly in Alzheimer's disease, Parkinson's disease, and cerebral stroke. Depression is one of the most common neuropsychiatric symptoms in patients with Alzheimer's disease. Depressive symptoms that most strongly discriminate between Alzheimer's disease patients with (major depression) and without (minor depression) sad moods are guilty ideation, suicidal ideation, loss of energy, insomnia, weight loss, psychomotor retardation /agitation, poor concentration, and loss of interest [8].

Patients with Alzheimer's disease are more likely to report a diminished ability to concentrate or indecisiveness and are less likely to experience sleep disturbances and feelings of worthlessness or excessive guilt during their major depressive episodes [9]. Among the various neuropsychiatric symptoms, depression frequently occurs in the preclinical phase of Alzheimer's disease and is considered to be one of the predictors of conversion to dementia in the stage of MCI [5].

Depressive patients with Parkinson's disease develop depressive mood change, loss of interest, and feelings of hopelessness [10]. Diminished ability to concentrate is also seen in parkinsonian patients with depression. Psychiatric features of guilt, self-reproach, or feelings of guilt and punishment are occasionally manifested in depression in Parkinson's disease. Anxiety, irritability, suicidal ideation, and depressive delusions are less frequent in Parkinson's patients with depression when compared to endogenous depressives. In addition, circadian rhythm of mood and manic state are exceptional. Somatic complaints such as fatigue, constipation, headache, insomnia, loss of appetite, dizziness, and abnormal sweating are frequent in patients with Parkinson's disease and depression.

The concept of vascular depression was proposed because of the comorbidity of depression and vascular disease [11]. Therefore, the diagnostic criteria for vascular depression require a major depression associated with evidence of confluent or diffuse vascular lesions in the subcortical regions seen on neuroimaging. Disruptions of the prefrontal systems or their modulating pathway are hypothesized to cause depressive mood in cerebrovascular disorders. Clinical symptoms of vascular depression are characterized by greater disability and higher risk for poorer outcomes, which may be related in part to executive dysfunction and consequent disability. Patients with late-life depression have significant impairment in executive functioning.

Poststroke depression (PSD) is a complication that occurs in patients with cerebral stroke. It has been reported that stroke in the left hemisphere causes depression more frequently than that in the right hemisphere [12]. Magnetic resonance imaging (MRI)-defined vascular depression is late-onset depression with mild infarction and rather intense white matter abnormalities in MRI [13].

Hallucinations and Delusions

Visual hallucination is usually one of the symptoms of delirium, caused by acute cerebral dysfunctions or physical illnesses. Hallucinosis could be caused by a localized brain lesion, especially in the brainstem or occipital lobe. Visual hallucination is the most common type of hallucinations in cerebral disorders. Organic hallucinations are frequently accompanied by illusions and delusional misidentifications. Delusional elaboration of hallucination also may occur in elderly patients. Charles Bonnet syndrome is nonorganic hallucination in the elderly, characterized by visual impairment, vivid visual hallucination, and illusion without any other psychotic symptoms. A special type of auditory hallucination, namely, musical hallucination, may occur in geriatric patients with auditory disturbance.

Psychiatric symptoms develop usually in the advanced stage of Parkinson's disease during long-term treatment with dopaminergic drugs. Recurrent episodes of visual hallucination and illusion are characteristic features of drug-induced psychiatric symptoms of Parkinson's disease. In approximately half the parkinsonian patients, hallucinations are accompanied by cognitive impairments [10].

Recently, visual hallucinations and delusions are considered to be characteristic clinical features of "dementia with Lewy bodies." Visual hallucination and other perceptual disorders, including misidentification syndrome and visual agnosia, are common symptoms in this disorder. Characteristic delusions, such as Capgras syndrome and "phantom boarders," occasionally occur in patients in their old age. Delusions of persecution, especially delusion of theft, are frequently encountered in the early stage of Alzheimer's disease. Delusions caused by cerebral diseases are usually poorly systematized and are occasionally accompanied by confabulation.

Behavioral and Personality Changes

Behavioral and personality changes characterized by disturbances of mood, volition, and cognition could be caused by chronic brain disorders [14]. Agitation, psychomotor retardation, apathy, and stereotyped behavior are common types of behavioral changes in chronic neuropsychiatric disorders. Aggression, screaming, restlessness, wandering, culturally inappropriate behavior, sexual disinhibition, hoarding, cursing, and shadowing are common behavioral disturbances in patients with dementia. Current pharmacologic treatments or sociopsychological interventions may ameliorate behavioral symptoms significantly.

Personality change is characterized by significant alterations of habitual patterns of behavior. It is usually accompanied by impairment of cognition and volition and by change of mood in cerebral disorders. Irritability, apathy, and exaggerated emotionality are common behavioral changes in various neurological disorders. Personality disorder frequently occurs, especially in the advanced stages of neurodegenerative disorders or vascular dementia.

Delirium

Delirium is a psychiatric state that is characterized clinically by transient disturbances of consciousness and attention, perception, memory, thinking, psychomotor behavior, and emotion. Visual hallucination and disturbance of sleep–wake rhythms occur frequently [15]. Acute cerebral damage, physical illnesses, and withdrawal of psychoactive substances of abuse, including alcohol, cause delirium. Complete recovery could be expected if the causal disorders or dysfunction diminished. During recovery from delirium, mild neuropsychiatric symptoms, such as disturbance of memory and attention, may continue for a long period, even for several months.

Persistent Cognitive Impairment (Dementia)

Persistent cognitive impairment is a core symptom of cerebral disorders. Brain diseases, for the most part, cause cognitive decline in the advanced stage. Therefore, persistent cognitive impairment could be a clue for the diagnosis of cerebral disorders.

As well as impairment of memory, disturbances of attention, abstract thinking, judgment, calculation, language, and executive function are common clinical features of dementia.

Dementia of the Alzheimer Type

Dementia in Alzheimer's disease is clinically characterized by amnestic syndrome and neuropsychological symptoms, including aphasia, apraxia, and agnosia. Impairment of episodic memory is one of the most important criteria for the diagnosis of Alzheimer's disease [16]. It is characterized clinically by slowly progressive impairment of cognitive functions, occasionally accompanied by disturbance of mood, behavior, and psychiatric symptoms, such as hallucination and delusion. The Mini-Mental State Examination reveals the disturbance of attention, impairment of recent memory, and disorientation in the earliest stage of Alzheimer's disease. Language abilities, such as naming and reading, are relatively spared until the advanced stages of the illness.

Neurodegenerative Dementias of Non-Alzheimer Type

Personality changes and language disturbances with less marked memory impairment are the main characteristics of cortical dementia in frontotemporal dementia. The early clinical features of frontotemporal dementia are changes of character and social behavior rather than impairment of memory and intellect. With the progression of the disease, impairment of cognitive functions, including memory, becomes obvious and slowly increases in severity. Stereotyped speech with a prominent reduction of vocabulary is conspicuous in the advanced stage of illness. Semantic dementia, as well as progressive nonfluent aphasia, is the characteristic clinical symptom of this type of dementia. Frontotemporal dementia with motor neuron disease is clinically characterized by the complication with motor neuron disease.

Subcortical dementia in progressive supranuclear palsy, corticobasal degeneration, Parkinson's disease, and Huntington's disease are characterized by peculiar "forgetfulness," psychomotor retardation, and mood changes. Progression of cognitive impairment with visual disturbance is a characteristic clinical feature of Creutzfeldt–Jakob disease, which causes a diffuse cortical degeneration with accentuation of occipital change. Progressive supranuclear palsy is clinically characterized by dementia, supranuclear ophthalmoplegia, and pseudobulbar palsy. Clinical characteristics of "subcortical dementia," namely, forgetfulness with psychomotor retardation, difficulty with complex problem solving and concept formation, and a relative absence of "cortical" features, including aphasia, apraxia, and agnosia, was originally described in this disorder.

Corticobasal degeneration is characterized clinically by cognitive impairment, rigidity, clumsiness, and "alien limb" phenomena.

Clinical features of dementia with Lewy bodies (DLB) are characterized by persistent cognitive impairment with fluctuation, recurrent visual hallucination, and parkinsonism [17]. It is still obscure what kind of factor causes the fluctuations of cognitive impairment and disturbance of consciousness.

Recently, it has been thought that the "dementia in Parkinson's disease (Parkinson disease dementia, PDD)" and DLB is essentially the same α-synucleinopathy in the spectrum of Lewy body disease [17, 18].

Vascular Cognitive Impairment

Cerebrovascular disorders may cause persistent cognitive impairment. After Alzheimer's disease, vascular dementia is the second most common disorder in the dementias of the elderly [19, 20]. Multiinfarction, and diffuse degeneration of the subcortical white matter, are the two main characteristic neuropathologies. Because hippocampal formation and adjacent structures are usually spared at the early stage of multiple cerebral infarctions, impairment of recent memory is not conspicuous in vascular cognitive impairment or vascular dementia until the advanced stage of illness. Executive dysfunction is conspicuous in comparison to memory impairment in the early stage of vascular dementia. Delirium occasionally intermingles with cognitive impairment in vascular dementia.

Conclusions

In general, almost all organic cerebral diseases cause psychiatric symptoms. Psychiatric symptoms caused by organic cerebral disorders are neuropsychiatric symptoms. Needless to say, neuropsychiatric symptoms and syndromes are the main target of neuropsychiatric studies. The main components of neuropsychiatric symptoms are cognitive impairment and disturbance of consciousness. Other neuropsychiatric symptoms, such as depression, anxiety, paranoid-hallucinatory states, and behavioral and personality changes, also commonly occur in the course of organic cerebral disorders. Mild neuropsychiatric symptoms could be the earliest manifestations of cerebral disorders. Cerebral diseases commonly cause neurological, neuropsychological, and psychiatric symptoms concurrently in the course of illness. Multiple neuropsychiatric symptoms commonly occur concurrently in the course of cerebral disorders. The organic factors should be carefully evaluated in the psychoses, especially in patients of older age. Clinicians who engage in the treatment of cerebral disorders or psychiatric disorders should have enough experience in the integrating neuroscience, that is, neuropsychiatry.

References

1. Lyketsos C (2006) Lessons from neuropsychiatry. J Neuropsychiatry Clin Neurosci 18:445–449
2. World Health Organization (1992) The ICD-10 classification of mental and behavioural disorders. Clinical descriptions and diagnostic guidelines. WHO, Geneva
3. Arciniegas DB, Kaufer DI et al (2006) Core curriculum for training in behavioral neurology and neuropsychiatry. J Neuropsychiatry Clin Neurosci 18:6–13
4. Petersen RC, Doody R, Kurz A et al (2001) Current concepts in mild cognitive impairment. Arch Neurol 58:1985–1992
5. Palmer K, Berger AK, Monastero R, Winblad B et al (2007) Predictors of progression from mild cognitive impairment to Alzheimer's disease. Neurology 68:1596–1602
6. Lyketsos CG, Lopez O, Jones B, Fitzpatrick A et al (2002) Prevalence of neuropsychiatric symptoms in dementia and mild cognitive impairment results from the cardiovascular health study. JAMA 288:1475–1483
7. Seignourel PJ, Kunik ME, Snow L et al (2008) Anxiety in dementia. A critical review. Clin Psychol Rev 28:1071–1082
8. Starkstein SE, Ingram L, Garau ML et al (2005) The overlap between apathy and depression in dementia. J Neurol Neurosurg Psychiatry 76:1070–1074
9. Zubenko G, Moosy J (1993) Major depression in primary dementia. Clinical and neuropathologic correlates. Arch Neurol 45:1182–1186
10. Miyoshi K, Ueki A, Nagano O (1996) Management of psychiatric symptoms of Parkinson's disease. Eur Neurol 36(Suppl 1):49–54
11. Alexopoulos GS, Meyers BS, Young RC et al (1997) Vascular depression hypothesis. Arch Gen Psychiatry 54:915–922
12. Robinson RG (2001) The neuropsychiatry of stroke. In: Miyoshi K, Shapiro C, Gaviria M, Morita Y (eds) Contemporary neuropsychiatry. Springer, Tokyo, pp 116–127
13. Krishnan KR, Hays JC, Blazer DG (1997) MRI-defined vascular depression. Am J Psychiatry 154:497–501
14. Finkel SI (1996) New focus on behavioral and psychological signs and symptoms of dementia. Int Psychogeriatr 8(Suppl 3):215–216
15. Trzepacz PT, Baker RW, Greenhouse J (1988) A symptom rating scale for delirium. Psychiatry Res 23:89–97
16. Dubois B, Feldman HH, Jacova C et al (2007) Research criteria for the diagnosis of Alzheimer's disease. Revising the NINCDS-ADRDA criteria. Lancet Neurol 6:734–746
17. McKeith IG, Dickson DW, Lowe J et al (2005) Diagnosis and management of dementia with Lewy bodies. Third report of the DLB consortium. Neurology 65:1863–1872
18. Kosaka K (1990) Diffuse Lewy body disease in Japan. J Neurol 237:197–207
19. O'Brien JT, Erkinjuntti T, Reisberg B et al (2003) Vascular cognitive impairment. Lancet Neurol 2:89–98
20. Román GC, Tatemichi TK, Erkinjuntti T et al (1993) Vascular dementia. Diagnostic criteria for research studies. Report of NINDS-AIREN international workshop. Neurology 43:250–260

Part II
Neuropsychiatric Syndromes

Thyroid–Brain Interactions in Neuropsychiatric Disorders

Robertas Bunevičius and Arthur J. Prange, Jr.

Abstract Thyroid hormones are important for the development and maturation of the brain as well as for the functioning of the mature brain. Most thyroid hormone-responsive genes are sensitive to thyroid hormones only during distinct periods of brain development, but some are also sensitive in the mature brain. A variety of factors influence the effects of thyroid hormones in the brain: availability of iodine; thyroid diseases and dysfunction; genetic variations that affect thyroid axis-related proteins, such as deiodinases, thyroid hormone transporters, and receptors; and timing of events. Interaction of these factors contributes to the development of the brain as well as to presentation of psychiatric symptoms and disorders in the mature brain. Clinical and subclinical thyroid dysfunction, thyroid autoimmunity, as well as individual genetic variations and mutations of thyroid axis-related proteins, may contribute not only to the presentation of psychiatric symptoms and disorders but also to response to psychiatric treatments. Better understanding of genomic and nongenomic mechanisms related to thyroid hormone metabolism in the brain opens new venues for finding new markers, new targets, and new agents for the treatment of mental disorders.

Keywords Brain development • Neuropsychiatric disorders • Thyroid hormones • Thyroid physiology

R. Bunevičius (✉)
Institute of Psychophysiology and Rehabilitation,
Kaunas University of Medicine, Vyduno 4, 00135 Palanga, Lithuania
e-mail: rob@ktl.mii.lt

A.J. Prange, Jr.
Department of Psychiatry, University of North Carolina at Chapel Hill,
Campus Box #7160, Chapel Hill, NC 27599-7160, USA
e-mail: ajprange@att.net

K. Miyoshi et al. (eds.), *Neuropsychiatric Disorders*,
DOI 10.1007/978-4-431-53871-4_2, © Springer 2010

Introduction

Thyroid hormones are important for the development and maturation of the brain as well as for functioning of the mature brain. Thyroid hormones influence brain gene expression. The majority of these genes are sensitive to thyroid hormones only during distinct periods of brain development, but some of them are also sensitive in the mature brain. Thyroid hormone deficiency during fetal and early postnatal life results in severe mental retardation and cretinism, while thyroid dysfunction in adult life results in mental symptoms, such as mood disorders and cognitive dysfunction. Although most psychiatric patients do not display overt thyroid dysfunction, many patients display lesser abnormalities. A variety of factors influence the effects of thyroid hormones in the brain: availability of iodine; thyroid diseases and dysfunction; genetic variations that affect proteins, such as deiodinases, thyroid hormone transporters, and receptors; and timing of events. Consideration of interaction of these factors contributes to better understanding of the presentation of psychiatric disorders as well as of the response to psychiatric treatments [1].

Thyroid Axis Hormone Secretion and Metabolism

Thyroid hormone secretion is controlled by pituitary thyrotropin, which is stimulated by hypothalamic thyrotropin-releasing hormone (TRH) and suppressed by negative feedback from serum thyroid hormones. In serum, more than 99% of thyroid hormones are bound to specific proteins and only free hormones are active. The thyroid gland secretes several hormones, including thyroxine (T_4), triiodothyronine (T_3), and metabolically inactive reverse T_3 (rT_3). The main secretion of the thyroid gland is T_4, and the thyroid gland is the only source of this hormone. In contrast, no more than 20% of the more biologically active hormone T_3 is secreted by the thyroid gland. The remainder of T_3 is produced in other tissues by removal of iodine from the T_4 molecule by enzymes called deiodinases, which exist in several forms and are located intracellularly. Type I deiodinase (D1) is located primarily in liver and kidney and is responsible for producing as much as 80% of T_3. Type II deiodinase (D2) is located primarily in brain glial cells, including astrocytes, and in muscles and mainly accounts for T_3 tissue concentrations. Type III deiodinase (D3) converts T_4 to inactive rT_3 and also degrades T_3. In the brain, D3 is located in neurons [1].

The major cause of disturbed thyroid hormone secretion is autoimmune thyroid disease (AITD), when autoantibodies against the normal elements of the thyroid axis are produced. Results of biopsy as well as autopsy show that up to 40% of women have AITD [2].There are two major forms of AITD: Graves' disease, a common cause of hyperthyroidism, and autoimmune thyroiditis, a common cause of hypothyroidism [3]. Other major causes of hyperthyroidism are toxic nodular goiters and adenomas; other major causes of hypothyroidism are treatments of thyroid disorders (radiation, thyroidectomy), thyroid dysgenesis, and iodine deficiency. In overt hyperthyroidism, thyroid hormone secretion is increased and thyrotropin secretion is suppressed. In overt hypothyroidism, thyroid hormone secretion is decreased and thyrotropin secretion is augmented. In subclinical thyroid dysfunction, only thyrotropin secretion, but not thyroid hormone secretion, is altered.

Circulating thyroid axis hormone concentrations in subjects with an unaffected thyroid gland show substantial interindividual variability, in which genetic variations play a major role. Genetic variation in deiodinase enzymes and thyrotropin receptors causes alteration in the balance of circulating thyroid hormones and their tissue concentrations, affecting thyroid hormone-related endpoints [4], including physiological consequences.

Thyroid Hormone Transport to the Brain

Thyroid hormones penetrate cell membranes and are responsible for the majority of genomic and nongenomic effects of thyroid hormones. Until recently it was presumed that cellular entry by free thyroid hormones was mediated via passive diffusion because of their lipophylic nature. Now it is recognized that thyroid hormones enter target cells using an energy-dependent transport mechanism that is mediated by the monocarboxylate transporter-8 (MCT8) and by other transporters such as the organic anion transporter protein 1c1 (OATP1c1). To enter the brain, thyroid hormones must cross the blood–brain barrier or the choroid-plexus–cerebrospinal fluid (CSF) barrier. OATP1c1 is a T_4-specific transporter; MCT8 may transport T_3 as well as T_4. In the brain, T_4 enters astrocytes, where it is converted to T_3 by local D2. T_3 generated in the astrocytes as well as T_3 from the general circulation is transported into neurons via MCT8, where, after completion of its action, it is degraded by D3 [5, 6] (Fig. 1).

Thyroid Hormone Receptors and Homeostasis in the Brain

The genomic action of T_3 is mediated via nuclear thyroid hormone receptors (TRs), which are members of the steroid/thyroid family. Human TRs are encoded by two genes and have alpha- and beta-receptor isoforms. TRs bind T_3 and, as ligand-inducible transcription factors, regulate expression of T_3-responsive target genes. TR alpha-1, beta-1, and beta-2 isoforms can be occupied by T_3, but the TR alpha-2 isoform cannot be occupied by T_3. TRs, whether or not occupied by T_3, bind to the DNA response elements, producing different effects on gene expression. Binding of T_3-occupied TRs leads to activation of the responsive gene; binding of T_3-unocupied TRs leads to suppression [7].

TRs are expressed in the brain before fetal thyroid hormone secretion. TR alpha-1 is the major isoform expressed in the brain during fetal development.

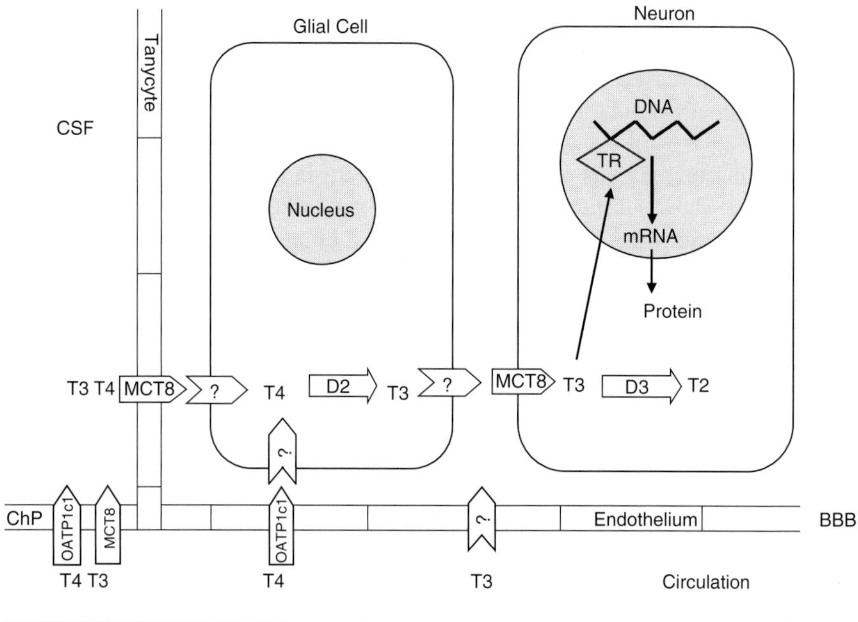

Fig. 1 Thyroid hormone delivery and metabolism in the brain. Thyroxine (*T_4*) is transported across the blood–brain barrier (*BBB*) via organic anion transporter protein 1c1 (*OATP1c1*) located in endothelium cells. Triiodothyronine (*T_3*) is transported via an unknown mechanism. From the cerebrospinal fluid (*CSF*), thyroid hormones are transported via monocarboxylate transporter-8 (*MCT8*) located in *tanycytes*. Choroid plexus (*ChP*) expresses both transporters OATP1c1 and MCT8. T_4 enters the glial cell via an unknown mechanism and is converted to T_3 by type II deiodinase (D2). T_3 exits the glial cell via an unknown mechanism and enters the neuron via MCT8. In the neuron, T_3 binds to nuclear thyroid receptor (*TR*) and acts as a transcription factor initiating protein synthesis, or is converted to inactive diiodothyronine (*T_2*) by type III deiodinase (D3)

Later, together with TR beta-1, it demonstrates different temporal and spatial distribution in the postnatal and mature brain, suggesting different expression of thyroid hormone-responsive genes in the developing versus the mature brain [3]. In the mature brain, thyroid hormones regulate expression of several genes that may affect mood and cognition, including genes for neurotrophins, such as nerve growth factor and brain-derived neurotrophic factor. By genomic and possibly nongenomic mechanisms, T_3 interacts with several important neurotransmitters such as serotonin and norepinephrine, which are crucial for mood regulation, and with acetylcholine, which is crucial for cognition [8].

A mutation in the TR beta gene that eliminates ligand binding is associated with thyroid hormone resistance syndrome, clinically presenting as a type of hypothyroidism with goiter, elevated serum thyroid hormone concentrations, and nonsuppressed thyrotropin concentrations [9]. Most affected children show attention-deficit disorder [10].

Regulation of thyroid hormone homeostasis in specific regions of the brain is achieved by temporal and spatial regulation of the deiodinase system. Expression of D3 in early gestation suppresses thyroid hormone activity in fetal tissues, maintaining proliferation and inhibiting differentiation. Later, expression of D2 activity initiates tissue differentiation. Deiodinase activity is different in specific regions of the brain. It also maintains brain thyroid hormone homeostasis in hyperthyroidism by increasing expression of D3 and suppressing expression of D2 and in hypothyroidism by increasing expression of D2 [5].

Fetal Thyroid Economy and Development of the Brain

During pregnancy, maternal thyroid hormone requirements increase by 50%. In the developing brain thyroid hormones regulate the process of differentiation such as axonal and dendrite proliferation, synapse formation, neural migration, and myelination [11]. In humans, thyroid hormone-dependent neurological development can be separated into several stages [5, 11, 12].

1. From conception to 16–20 weeks of pregnancy, before the onset of fetal thyroid hormone production, thyroid hormones are entirely derived from the mother. At this stage thyroid hormones influence neuronal proliferation and migration in the cerebral cortex, hippocampus, and medial ganglionic eminence.
2. From 16–20 weeks of gestation to birth, thyroid hormones are supplied from both the fetal and the maternal thyroid gland. At this stage, thyroid hormones influence neurogenesis, axonal and dendritic proliferation, synapse formation, glial cell differentiation, and the onset of myelination.
3. From birth, thyroid hormones are entirely derived from the infant's thyroid gland and still play an important role for the development of the brain. At this stage thyroid hormones influence gliogenesis, glial cell migration in the hippocampus, cerebellum, and cortex, as well as myelination.
4. After the second year of postnatal life, the effects of thyroid hormones are more related to physiological brain functioning than to brain development.

If thyroid hormone deficiency occurs, its timing is critical; this may be illustrated by the differences in neurological symptoms in endemic cretinism and in congenital hypothyroidism [5]. In endemic cretinism, maternal iodine deficiency causes both maternal hypothyroxinemia and fetal hypothyroidism, including fetal brain hypothyroidism, during the entire gestation. For the fetus, hypothyroidism is most severe early in gestation, before the fetal thyroid gland becomes active. This early hypothyroidism results in profound and irreversible mental retardation, deaf-mutism, spasticity, and ataxia, although thyroid function may be normal after birth.

In congenital hypothyroidism, fetal thyroid gland hypoplasia or aplasia is compensated by the maternal thyroid hormone secretion. Hypothyroidism occurs after birth. Neonates with congenital hypothyroidism in whom thyroid hormone replacement has not been started demonstrate symptoms of hypothyroidism and growth retardation together with mental retardation, spasticity, and speech and language deficits. Neurological deficits are less severe than in endemic cretinism [13]. Immediate thyroid hormone replacement prevents most neurological symptoms in neonatal hypothyroidism, although mild deficits in cognitive functioning persist [13].

Endemic cretinism may be prevented if administration of iodine is started in the first trimester. Despite knowledge of this simple remedy, iodine deficiency remains the most prevalent preventable cause of mental retardation worldwide [11]. Findings in iodine-deficient areas in China revealed a positive association of D2 polymorphisms with mental retardation [14]. This finding suggests an important interaction between environmental iodine deficiency and genetic variation, diminishing the enzymatic conversion of T_4 to T_3 in the brain.

In most parts of the world, dietary iodine is sufficient. Nevertheless, maternal hypothyroidism [15] or hypothyroxinemia [16], especially in early pregnancy, is associated with delay in infant neurodevelopment. Women who are unable to increase their production of T_4 early in pregnancy may constitute a population at risk for producing children with neurological disabilities [17]. On the other hand, maternal hyperthyroidism [18] may affect reactivity to stress in offspring [19].

MCT-8 Mutations and Neurodevelopment

It has been recognized recently that mutations in MCT8 affect T_3 transport into the neuron, causing isolated brain hypothyroidism with elevated serum T_3 concentrations [5, 6]. Clinical features of MCT8 mutations include severe mental retardation, axial hypotonia, absence of speech, and resemblance to patients with Allan–Herndon–Dudley syndrome (AHDS). In fact, MCT8 mutations were found in all families with AHDS, providing a molecular basis for this syndrome [20]. Apparently, when hypothyroidism is confined to the brain, the effects on brain development resemble those caused by systematic hypothyroidism. Although there are no effective treatments for patients with MCT8 mutation, the detection of this mutation is important for genetic counseling.

Hypothyroidism and Mental Function in Adults

In adults, hypothyroidism is frequently accompanied by symptoms such as diminished cognition, slow thought process, slow motor function, and drowsiness. Depression seems to be especially related to hypothyroidism; even subclinical hypothyroidism may affect mood [21]. Thyroid deficits are frequently observed in bipolar patients, especially in women with the rapid-cycling form of the disease [22]. In elderly patients, overt hypothyroidism may cause cognitive deficits that respond to thyroid hormone replacement. Both subclinical hypothyroidism and subclinical hyperthyroidism increase the risk for Alzheimer's disease, especially in women [23].

Treatment of Hypothyroidism

In hypothyroidism, replacement therapy with T_4 remains the treatment of choice and resolves most physical and psychological signs and symptoms in most patients. However, some patients do not feel entirely well despite adequate dosage of T_4 [24]. In T_4-treated patients it was found that reduced psychological well-being is associated with occurrence of polymorphism in the D2 encoding gene [25], as well as in the OATP1c1 encoding gene [26].

Thyroid hormone replacement with a combination of T_4 and T_3 in comparison to T_4 monotherapy differentially improves mental functioning in some but not all hypothyroid patients [27], and the majority of patients subjectively prefer combined treatment with T_4 and T_3 [28]. Two studies have evaluated whether D2 encoding gene polymorphism is associated with changes in psychological well-being after combined T_4 and T_3 treatment. One study reported only a trend toward improvement [29]. In a second study involving a very large sample, D2 encoding gene polymorphism was associated with improvement in psychological well-being after T_4 and T_3 treatment [25].

Hyperthyroidism and Mental Symptoms in Adults

The symptoms and signs of hyperthyroidism resemble those of primary mental disorders such as mania, depression, or anxiety. Overactivity of the adrenergic system caused by hyperthyroidism may explain the similarity between the clinical presentations of hyperthyroidism and mania or anxiety, as well as the precipitating role of hyperthyroidism in the development of mania or anxiety [30]. It also may explain the increased sense of well-being in persons in early stages of hyperthyroidism [31, 32].

The relationship between hyperthyroidism and depression is less clear. As already discussed, depression is usually linked to hypothyroidism, not hyperthyroidism. However, prolonged hyperthyroidism might exhaust noradrenergic transmission and thus contribute to depression. Noradrenergic exhaustion might well occur in patients with hyperthyroidism who have bipolar disorder. In the initial phase of hyperthyroidism, thyroid hormone stimulation of the noradrenergic system may cause mania; later, when noradrenergic neurotransmission is exhausted, it may contribute to depression [33].

Treatment of Hyperthyroidism

Mental symptoms and disorders secondary to hyperthyroidism should be treated in the first instance by restoring euthyroidism. Treatment with a beta-adrenergic antagonist drug in combination with antithyroid therapy remains the treatment of choice for the entire spectrum of mental symptoms caused by hyperthyroidism [34]. The majority of mental disorders and mental symptoms usually resolve once euthyroidism has been regained.

The use of beta-adrenergic antagonist drugs is part of the standard treatment of hyperthyroidism. These drugs quickly relieve many symptoms, including mental symptoms, and they do not interfere with endocrine diagnostic tests. Among these drugs, propranolol and metoprolol have the highest lipid solubility and cross the blood–brain barrier most readily [35].

Low T_3 Syndrome in Mental Disorders

A decrease in serum T_3 concentration and a parallel increase in rT_3 concentration are common findings in many illnesses, in trauma, in starvation, and after surgical operations. These changes in thyroid axis function, taken together, are referred to as the low T_3 syndrome. Low T_3 syndrome has also been called euthyroid sick syndrome, tending to minimize its clinical significance. An alternative designation, which does not presume metabolic significance, is nonthyroidal illness syndrome [36].

A principal mechanism underlying low serum concentration of T_3 in patients with nonthyroidal illness syndrome is reduced activity of the D1 enzyme in liver. Increased concentration of cytokines, such as interleukin-6 and tumor necrosis factor-alpha, are responsible for the impaired expression of hepatic D1. Other mechanisms involved in the pathogenesis of the syndrome include a decrease in concentration of thyroid hormone-binding proteins and decreased secretion of TRH [36].

Low T_3 syndrome can play a significant role in development of cognitive dysfunction, e.g., delirium, in patients with Alzheimer's disease after surgical interventions [37]. It also has been described in other mental disorders such as major depression [38] and schizophrenia [39].

Thyroid Autoimmunity and Mood Disorders

AITD is frequently related to thyroid dysfunction, and even marginal thyroid dysfunction may be associated with mood and anxiety disorders. However, a large epidemiological study found no association between overt or subclinical thyroid gland dysfunction and the presence of depression or anxiety disorders [40]. An association between AITD and depression was reported in primary care patients [41] and in pregnant women [42].

It may be that it is not thyroid gland dysfunction per se, but rather thyroid autoimmune processes, that frequently cause thyroid gland dysfunction [43], is responsible for comorbidity with mood disorders. Involvement of AIT in brain functioning was found in several neuroimaging studies. Euthyroid patients with autoimmune thyroiditis were compared to euthyroid patients without autoimmune thyroiditis. The former group showed more brain perfusion abnormalities, anxiety, and depression [44]. Neuroimaging abnormalities were similar to those observed in Hashimoto's encephalopathy, an infrequent but life-threatening acute brain syndrome caused by AITD. These findings suggest a higher than expected involvement of the brain in AITD [45].

Thyroid Function in Mood Disorders

Although most overtly hypothyroid or hyperthyroid patients show mental deficits, predominantly depression, most depressed patients are euthyroid; however, some show transient hyperthyroxinemia [46], which may indicate involvement of the thyroid axis in a restorative effort. A small proportion of patients with recognized major depression demonstrate subclinical hypothyroidism, of which an exaggerated thyrotropin response to TRH injection is a most sensitive characteristic. At the same time, a quarter to a third of depressed patients demonstrate a blunted thyrotropin response to TRH [43], which is believed to be a biological marker of depression and may indicate exhaustion of a compensatory effort in euthyroid patients and early stages of the low T_3 syndrome. Basal thyrotropin levels in major depression are usually normal or low normal. Recovery from depression, similar to recovery from other nonthyroid illness, results in normalization of thyrotropin secretion as well as in normalization of thyroid hormone concentration in serum and in the cerebrospinal fluid (CSF) [46]. Thyroid hormone metabolism in brain undergoes a specific change in depressed patients during recovery, and increasing T_3 concentrations may be a precondition for the recovery process [47].

Thyroid Abnormalities and Schizophrenia

An increased prevalence of thyroid function abnormalities was reported in families of patients with schizophrenia [48], suggesting a possible genetic linkage of the two disorders. It was reported that polymorphism of the human opposite paired (HOPA) gene, which is located on chromosome X, is linked to both hypothyroidism and schizophrenia [49].

Elevated T_4 concentrations [50] or low T_3 concentrations [39] are found in schizophrenia. Higher thyroid hormone concentrations predict better response to treatment. Clinical response to treatment usually correlates with normalization of thyroid hormone concentrations [50].

Thyroid Axis Hormones in Treatment of Mental Disorders

Thyroid Hormones

A significant proportion of depressed patients do not respond to standard drug treatment. Even patients who do respond need weeks to achieve full remission. This delay pertains to both groups of standard antidepressants, tricyclics (TCAs) and selective serotonin reuptake inhibitors (SSRIs). The delay prolongs both the morbidity of symptoms and the risk of mortality through suicide [51].

Thyroid hormones may provide an ancillary treatment because many connections between the thyroid axis and depression are known. Both TCAs and SSRIs increase brain D2 activity, which is responsible for local production of T_3 [47]. As an ancillary treatment, T_3 has been used in two ways: to accelerate the antidepressant drug from the beginning of treatment; and later to convert to responders patients whose response to drug has been inadequate. There is conclusive evidence that T_3 can accelerate the effects of TCAs [52]. There is also conclusive evidence that T_3 can convert TCA nonresponders to responders [53].

SSRIs have mainly replaced TCAs as the first-line treatment of depression. The ancillary use of T_3 with SSRIs is controversial. Recent meta-analyses found that differences in response and remission rates were insignificant in T_3 versus placebo supplementation. However, the authors concluded that SSRI and T_3 therapy may be effective in some subgroups of depressed patients, including patients with atypical depression and patients with functional D1 encoding gene polymorphism [54]. Depressed patients who have lower genetically determined T_4 conversion to T_3 may be more likely to benefit from T_3 supplementation [55]. The antidepressant effect of T_3 augmentation of SSRIs correlates with significant changes in the brain bioenergetic metabolism [56], suggesting that T_3 is an important factor regulating bioenergetic processes in the brain and that these processes are related to the manifestation and treatment of depressive disorders. Direct comparison of two treatment approaches augmenting the antidepressive effects of TCA showed that addition of T_3 is more beneficial than addition of T_4 [57].

Thyrotropin-Releasing Hormone

Thyrotropin-releasing hormone (TRH) was the first hormone described as a product of brain tissue. It is suggested [58] that TRH neurons compose a homeostatic system organized into four anatomical components: (1) the hypothalamic–pituitary–endocrine system; (2) the brainstem–midbrain–spinal cord system; (3) the limbic–cortical system; and (4) the chronobiological system. Later an even broader concept proposed "the TRH-immune system homeostatic hypothesis" [59]. Emphasis was given to the state-dependent and normalizing effects of TRH.

Some clinical reports, although not all, show that a single intravenous injection of TRH produces a prompt, albeit partial and brief, relief of symptoms in depressed patients. Consistent with the state-dependent concept is the finding that TRH also may cause improvement in manic patients [60]. TRH has yet to find broad acceptance as a treatment modality. However, one TRH congener, taltirelin, is available in Japan for the treatment of spinocerebellar degeneration. Also in Japan an intravenous formulation of TRH is available for the treatment of head injury and disturbances of consciousness. The recent finding that there are at least two types of TRH receptors [59] may give added impetus to the search for other TRH-related drugs.

Conclusion

Thyroid hormone action in the brain is determined by a complex of factors, including circulating concentrations of thyroid hormones; availability of free hormone; activity of thyroid hormone transporters, deiodinase enzymes, and TRs; thyroid autoimmunity; and, finally, timing of hormone action and the availability of iodine in the diet. Individual genetic variations and mutations of thyroid axis-related proteins may also contribute to presentation of psychiatric disorders, as well as to response to psychiatric treatments. Better understanding of genomic and nongenomic mechanisms related to thyroid hormone metabolism in the brain opens new venues for finding new markers, new targets, and new compounds for the treatment of mental symptoms and disorders.

Acknowledgments The authors thank the Hope for Depression Research Foundation (HDRF) and the Institute of the Study of Affective Neuroscience (ISAN) for research support.

References

1. Bunevicius R (2009) Thyroid disorders in mental patients. Curr Opin Psychiatry 22:391–395
2. Weetman AP (2004) Autoimmune thyroid disease. Autoimmunity 37:337–340
3. Pedersen IB, Knudsen N, Jorgensen T et al (2003) Thyroid peroxidase and thyroglobulin autoantibodies in a large survey of populations with mild and moderate iodine deficiency. Clin Endocrinol (Oxf) 58:36–42
4. Peeters RP, van der Deure WM et al (2006) Genetic variation in thyroid hormone pathway genes; polymorphisms in the TSH receptor and the iodothyronine deiodinases. Eur J Endocrinol 155:655–662
5. Williams GR (2008) Neurodevelopmental and neurophysiological actions of thyroid hormone. J Neuroendocrinol 20:784–794
6. Suzuki T, Abe T (2008) Thyroid hormone transporters in the brain. Cerebellum 7:75–83
7. Yen PM (2005) Genomic and nongenomic actions of thyroid hormones. In: Braverman LE, Utiger RD (eds) Warner and Ingbar's the thyroid: a fundamental and clinical text, 9th edn. Lippincott Williams & Wilkins, Philadelphia
8. Lifschytz T, Segman R, Shalom G et al (2006) Basic mechanisms of augmentation of antidepressant effects with thyroid hormone. Curr Drug Targets 7:203–210

9. Refetoff S, Dumitrescu AM (2007) Syndromes of reduced sensitivity to thyroid hormone: genetic defects in hormone receptors, cell transporters and deiodination. Best Pract Res Clin Endocrinol Metab 21:277–305
10. Hauser P, Zametkin AJ, Martinez P et al (1993) Attention deficit-hyperactivity disorder in people with generalized resistance to thyroid hormone. N Engl J Med 328:997–1001
11. de Escobar GM, Obregon MJ (2004) del Rey FE (2004) Maternal thyroid hormones early in pregnancy and fetal brain development. Best Pract Res Clin Endocrinol Metab 18:225–248
12. Bernal J, Guadano-Ferraz A, Morte B (2003) Perspectives in the study of thyroid hormone action on brain development and function. Thyroid 13:1005–1012
13. Zoeller RT, Rovet J (2004) Timing of thyroid hormone action in the developing brain: clinical observations and experimental findings. J Neuroendocrinol 16:809–818
14. Guo TW, Zhang FC, Yang MS et al (2004) Positive association of the DIO2 (deiodinase type 2) gene with mental retardation in the iodine-deficient areas of China. J Med Genet 2004(41):585–590
15. Haddow JE, Palomaki GE, Allan WC et al (1999) Maternal thyroid deficiency during pregnancy and subsequent neuropsychological development of the child. N Engl J Med 341:549–555
16. Pop VJ, Brouwers EP, Vader HL et al (2003) Maternal hypothyroxinaemia during early pregnancy and subsequent child development: a 3-year follow-up study. Clin Endocrinol (Oxf) 59:280–281
17. de Escobar GM, Obregón MJ, del Rey FE (2007) Iodine deficiency and brain development in the first half of pregnancy. Public Health Nutr 10:1554–1570
18. Bunevicius R, Kusminskas L, Mickuviene N et al (2009) Depressive disorder and thyroid axis functioning during pregnancy. World J Biol Psychiatry 10(4):324–329
19. Zhang L, Hernandez VS, Medina-Pizarro M et al (2008) Maternal hyperthyroidism in rats impairs stress coping of adult offspring. Neurosci Res 86:1306–1315
20. Visser WE, Friesema EC, Jansen J et al (2008) Thyroid hormone transport in and out of cells. Trends Endocrinol Metab 19:50–56
21. Haggerty JJ Jr, Prange AJ Jr (1995) Borderline hypothyroidism and depression. Annu Rev Med 46:37–46
22. Bauer M, Goetz T, Glenn T et al (2008) The thyroid–brain interaction in thyroid disorders and mood disorders. J Neuroendocrinol 20:1101–1114
23. Tan ZS, Beiser A, Vasan RS et al (2008) Thyroid function and the risk of Alzheimer disease: the Framingham study. Arch Intern Med 168:1514–1520
24. Saravanan P, Chau WF, Roberts N et al (2002) Psychological well-being in patients on 'adequate' doses of L-thyroxine: results of a large, controlled community-based questionnaire study. Clin Endocrinol (Oxf) 57:577–585
25. Panicker V, Saravanan P, Vaidya B et al (2009) Common variation in the DIO2 gene predicts baseline psychological well-being and response to combination thyroxine plus triiodothyronine therapy in hypothyroid patients. J Clin Endocrinol Metab 94:1623–1629
26. van der Deure WM, Appelhof BC, Peeters RP et al (2008) Polymorphisms in the brain-specific thyroid hormone transporter OATP1C1 are associated with fatigue and depression in hypothyroid patients. Clin Endocrinol (Oxf) 69:804–811
27. Bunevicius R, Kazanavicius G, Zalinkevicius R et al (1999) Effects of thyroxine as compared with thyroxine plus triiodothyronine in patients with hypothyroidism. N Engl J Med 340:424–429
28. Escobar-Morreale HF, Botella-Carretero JI, Escobar del Rey F et al (2005) Review: Treatment of hypothyroidism with combinations of levothyroxine plus liothyronine. J Clin Endocrinol Metab 90:4946–4954
29. Appelhof BC, Peeters RP, Wiersinga WM et al (2005) Polymorphisms in type 2 deiodinase are not associated with wellbeing, neurocognitive functioning and preference for combined T_4/T_3 therapy. J Clin Endocrinol Metab 90:6296–6299

30. Mason GA, Bondy SC, Nemeroff CB et al (1987) The effects of thyroid state on beta-adrenergic and serotonergic receptors in rat brain. Psychoneuroendocrinology 12:261–270
31. Grabe HJ, Volzke H, Ludemann J et al (2005) Mental and physical complaints in thyroid disorders in the general population. Acta Psychiatr Scand 112:286–293
32. Samuels MH, Schuff KG, Carlson NE et al (2008) Health status, mood, and cognition in experimentally induced subclinical thyrotoxicosis. J Clin Endocrinol Metab 93:1730–1736
33. Bunevicius R, Velickiene D, Prange AJ Jr (2005) Mood and anxiety disorders in women with treated hyperthyroidism and ophthalmopathy caused by Graves' disease. Gen Hosp Psychiatry 27:133–139
34. Trzepacz PT, McCue M, Klein I et al (1988) Psychiatric and neuropsychological response to propranolol in Graves' disease. Biol Psychiatry 23:678–688
35. Bunevicius R, Prange AJ Jr (2006) Psychiatric manifestations of Graves' hyperthyroidism: pathophysiology and treatment options. CNS Drugs 20:897–909
36. Bunevicius R (2009) Low triiodothyronine syndrome and depression in patients with chronic heart failure. In: Iervasi G, Pingitore A (eds) Thyroid and heart failure: from pathophysiology to clinics. Springer, Milan
37. Mafrica F, Fodale V (2008) Thyroid function, Alzheimer's disease and postoperative cognitive dysfunction: a tale of dangerous liaisons? J Alzheimers Dis 14:95–105
38. Premachandra BN, Kabir MA, Williams IK (2006) Low T_3 syndrome in psychiatric depression. J Endocrinol Invest 29:568–572
39. Yazici K, Yazici AE, Taneli B (2002) Different neuroendocrine profiles of remitted and non-remitted schizophrenic patients. Prog Neuropsychopharmacol Biol Psychiatry 26:579–584
40. Engum A, Bjoro T, Mykletun A et al (2002) An association between depression, anxiety and thyroid function: a clinical fact or an artefact? Acta Psychiatr Scand 106:27–34
41. Bunevicius R, Peceliuniene J, Mickuviene N et al (2007) Mood and thyroid immunity assessed by ultrasonographic imaging in a primary health care. J Affect Disord 97:85–90
42. Pop VJ, Wijnen HA, Lapkiene L et al (2006) The relation between gestational thyroid parameters and depression: a reflection of the downregulation of the immune system during pregnancy? Thyroid 16:485–492
43. Bunevicius R, Lasas L, Kazanavicius G et al (1996) Pituitary responses to thyrotropin releasing hormone stimulation in depressed women with thyroid gland disorders. Psychoneuroendocrinology 21:631–639
44. Zettinig G, Asenbaum S, Fueger BJ et al (2003) Increased prevalence of subclinical brain perfusion abnormalities in patients with autoimmune thyroiditis: evidence of Hashimoto's encephalitis? Clin Endocrinol (Oxf) 59:637–643
45. Chong JY, Rowland LP, Utiger RD (2003) Hashimoto encephalopathy: syndrome or myth? Arch Neurol 60:164–171
46. Kirkegaard C, Faber J (1991) Free thyroxine and 3, 3', 5'-triiodothyronine levels in cerebrospinal fluid in patients with endogenous depression. Acta Endocrinol (Copenh) 124:166–172
47. Baumgartner A (2000) Thyroxine and the treatment of affective disorders: an overview of the results of basic and clinical research. Int J Neuropsychopharmacol 3:149–165
48. DeLisi LE, Boccio AM, Riordan H et al (1991) Familial thyroid disease and delayed language development in first admission patients with schizophrenia. Psychiatry Res 38:39–50
49. Philibert RA, Sandhu HK, Hutton AM et al (2001) Population-based association analyses of the HOPA12bp polymorphism for schizophrenia and hypothyroidism. Am J Med Genet 105:130–134
50. Baumgartner A, Pietzcker A, Gaebel W (2000) The hypothalamic-pituitary-thyroid axis in patients with schizophrenia. Schizophr Res 44:233–243
51. Jick H, Kaye JA, Jick SS (2004) Antidepressants and the risk of suicidal behaviors. JAMA 292:338–343
52. Altshuler LL, Bauer M, Frye MA et al (2001) Does thyroid supplementation accelerate tricyclic antidepressant response? A review and meta-analysis of the literature. Am J Psychiatry 158:1617–1622

53. Aronson R, Offman HJ, Joffe RT et al (1996) Triiodothyronine augmentation in the treatment of refractory depression. A meta-analysis Arch Gen Psychiatry 53:842–848
54. Papakostas GI, Cooper-Kazaz R, Appelhof BC et al (2009) Simultaneous initiation (coinitiation) of pharmacotherapy with triiodothyronine and a selective serotonin reuptake inhibitor for major depressive disorder: a quantitative synthesis of double-blind studies. Int Clin Psychopharmacol 24:19–25
55. Cooper-Kazaz R, van der Deure WM, Medici M et al (2009) Preliminary evidence that a functional polymorphism in type 1 deiodinase is associated with enhanced potentiation of the antidepressant effect of sertraline by triiodothyronine. J Affect Disord 116:113–116
56. Iosifescu DV, Bolo NR, Nierenberg AA et al (2008) Brain bioenergetics and response to triiodothyronine augmentation in major depressive disorder. Biol Psychiatry 63:1127–1134
57. Joffe RT, Singer W (1990) A comparison of triiodothyronine and thyroxine in the potentiation of tricyclic antidepressants. Psychiatry Res 32:241–251
58. Gary KA, Sevarino KA, Yarbrough GG et al (2003) The thyrotropin-releasing hormone (TRH) hypothesis of homeostatic regulation: Implications for TRH-based therapeutics. J Pharmacol Exp Ther 305:410–416
59. Kamath J, Yarbrough GG, Prange AJ Jr et al (2009) The thyrotropin-releasing hormone (TRH)-immune system homeostatic hypothesis. Pharmacol Ther 121:20–28
60. Yarbrough GG, Kamath J, Winokur A et al (2007) Thyrotropin-releasing hormone (TRH) in the neuroaxis: therapeutic effects reflect physiological functions and molecular actions. Med Hypotheses 69:1249–1256

Lack of Insight and Awareness in Schizophrenia and Neuropsychiatric Disorders

James Gilleen, Kathryn Greenwood, and Anthony S. David

Abstract Lack of insight or awareness of illness is a major problem in the management of patients with a range of neuropsychiatric disorders. Insight in schizophrenia has been extensively studied over the past 20 years, and much is known about its clinical associations. In this chapter, we review the literature on insight in schizophrenia and go on to describe the results of a study in which awareness of illness and impairment was compared in three clinical groups matched for premorbid IQ: patients with schizophrenia, Alzheimer's disease, and brain injury. We considered performance and awareness across a number of domains: social behavior, psychopathology, and executive function. Awareness was measured by different methods including clinician ratings and discrepancy scores between patients' own ratings and their relatives' ratings using the Dysexecutive Questionnaire. All groups showed varying levels of deficit in each domain as well as varying levels of awareness. The Alzheimer group showed the most severe lack of awareness of cognitive and behavioral problems, followed by the brain-injured and schizophrenia patients. Low mood was associated with better insight in all groups. We conclude that insight is multidimensional and domain specific but that it also has associations which are common across domains and disorders.

Keywords Alzheimer's disease • Awareness • Brain injury • Insight • Schizophrenia

---

J. Gilleen, K. Greenwood, and A.S. David (✉)
Department of Psychiatry, Section of Cognitive Neuropsychiatry,
Institute of Psychiatry, King's College London,
PO Box 68, London SE5 8AF, UK
e-mail: antony.david@kcl.ac.uk

K. Miyoshi et al. (eds.), *Neuropsychiatric Disorders*,
DOI 10.1007/978-4-431-53871-4_3, © Springer 2010

Introduction

The terms "anosognosia," "insight," "lack of awareness," and even "denial" are often used synonymously to describe a collection of attitudes and behaviors directed at one's illness. Anosognosia is generally used to convey lack of awareness of specific functions seen after brain injury, such as hemiplegia. In contrast, insight and lack of awareness are typically used to describe the phenomena in psychiatric disorders, such as schizophrenia, and in neurological conditions, such as Alzheimer's disease (AD), where the awareness in question refers to that of being ill in general and, more specifically, the capacity to judge impairment of memory, or finally, the content of symptoms, such as delusions and hallucinations, as not being real [1, 2]. These terms, therefore, differ regarding the *object*(s) of insight to which they refer [3]. This distinction is crucial because awareness of an objective obvious deficit such as hemiplegia would seem to be different in kind from that of an objectively verifiable but invisible deficit such as amnesia, which is different again from a subjective experience such as a hallucination.

Within the schizophrenia field there has been an attempt to fractionate insight into different components or *dimensions* of awareness, which may, to some degree, be independent (e.g. [1, 4–6]). David [1] proposed three dimensions: recognition of having a mental illness, compliance with treatment, and the ability to label unusual events as pathological. Amador et al. [6] split insight into five components: four relate to (un)awareness of having a mental disorder, of the effects of medication, of consequences of illness, and of specific symptoms, and the fifth or final component is the attribution of symptoms to illness. Popular measures of insight include the Schedule for the Assessment of Insight – Expanded Version (SAI-E) [7, 8]; the semistructured interview: Scale to Assess Unawareness of Mental Disorder (SUMD) [6]; the simple clinician-rated Insight and Treatment Attitudes Questionnaire (ITAQ) [9]; and the Birchwood self-report Insight Scale (IS) [10]. All these scales have reasonably good intercorrelation [8]. Many authors have used a single item from general psychopathology schedules, and others, particularly in the dementia and brain injury fields, have made use of patient–carer discrepancy questionnaires such as the Patient Competency Rating Scale (PCRS) [11] and the Dysexecutive Questionnaire (DEX) [12].

Insight into Psychiatric Disorders (Schizophrenia)

Theories seeking to explain awareness in neuropsychiatric conditions broadly fall into three categories. Lack of awareness is conceptualized as a direct manifestation of psychiatric symptomatology (or a symptom in itself), a function of general or specific neuropsychological (e.g., executive) impairment, or a motivated response to a mental disorder to preserve self-esteem and protect against low mood.

Awareness and Symptomatology

Before the early nineteenth century, it would have been seen as a logical contradiction in terms to talk of "insight" into psychiatric symptoms such as delusions, yet at around this time, early French "alienists" began to acknowledge the concept of "partial" insanity, wherein "madness" could be accompanied by lucidity, indicating that some aspects of mental function could be "deranged" while others were preserved [3, 13]. It seems intuitive that awareness would be associated with severity of psychopathology, such that increased severity of delusions and hallucinations would necessarily by their very nature leave the sufferer unaware that their experiences were not real. Several studies have shown a relationship between awareness and global psychopathology in schizophrenia [4, 14–20], whereas others have found associations only with positive symptoms [21–27], or only with negative symptoms [28–31], or with both positive and negative symptoms (e.g., [32]). Other studies find awareness to be associated with specific symptoms such as "formal thought disorder" [33, 34], "degree of grandiosity" [35], or with degree of "unusual thought content" (equivalent to delusions), as measured by the Brief Psychiatric Rating Scale [20, 36].

In an effort to clarify the relationship of awareness and psychopathology, Mintz et al. [32] conducted a meta-analysis of 40 relevant studies and found small negative associations between awareness and global, positive, and negative symptoms, accounting for 7.2%, 6.3%, and 5.2% of the variance in awareness, respectively. This finding would strongly suggest that symptomatology plays only a small part in the degree of awareness displayed by schizophrenia patients. It must therefore be concluded that insight is related to psychopathology: as one increases, the other tends to decrease. Nevertheless the association is weak cross sectionally and variable longitudinally. In other words, lack of awareness or poor insight is more than "just psychopathology" [37].

Several studies have shown that schizophrenia patients present with less awareness than patients with other diagnoses such as bipolar disorder and major depressive disorder [17, 38] and schizo-affective disorder and mood disorder with and without psychosis ([39]; but see [40, 41]), or with similar levels of awareness as bipolar patients but less awareness than patients with unipolar affective disorder [42, 43]. However, others have found no significant differences between different patient groups [4, 30, 34, 44, 45].

Clinical and Demographic Factors

There is little consistency across studies regarding reliable sociodemographic predictors of awareness in schizophrenia (see [3]). For example, age and gender do not appear to be associated with level of awareness, nor does awareness appear to be related to level of education [6]. Studies that report positive findings have occasionally done so in opposite directions, for example, duration of illness and awareness [46, 47].

Age has been found to associate with awareness in only a few studies [6, 22, 23, 42]. A meta-analysis reported that age at onset of the disorder moderated the relationship between awareness and symptom clusters [32], such that acute patient status was also found to act as a moderator variable between awareness and positive symptoms; acutely ill patients were least aware.

Awareness and Neurocognition

Several studies have suggested a relationship between intelligence (IQ) and awareness in schizophrenia [48], whereas others claim a more specific association with executive functioning [15, 18], particularly as assessed using the Wisconsin Card Sorting Test (WCST). The WCST is generally thought to be a measure of set-shifting ability, where impairment has been hypothesized to be analogous to patients' inability to shift from an previously established "set" (that of being well) to a more accurate, postmorbid "set" (of being ill). Cooke et al. [49] examined 29 studies that included a measure of WCST performance and awareness and found 11 studies reported no association between any WCST measure and awareness; 9 studies found all WCST measures correlated with awareness; and 9 found some but not all WCST measures correlated with awareness. All findings were in the anticipated direction, with lower awareness being associated with poorer WCST performance. In total, 12 of the 29 studies reported a correlation between "perseverative errors" and awareness and 9 between "sets achieved" and awareness. It has been suggested that cognitive perseveration may underlie patients "perseverating in denial of illness despite evidence to the contrary" [50], but the evidence remains contradictory [51]. The most comprehensive and quantitative systematic review and meta-analysis of work in this area [52], however, suggests that WCST performance has more in common with awareness than other measures such as IQ, or memory, with 13 studies creating a pooled effect size of $r=0.23$.

Neuroimaging

As interest in awareness has grown, so has the use of magnetic resonance imaging (MRI) as an investigative tool. The findings to date suggest an association between poor insight and reduced total brain volume [53, 54], frontal lobe atrophy [31], reduced frontal lobe volume [55, 56], reduced cingulate gyrus and temporal lobe grey matter volume [56], and ventricular enlargement [14]. There is, however, some inconsistency in these findings, much study variation in the location of brain–insight correlates, and in some instances a failure to identify any brain abnormalities associated with poor insight [57]. One explanation for this inconsistency could be measurements or voxel-based morphometry (VBM) methods of analysis. In some studies, a single insight assessment item has been used [44, 58], while in others insight schedules were employed [19, 59]. Shad et al. [59] investigated SUMD scores and brain volume in 14 patients with schizophrenia and found lower awareness of current symptoms to be associated with lower right dorsolateral prefrontal cortex volume, although misattribution of current symptoms was associated with higher right medial orbitofrontal cortex volume. Cooke et al. [60] used VBM in a different but overlapping sample reported earlier [56] and found temporal and parietal grey matter reductions to be correlated with various insight dimensions. Finally, Morgan et al. [109] also used VBM methods in a large sample of first-episode psychosis patients and found deficits, particularly with respect to attribution of symptoms in the cingulate cortex, perhaps related to the midline cerebral system for self-processing [61], as well as right posterior deficits, reminiscent of regions implicated in neurological cases of anosognosia of hemiplegia and neglect [62]. Damage to any of these putative systems could potentially account for impaired self-awareness. Research in other psychiatric disorders is needed before we can say whether these findings are disorder specific.

Mood

One of the more reliable findings in the literature is the positive correlation between awareness and low mood or depression (and between elevated mood and lack of awareness [41]), which has been shown across different patient groups [3, 63]. Although findings are variable, many studies have reported that increased awareness in schizophrenia is associated with greater depressive symptoms [25, 34, 47, 64–69], including a meta-analysis [32]. In this way, low awareness of symptoms and illness is conceptualized as a form of denial to maintain self-esteem and preclude the psychological consequences of acknowledging one has a mental illness.

A critical question is this: Does a depressive mood ensue from awareness of illness, or does a depressive mood foster a more self-critical attitude? The framework of "depressive realism" may help explain this association (see [70]). On the other hand, Rathod et al. [71] reported that patients undergoing cognitive-behavioral therapy (CBT) intervention to improve awareness became depressed subsequent to gaining awareness, but this result was not found in an earlier study [72].

Insight and Awareness in Alzheimer's Disease

Alzheimer's disease (AD) can be characterized by a deterioration in memory and self-care as well as behavioral and mood disturbance. Despite the severity of their impairments, Alzheimer's patients often show profound unawareness of their deficits [73], even at the earliest stages [74]. Understanding awareness in dementia has important implications [63, 75], as it has been found to be associated with greater perceived burden of care by their carers [76], delayed diagnosis [77], and poorer outcome after rehabilitative treatment [78].

Awareness has been shown to worsen with disease progression [79] and has been found to be associated more frequently with damage to certain anatomical sites, for example, right frontal and parietal lobes [80–82], which are also often found to be associated with anosognosia following brain injury (see [80]). Other studies have found awareness to worsen with disease severity [83], although some have not [84, 85]. Similarly, although some studies have found an association between "frontal"/executive performance and awareness [86, 87], others have not [88, 89].

Less commonly, unawareness is conceived as being a defense mechanism against the knowledge and consequences of illness. As already noted with respect to schizophrenia, defensive denial is proposed to serve to defend Alzheimer's patients from depression, and indeed patients with less insight show less depressive symptomatology [82, 83, 90, 91], but again other studies have not shown this [77, 84, 92], and the direction of causality of this effect is debatable.

Insight and Awareness in Brain Injury

Disturbances to awareness of functional impairments are common sequelae of brain injury [93] and have been suggested to be present, to some level, in between 76% and 97% of postacute patients with brain injury and up to 45% of individuals with moderate to severe brain injury [94]. Such individuals may have multiple medical, physical, and cognitive limitations of which they are often unaware. Brain injury patients may exhibit global deficits in awareness of mental disorder or more circumscribed lack of awareness of specific deficits such as hemiparesis, object agnosia [80], and hemispatial neglect [62]. Paradoxically, patients are often unaware of even the grossest impairments in functioning but may be aware of more minor impairments; and just as seen with delusions in schizophrenia, false beliefs of unimpaired functioning can persist despite overwhelming contradictory evidence.

As a consequence of lack of awareness, patients with brain injury may not be capable of monitoring their own behavior or comprehending the impact of the consequences of their deficits on day-to-day life. Moreover, unawareness has been shown to greatly impede rehabilitation [94] and is associated with lower vocational and residential status [95, 96] (see also [97] for a review of studies pertaining to employment outcome), "less favorable outcome" [98], and perpetuation of socially inappropriate behaviors [99], and has been shown to be associated with increased burden for the respective carer [84]. Therefore, understanding the nature of awareness could have profound benefits for patient prognosis and carer quality of life.

Direct Comparison of Insight and Awareness in Patients with Schizophrenia, AD, and Brain Injury

Most studies of awareness investigate a single patient population. Is there a case for comparing different patient groups on the same measures [100, 101]? As well as perhaps revealing more about the nature of awareness per se, doing so also allows us to observe how awareness may differ in these different groups where pathology is a known factor. By contrasting different patient groups, it may be possible to better elucidate which mechanisms subserve awareness, or alternatively it may reveal that patients from different clinical groups show lack of awareness for different reasons.

Just as patients with schizophrenia have, in addition to their core symptoms, cognitive impairments and behavioral and social deficits, so patients with AD and brain injury may have a range of psychopathologies about which they may or may not have degrees of awareness. Comparison within – as well as between – groups may have important theoretical implications. For example, if patient groups with widely divergent pathologies (e.g., Alzheimer and schizophrenia patients) both have memory deficits, then we can ask whether the same factors associated with awareness of these are consistent across the groups (e.g., [102, 103] for awareness of cognitive deficits in schizophrenia). If the answer is broadly affirmative, it suggests that a common cognitive structure of awareness pertains, and this in turn can prompt overarching cognitive models that need not be overly concerned with diagnosis. Furthermore, if, say, awareness of psychopathology is relatively independent of awareness into cognitive deficits (the correlation was nonsignificant in one recent study [102], regardless of diagnosis), it points to modularity in awareness. Modularity of "awarenesses" is perhaps the most likely pattern from the neurological literature [79] (Fig. 1). Such modularity has seldom

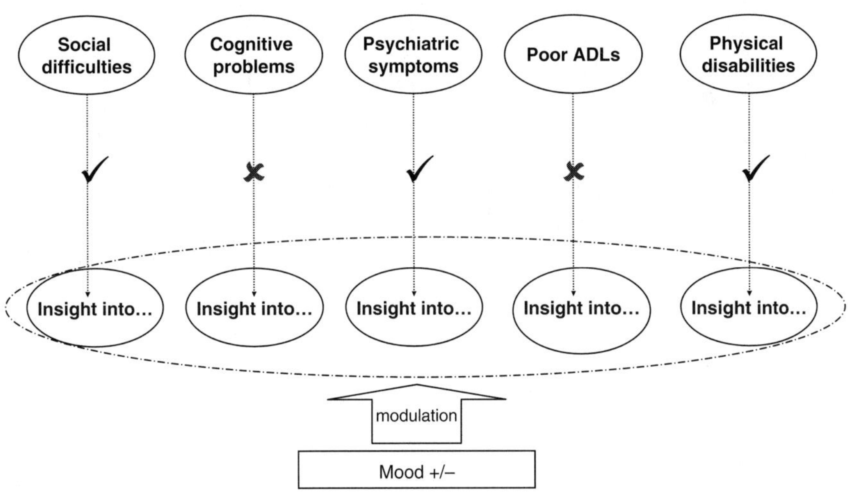

Fig. 1 Model of multiple, modality-specific awareness systems (modularity), each of which may or may not be impaired, but with general modulation by factors such as mood. In this theoretical example, insight is preserved into social difficulties, psychiatric symptoms, and physical disability but not cognitive problems and poor activities of daily living (*ADLs*)

been tested using broad domains such as psychopathology and behavioral problems (alongside neuropsychological impairments). Where it has, as in the large pan-European brain injury study [104], considerable within-diagnosis heterogeneity was found. Similarly, in the dementia field different levels of awareness have been noted by contrasting behavior with cognition [63, 73, 75, 105].

Participants

We recently conducted a study in which we compared different aspects of awareness in three different neuropsychiatric populations: schizophrenia, brain injury, and probable AD (Table 1). The former were mostly subacute, chronic, and treated outpatients plus some inpatients at the Maudsley Hospital, London; the Alzheimer group were locally dwelling subjects identified as part of a larger cohort study. The brain injury patients were a heterogeneous group with a mixture of traumatic, hypoxic, and vascular etiologies and with behavioral problems. We were keen to address to what extent awareness in the same domain differed between neuropsychiatric patient groups and whether differences could be measured using standard scales.

Naturally, the patients were not matched on factors such as age and length of illness. We contend that for the purposes of making inferences about the pattern of awareness deficits in different pathological groups and contrasting profiles of awareness within groups, this distinction is not critical. We acknowledge, however, that there may be subtle period- and age-related effects regarding social influences in accepting illness that require further study.

Table 1 Demographic and insight data on clinical groups

Variable	Schizophrenia	Brain injury	Alzheimer's
Mean (SD)	*n*=31	*n*=26	*n*=27
Age, years	38.3 (10.4)	40.0 (12.1)	82.4 (4.3)
Sex, M/F	16/15	22/4	14/13
Premorbid IQ (NART)	102.3 (12.8)	102.2 (13.8)	109.1 (12.8)
SAI-E	11.2 (7.15)	15.4 (5.7)	7.0 (6.4)
SUMD awareness of mental illness	3.37 (1.6)	1.92 (1.43)	4.04 (1.4)
DEX discrepancy scores[a] (mean and range)	2.48 (–33 to 31)	–14.76 (–55 to 15)	–25.96 (–62 to 13)

NART National Adult Reading Test (estimate of premorbid IQ); *SAI-E* Schedule for the Assessment of Insight–Expanded; *SUMD* Scale to Assess Unawareness of Mental Disorder

[a]Self-rating of difficulties minus informant rating of difficulties yielding a negative score. The more negative, the greater the discrepancy (greater patient unawareness)

Methods

The groups were compared on measures of estimated premorbid IQ (NART) and clinician-rated and patient–carer-rated awareness scales. All were rated on the SAI-E, and the SUMD (it was found that the awareness of mental illness was the most useful item from the scale; many Alzheimer patients were on no medication), and the DEX (see Table 1).

The DEX from the Behavioural Assessment of the Dysexecutive Syndrome (BADS) [106] was originally designed for use with brain injury populations; however, questions concerning functioning apply equally well to dementia and schizophrenia patients. It is a 20-item measure of functioning that addresses problems such as impulsivity, apathy, distractibility, unconcern for social rules, and difficulties with abstract thinking. Informants rate patient functioning, and the patient rates him/herself on the scales, and the difference between patient and informant scores creates a discrepancy score; the greater and more negative the discrepancy between the scores, the greater the unawareness of the patient. Items are scored on a 5-point scale from 0 (never) to 4 (very often). Hence, DEX discrepancy scores can range from –80 to +80. A score of 0 indicates perfect awareness in that the patient agrees with the level of impairment scored by the respective informant.

The validity of the discrepancy index to measure insight and awareness may be questioned because it assumes that the informant is the "gold standard." Informants may overestimate deficits (e.g., because of their own frustration or inability to cope) or underestimate them (e.g., because they are hidden, or because the informant wishes to protect the person they care for). Correlation with clinician ratings may be poor (see [63, 75]). Nevertheless, the methodology has been found to be valuable and consistently shows underestimation of deficits by patients in relationship to informal caregivers.

Results

Between-Group Contrasts

Across the groups, patient and informant ratings of behavioral problems, as measured by the total DEX score, were highly discrepant in the brain injury and AD groups (see Table 1; Fig. 2), representing low awareness of behavioral impairments, but this was much less so in the schizophrenia group, suggesting that patients exhibit different levels of unawareness of behavioral deficits. Importantly, ratings made by either patients or informants in any patient group were not grossly at ceiling or floor, but varied somewhat, suggesting that these scales provided sensitivity in measuring behavioral impairment and, in turn, awareness.

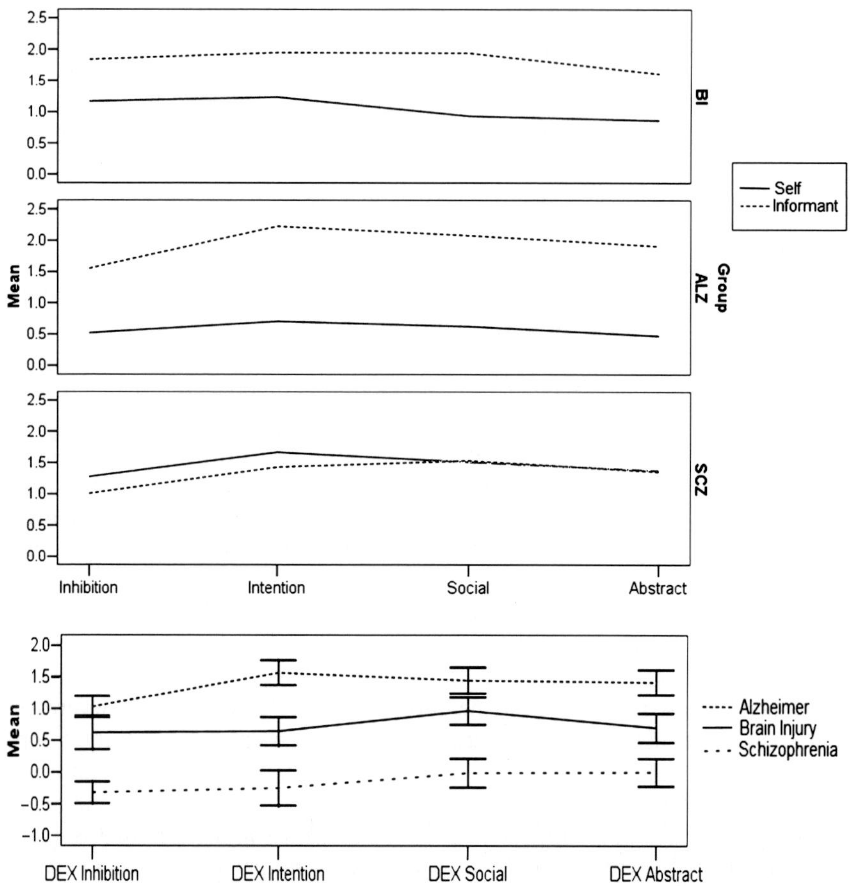

Fig. 2 Graphs show mean Dysexecutive Questionnaire (DEX) self and informant subfactor scores (per individual item) paneled according to patient group. Zero scores reflect the absence of problems. The *lower panel* shows the resultant DEX discrepancy scores for the three groups. For ease of presentation, the sign of the discrepancy score has been reversed so that a more positive value indicates greater discrepancy (i.e., less patient awareness). *BI* brain injury; *ALZ* Alzheimer's; *SCZ* schizophrenia

It was also of interest to see in what dimensions awareness between behavioral domains may differ, and whether there is an extant hierarchy of awareness (i.e., more awareness of motor/sensory versus executive and social cognitive deficits). Comparison of subfactor scores between groups can also reveal whether there are different "profiles" of awareness in different patient groups. From Fig. 2 it can be seen that both the brain injury and Alzheimer groups rated themselves as having few problems with executive functioning including inhibition, intentionality, social interactions, and abstract reasoning. The two groups differed in that the informants in the Alzheimer group rated these patients as having particular problems in intentional behavior, that is, apathy. Comparatively, the schizophrenia group rated themselves as lower functioning, but their ratings were concordant with the informants' view across all subdomains; this reflects good awareness of behavioral problems. The lower panel shows that this results in lowest awareness for the Alzheimer group, and greatest awareness for the schizophrenia group, but also that there is no consistent profile across patients, failing to support the notion of a hierarchy of awareness.

Pooled Patient Analysis

The entire patient sample was pooled ($n=84$), and Pearson correlational analyses were performed between the awareness and other clinical and symptoms ratings. The DEX discrepancy score correlated with clinician-rated insight (SAI-E) at 0.321 ($P<0.001$) and self-rated depression on the Beck Depression Inventory at $r=0.562$ ($P<0.001$) (Fig. 3); SAI-E also correlated with BDI at $r=0.239$ ($P<0.05$). That is to say, as the discrepancy score became closer to zero or positive, indicating good awareness, so did depression scores increase. DEX scores were correlated significantly negatively with overall psychopathology as measured by the BPRS ($r=-0.570$, $P<0.001$); that is, as the discrepancy became smaller (i.e., awareness increased), so depressive symptoms became worse.

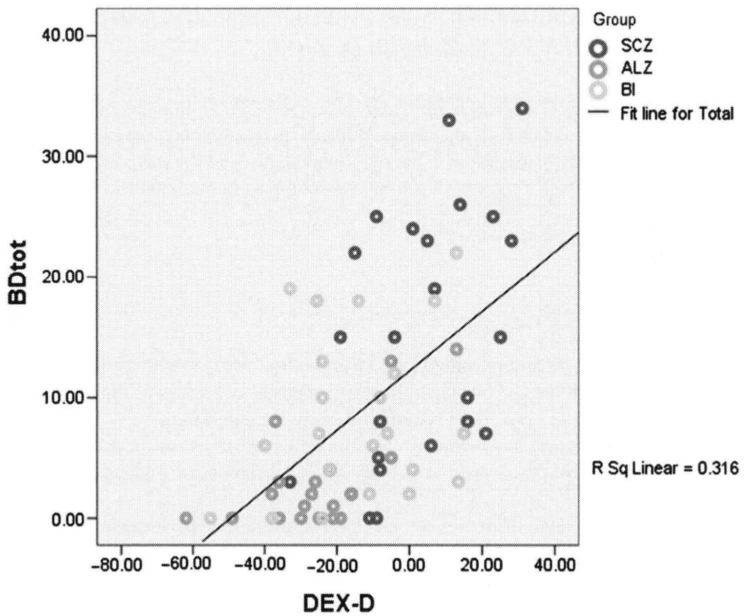

Fig. 3 Scatterplot shows the correlation between DEX discrepancy scores (*DEX-D*) and total Beck Depression scores (*BDtot*) for the three patient groups: schizophrenia (*SCZ*), Alzheimer's (*ALZ*), and brain injury (*BI*). The *regression line* shows that increasing awareness is associated with increasing depression scores

Summary and Conclusions

In summary, insight or awareness in psychiatric disorders such as schizophrenia and neuropsychiatric conditions may be multiply determined, although broadly speaking there is converging evidence for key etiological factors, such as executive function and positive psychopathology, with mood playing a mediating role. Insight is an important indicator of prognosis and outcome. In the data we present here, patients with chronic schizophrenia show good awareness of their functional and executive problems compared to patients with brain injury and AD, despite being mostly unaware of their mental illness and being mostly unable to reattribute their symptoms to mental illness. Pooling the neuropsychiatric patients together showed that overall awareness, as measured by the DEX discrepancy, correlated inversely with symptom severity and positively with mood (worse symptoms, worse awareness; lower mood, better awareness). These results are generally in favor of modularity of awareness with a degree of consistency regardless of diagnosis [107, 108]. We propose, tentatively, that the pattern is consistent with the existence of a common *cognitive* architecture for awareness of psychopathologies that may be disrupted following varied neurophysiological and neuroanatomical dysfunction – as in brain injury, schizophrenia, and AD. This concept would go against focal localization of such an architecture but instead points to a somewhat distributed, or multiple, function-specific system or systems. However, such a system (or systems) appears to rely on general support systems, such as executive processing, and may be modulated by generalized factors such as mood.

Acknowledgments James Gilleen was supported by an MRC Ph.D. Studentship. We are grateful to Prof. Simon Lovestone for facilitating access to his Alzheimer cohort; Laura Bach helped with recruitment of brain injury patients, and Sandra Randell provided secretarial support. We are grateful to all the patients and carers who generously took part in our studies.

References

1. David AS (1990) Insight and psychosis. Br J Psychiatry 156:798–808
2. Amador XF, David AS (eds) (2004) Insight and psychosis: awareness of illness in schizophrenia and related disorders, 2nd edn. Oxford University Press, Oxford
3. Markova IS (2005) Insight in psychiatry. Cambridge University Press, Cambridge
4. David A, Buchanan A, Reed A et al (1992) The assessment of insight in psychosis. Br J Psychiatry 161:599
5. Amador XF, Strauss DH, Yale SA et al (1991) Awareness of illness in schizophrenia. Schizophr Bull 17:113–132
6. Amador XF, Strauss DH, Yale SA et al (1993) Assessment of insight in psychosis. Am J Psychiatry 150:873–879
7. Kemp R, David AS (1997) Insight and compliance. In: Blackwell B (ed) Treatment compliance and the therapeutic alliance. Harwood, Amsterdam
8. Sanz M, Constable G, Lopez-Ibor I et al (1998) A comparative study of insight scales and their relationship to psychopathological and clinical variables. Psychol Med 28:437–446

9. McEvoy JP, Apperson LJ, Appelbaum PS et al (1989) Insight in schizophrenia. Its relationship to acute psychopathology. J Nerv Ment Dis 177:43–47
10. Birchwood M et al (1994) A self-report Insight Scale for psychosis: reliability, validity and sensitivity to change. Acta Psychiatr Scand 89:62–67
11. Prigatano GP, Fordyce DJ (1986) Cognitive dysfunction and psychosocial adjustment after brain injury. In: Prigatano GP, Fordyce DJ (eds) Neuropsychological rehabilitation after brain injury. John Hopkins University Press, Baltimore, pp 96–118
12. Burgess PW, Alderman N, Evans J et al (1998) The ecological validity of tests of executive function. J Int Neuropsychol Soc 4:547–558
13. Berrios GE (2004) Insight: a conceptual history. In: Amador XF, David AS (eds) Insight and psychosis: awareness of illness in schizophrenia and related disorders, 2nd edn. Oxford University Press, Oxford
14. Takai A, Uematsu M, Ueki H et al (1992) Insight and its related factors in chronic schizophrenic patients: a preliminary study. Eur J Psychiatry 6:159–170
15. Young DA, Davila R, Scher H (1993) Unawareness of illness and neuropsychological performance in chronic schizophrenia. Schizophr Res 10:117–124
16. Kemp RA, Lambert TJ (1995) Insight in schizophrenia and its relationship to psychopathology. Schizophr Res 18:21–28
17. Fennig S, Everett E, Bromet EJ et al (1996) Insight in first-admission psychotic patients. Schizophr Res 22:257–263
18. Young DA, Zakzanis KK, Bailey C et al (1998) Further parameters of insight and neuropsychological deficit in schizophrenia and other chronic mental disease. J Nerv Ment Dis 186:44–50
19. Rossell SL, Coakes J, Shapleske J et al (2003) Insight: its relationship with cognitive function, brain volume and symptoms in schizophrenia. Psychol Med 33:111–119
20. Keshavan MS, Rabinowitz J, DeSmedt G et al (2004) Correlates of insight in first episode psychosis. Schizophr Res 70:187–194
21. Almeida OP, Levy R, Howard RJ et al (1996) Insight and paranoid disorders in late life (late paraphrenia). Int J Geriatr Psychiatry 11:653–658
22. Kim Y, Sakamoto K, Kamo T et al (1997) Insight and clinical correlates in schizophrenia. Compr Psychiatry 38:117–123
23. Lysaker PH, Bell MD, Bryson G et al (1998) Neurocognitive function and insight in schizophrenia: support for an association with impairments in executive function but not with impairments in global function. Acta Psychiatr Scand 97:297–301
24. Schwartz RC (1998) Symptomatology and insight in schizophrenia. Psychol Rep 82:227–233
25. Carroll A, Fattah S, Clyde Z et al (1999) Correlates of insight and insight change in schizophrenia. Schizophr Res 35:247–253
26. McCabe R, Quayle E, Beirne AD et al (2002) Insight, global neuropsychological functioning, and symptomatology in chronic schizophrenia. J Nerv Ment Dis 190:519–525
27. Olfson M, Marcus SC, Wilk J et al (2006) Awareness of illness and nonadherence to antipsychotic medications among persons with schizophrenia. Psychiatr Serv 57:205–211
28. Macpherson R, Jerrom B, Hughes A (1996) Relationship between insight, educational background and cognition in schizophrenia. Br J Psychiatry 168:718
29. Collins AA, Remington GJ, Coulter K et al (1997) Insight, neurocognitive function and symptom clusters in chronic schizophrenia. Schizophr Res 27:37–44
30. Cuesta MJ, Peralta V, Zarzuela A (2000) Reappraising insight in psychosis. Multi-scale longitudinal study. Br J Psychiatry 177:233–240
31. Laroi F, Fannemel M, Ronneberg U et al (2000) Unawareness of illness in chronic schizophrenia and its relationship to structural brain measures and neuropsychological tests. Psychiatry Res 100:49–58
32. Mintz AR, Dobson KS, Romney DM (2003) Insight in schizophrenia: a meta-analysis. Schizophr Res 61:75–88

33. Baier M, DeShay E, Owens K et al (2000) The relationship between insight and clinical factors for persons with schizophrenia. Arch Psychiatr Nurs 14:259–265
34. Smith TE, Hull JW, Israel LM et al (2000) Insight, symptoms, and neurocognition in schizophrenia and schizoaffective disorder. Schizophr Bull 26:193–200
35. Heinrichs DW, Cohen BP, Carpenter WT Jr (1985) Early insight and the management of schizophrenic decompensation. J Nerv Ment Dis 173:133–138
36. Overall JE, Gorham D (1962) The Brief Psychiatric Rating Scale. Psychol Rep 10:799–812
37. David AS (2004) The clinical importance of insight. In: Amador XF, David AS (eds) Insight and psychosis: awareness of illness in schizophrenia and related disorders. Oxford University Press, Oxford
38. Michalakeas A, Skoutas C, Charalambous A et al (1994) Insight in schizophrenia and mood disorders and its relation to psychopathology. Acta Psychiatr Scand 90:46–49
39. Amador XF et al (1994) Awareness of illness in schizophrenia and schizoaffective and mood disorders. Arch Gen Psychiatry 51:826–836
40. Varga M, Magnusson A, Flekkoy K et al (2007) Clinical and neuropsychological correlates of insight in schizophrenia and bipolar I disorder: does diagnosis matter? Compr Psychiatry 28:583–591
41. Ghaemi SN, Rosenquist KJ (2004) Is insight in mania state-dependent?: a meta-analysis. J Nerv Ment Dis 192:771–775
42. Weiler MA, Fleisher MH, Arthur-Campbell D (2000) Insight and symptom change in schizophrenia and other disorders. Schizophr Res 45:29–36
43. Pini S, Cassano GB, Dell'Osso L et al (2001) Insight into illness in schizophrenia, schizoaffective disorder, and mood disorders with psychotic features. Am J Psychiatry 158:122–125
44. David A, van Os J, Jones P et al (1995) Insight and psychotic illness. Cross-sectional and longitudinal associations. Br J Psychiatry 167:621–628
45. Arduini L, Kalyvoka A, Stratta P et al (2003) Insight and neuropsychological function in patients with schizophrenia and bipolar disorder with psychotic features. Can J Psychiatry 48:338–341
46. Marks KA, Fastenau PS, Lysaker PH et al (2000) Self-Appraisal of Illness Questionnaire (SAIQ): relationship to researcher-rated insight and neuropsychological function in schizophrenia. Schizophr Res 45:203–211
47. Pyne JM, Bean D, Sullivan G (2001) Characteristics of patients with schizophrenia who do not believe they are mentally ill. J Nerv Ment Dis 189:146–153
48. David AS (1999) To see ourselves as others see us. Aubrey Lewis's insight. Br J Psychiatry 174:210–216
49. Cooke MA, Peters ER, Kuipers E et al (2005) Disease, deficit or denial? Models of poor insight in psychosis. Acta Psychiatr Scand 112:4–17
50. Lysaker P, Bell M (1994) Insight and cognitive impairment in schizophrenia. Performance on repeated administrations of the Wisconsin Card Sorting Test. J Nerv Ment Dis 182:656–660
51. Morgan KD, David AS (2004) Neuropsychological studies of insight in patients with psychotic disorders. In: Insight and psychosis: awareness of illness in schizophrenia and related disorders. Oxford University Press, Oxford
52. Aleman A, Agrawal N, Morgan KD et al (2006) Insight in psychosis and neuropsychological function: meta-analysis. Br J Psychiatry 189:204–212
53. Flashman LA, McAllister TW, Andreasen NC et al (2000) Smaller brain size associated with unawareness of illness in patients with schizophrenia. Am J Psychiatry 157:1167–1169
54. McEvoy JP, Johnson J, Perkins D et al (2006) Insight in first-episode psychosis. Psychol Med 36:1385–1393
55. Flashman LA, McAllister TW, Johnson SC et al (2001) Specific frontal lobe subregions correlated with unawareness of illness in schizophrenia: a preliminary study. J Neuropsychiatry Clin Neurosci 13:255–257
56. Sapara A, Cooke M, Fannon D et al (2007) Prefrontal cortex and insight in schizophrenia: a volumetric MRI study. Schizophr Res 89:22–34

57. Bassitt DP, Neto MRL, de Castro CC et al (2007) Insight and regional brain volumes in schizophrenia. Eur Arch Psychiatry Clin Neurosci 257:58–62
58. Ha TH, Youna T, Ha K et al (2004) Grey matter abnormalities in paranoid schizophrenia and their clinical correlations. Psychiatry Res Neuroimaging 132:251–260
59. Shad MU, Muddasani S, Keshavan MS (2006) Prefrontal subregions and dimensions of insight in first-episode schizophrenia: a pilot study. Psychiatry Res 146:35–42
60. Cooke MA, Fannon D, Kuipers E et al (2008) Neurological basis of poor insight in psychosis: a voxel-based MRI study. Schizophr Res 103:40–51
61. Schmitz TW, Johnson SC (2007) Relevance to self: a brief review and framework of neural systems underlying appraisal. Neurosci Biobehav Rev 31:585–596
62. Berti A, Bottini G, Gandola M et al (2005) Shared cortical anatomy for motor awareness and motor control. Science 309:488–491
63. Clare L (2004) Awareness in early-stage Alzheimer's disease: a review of methods and evidence. Br J Clin Psychol 43:177–196
64. Smith TE, Hull JW, Santos L (1998) The relationship between symptoms and insight in schizophrenia: a longitudinal perspective. Schizophr Res 33:63–67
65. Moore O, Cassidy E, Carr A et al (1999) Unawareness of illness and its relationship with depression and self-deception in schizophrenia. Eur Psychiatry 14:264–269
66. Iqbal Z, Birchwood M, Chadwick P et al (2000) Cognitive approach to depression and suicidal thinking in psychosis. 2. Testing the validity of a social ranking model. Br J Psychiatry 177:522–528
67. White R, Bebbington P, Pearson J et al (2000) The social context of insight in schizophrenia. Soc Psychiatry Psychiatr Epidemiol 35:500–507
68. Schwartz RC (2001) Self-awareness in schizophrenia: its relationship to depressive symptomatology and broad psychiatric impairments. J Nerv Ment Dis 189:401–403
69. Mutsatsa SH, Joyce EM, Hutton SB et al (2006) Relationship between insight, cognitive function, social function and symptomatology in schizophrenia: the West London first episode study. Eur Arch Psychiatry Clin Neurosci 256:356–363
70. Ghaemi SN (2007) Feeling and time: the phenomenology of mood disorders, depressive realism, and existential psychotherapy. Schizophr Bull 33:122–130
71. Rathod S, Kingdon D, Smith P et al (2005) Insight into schizophrenia: the effects of cognitive behavioural therapy on the components of insight and association with sociodemographics: data on a previously published randomised controlled trial. Schizophr Res 74:211–219
72. Kemp R, Kirov G, Everitt B et al (1998) Randomised controlled trial of compliance therapy: 18-month follow-up. Br J Psychiatry 172:413–419
73. Vasterling JJ, Seltzer B, Foss JW et al (1995) Unawareness of deficit in Alzheimer's disease. Domain-specific differences and disease correlates. Neuropsychiatry Neuropsychol Behav Neurol 8:26–32
74. Starkstein SE, Chemerinski E, Sabe L et al (1997) Prospective longitudinal study of depression and anosognosia in Alzheimer's disease. Br J Psychiatry 171:47–52
75. Clare L (2004) The construction of awareness in early-stage Alzheimer's disease: a review of concepts and models. Br J Clin Psychol 43:155–175
76. Seltzer B, Vasterling JJ, Hale MA et al (1995) Unawareness of memory deficit in Alzheimer's disease relation to mood and other disease variables. Neuropsychiatry Neuropsychol Behav Neurol 8:176–181
77. Derouesne C, Thibault S, Lagha-Pierucci S et al (1999) Decreased awareness of cognitive deficits in patients with mild dementia of the Alzheimer type. Int J Geriatr Psychiatry 14:1019–1030
78. Koltai DC, Welsh-Bohmer KA, Schmechel DE (2001) Influence of anosognosia on treatment outcome among dementia patients. Cogn Rehabil Dement 3:455–475
79. McGlynn SM, Schacter DL (1989) Unawareness of deficits in neuropsychological syndromes. J Clin Exp Neuropsychol 11:143–205
80. Laroi F, Barr WB, Keefe RSE (2004) The neuropsychology of insight in psychiatric and neurological disorders. In: Amador X, David A (eds) Insight and psychosis: awareness of illness in schizophrenia and related disorders. Oxford University Press, Oxford

81. Vogel A, Hasselbalch SG, Gade A et al (2005) Cognitive and functional neuroimaging correlate for anosognosia in mild cognitive impairment and Alzheimer's disease. Int J Geriatr Psychiatry 20:238–246
82. Harwood DG, Sultzer DL, Wheatley MV (2000) Impaired insight in Alzheimer disease: association with cognitive deficits, psychiatric symptoms, and behavioral disturbances. Neuropsychiatry Neuropsychol Behav Neurol 13:83–88
83. Feher EP, Mahurin RK, Inbody SB et al (1991) Anosognosia in Alzheimer's disease. Neuropsychiatry Neuropsychol Behav Neurol 4:136–146
84. DeBettignies BH, Mahurin RK, Pirozzolo FJ (1990) Insight for impairment in independent living skills in Alzheimer's disease and multi-infarct dementia. J Clin Exp Neuropsychol 12:355–363
85. Michon A, Deweer B, Pillon B et al (1994) Relation of anosognosia to frontal lobe dysfunction in Alzheimer's disease. J Neurol Neurosurg Psychiatry 57:805–809
86. Auchus AP, Goldstein FC, Green J et al (1994) Unawareness of cognitive impairments in Alzheimer's disease. Neuropsychiatry Neuropsychol Behav Neurol 7:25–29
87. Lopez OL, Becker JT, Somsak D et al (1994) Awareness of cognitive deficits and anosognosia in probable Alzheimer's disease. Eur Neurol 34:277–282
88. Dalla Barba G, Parlato V, Iavarone A et al (1995) Anosognosia, intrusions and frontal functions in Alzheimer's disease and depression. Neuropsychologia 33:247–259
89. Migliorelli R, Teson A, Sabe L et al (1995) Prevalence and correlates of dysthymia and major depression among patients with Alzheimer's disease. Am J Psychiatry 152:37–44
90. Sevush S (1999) Relationship between denial of memory deficit and dementia severity in Alzheimer disease. Neuropsychiatry Neuropsychol Behav Neurol 12:88–94
91. Feher EP, Larrabee GJ, Sudilovsky A et al (1994) Memory self-report in Alzheimer's disease and in age-associated memory impairment. J Geriatr Psychiatry Neurol 7:58–65
92. Zanetti O, Vallotti B, Frisoni GB et al (1999) Insight in dementia: when does it occur? Evidence for a nonlinear relationship between insight and cognitive status. J Gerontol B Psychol Sci Soc Sci 54:100–106
93. Prigatano GP, Altman IM (1990) Impaired awareness of behavioral limitations after traumatic brain injury. Arch Phys Med Rehabil 71:1058–1064
94. Sherer M, Boake C, Levin E (1998) Characteristics of impaired awareness after traumatic brain injury. J Int Neuropsychol Soc 4:380–387
95. Trudel TM, Tryon WW, Purdum CM (1998) Awareness of disability and long-term outcome after traumatic brain injury. Rehabil Psychol 43:267–281
96. Sherer M, Hart T, Nick TG et al (2003) Early impaired self-awareness after traumatic brain injury. Arch Phys Med Rehabil 84:168–176
97. Wise K, Ownsworth T, Fleming J (2005) Convergent validity of self-awareness measures and their association with employment outcome in adults following acquired brain injury. Brain Inj 19:765–775
98. Bergquist TF, Jacket MP (1993) Awareness and goal setting with the traumatically -brain injured. Brain Inj 7:275–282
99. Prigatano GP (2005) Disturbances of self-awareness and rehabilitation of patients with traumatic brain injury: a 20-year perspective. J Head Trauma Rehabil 20:19–29
100. Banks SJ, Weintraub S (2009) Generalized and symptom-specific insight in behavioral variant frontotemporal dementia and primary progressive aphasia. J Neuropsychiatry Clin Neurosci 21:299–306
101. O'Keeffe FM, Murray B, Coen RF et al (2007) Loss of insight in frontotemporal dementia, corticobasal degeneration and progressive supranuclear palsy. Brain 130:753–764
102. Medalia A, Lim RW (2004) Self-awareness of cognitive functioning in schizophrenia. Schizophr Res 71:331–338
103. Kircher TTJ, Koch K, Stottmeister F et al (2007) Metacognition and reflexivity in patients with schizophrenia. Psychopathology 40:254–260
104. Teasdale TW, Christensen AL, Willmes K et al (1997) Subjective experience in brain injured patients and their close relatives: a European Brain Injury Questionnaire study. Brain Inj 11:543–564

105. Vasterling JJ, Seltzer B, Watrous WE (1997) Longitudinal assessment of deficit unawareness in Alzheimer's disease. Neuropsychiatry Neuropsychol Behav Neurol 10:197–202
106. Burgess PW, Alderman N, Emslie H, Evans JJ, Wilson BA (1996) The dysexecutive questionnaire. In: Wilson BA, Alderman N, Burgess PW, Emslie H, Evans JJ (eds) Behavioural assessment of the Dysexecutive Syndrome. Thames Valley Test Company, Bury St. Edmunds, UK
107. Bayard S, Capdevielle D, Boulenger JP et al (2009) Dissociating self-reported cognitive complaint from clinical insight in schizophrenia. Eur Psychiatry 24:251–258
108. Flashman LA, Roth RM, McAllister TW et al (2007) Dissociation of awareness of different components of illness in schizophrenia. J Neuropsychiatry Clin Neurosci 19:221–222
109. Morgan KD, Dazzan P, Morgan C et al (2010). Insight, grey matter and cognitive function in first-onset psychosis, Brit J Psychiat (in press).

Visual Hallucinations in Neurodegenerative Disorders

Spyridon Papapetropoulos and Blake K. Scanlon

Abstract Neuropsychiatric symptoms, such as hallucinations, are common in neurodegenerative disorders and primarily in Parkinson's disease, where they contribute significantly to disease morbidity and caregiver burden, eventually leading to early nursing home placement. As the average life expectancy in developed nations continues on an upward trend, the incidence of neurodegenerative disease and their neuropsychiatric complications follows in parallel. This review provides an overview of synucleinopathies, tauopathies, prion diseases, and heredodegenerative disorders in which visual hallucinations (VH) are present. Epidemiological information along with factors associated with symptom presentation is outlined. The clinical characteristics of visual disturbances and their impact on disease management are discussed. Relevant treatment options for VH in each neurodegenerative syndrome are also reviewed.

Keywords Alzheimer's disease • Dementia with Lewy bodies • Neurodegenerative disorders • Parkinson's disease • Visual hallucinations

Introduction

Neurodegenerative diseases are characterized by progressive decline in the structure, activity, and function of the central nervous system. Neuronal dropout usually results in disruption of multiple pathways, regional neurotransmitter

---

S. Papapetropoulos (✉) and B.K. Scanlon
Department of Neurology, University of Miami Miller School of Medicine,
1536 9th Avenue, Miami, FL 33136, USA
e-mail: spapapetropoulos@med.miami.edu

S. Papapetropoulos
Biogen Idec, 14 Cambridge Center, Bio 6A, 6th Floor,
Cambridge, MA 02142, USA

B.K. Scanlon
Department of Psychology, University of Miami,
5665 Ponce de Leon Blvd., Coral Gables, FL 33146, USA

K. Miyoshi et al. (eds.), *Neuropsychiatric Disorders*,
DOI 10.1007/978-4-431-53871-4_4, © Springer 2010

deficits, and neurochemical imbalance. As a result, distinctive phenotypic expressions are grouped into disease clinicopathological entities [Alzheimer's disease (AD), Parkinson's disease (PD), etc.]. Clinicians recognize this distinctive set of progressive signs and symptoms and, on pathological examination, the pathologist reports lesions in brain regions that underpin these signs and symptoms.

Neuropsychiatric manifestations are very prevalent and an integral part of the symptom/sign pattern of neurodegenerative diseases. Most importantly, they significantly add to disease morbidity, caregiver burden, and deteriorating health-related quality of life. Although the mechanism remains unknown, it is hypothesized that neuropsychiatric symptoms may be primary and an integral part of the neurodegenerative process, secondary to medication or comorbid conditions affecting the dysregulated and susceptible system, or simply reactive phenomena.

The pattern recognition approach to disease has been palliative, and there has been no knowledge of the causes of the damage. Advances in molecular genetics and immune-based histopathology techniques have allowed a classification system of neurodegenerative diseases based on protein accumulation. Microtubule-associated tau is one protein that has important functions in healthy neurons but which forms insoluble deposits in diseases now known collectively as tauopathies. Tauopathies encompass more than 20 clinicopathological entities, including AD, the most common tauopathy, progressive supranuclear palsy (PSP), frontotemporal dementia (FTD), corticobasal degeneration, and postencephalitic parkinsonism. The term synucleinopathies refers to a certain subset of neurodegenerative diseases with a similar pathological lesion pattern consisting of insoluble alpha-synuclein in selected neuronal and glial cells. Accumulation of alpha-synuclein is seen in dementia with Lewy bodies (DLB), PD, and multiple systems atrophy (MSA). A smaller subset of neurodegenerative diseases is genetically determined and can be collectively grouped into the heredodegenerative category. This review focuses on one of the most common neuropsychiatric symptoms in neurodegenerative disorders: the characteristics, etiology, and treatment of visual hallucinations (VH) are discussed in the most common neurodegenerative disorders.

Visual Hallucinations in Synucleinopathies

Dementia with Lewy Bodies

Epidemiology

Dementia with Lewy bodies (DLB) is frequently recognized as the second most common degenerative dementia [1]. Although extensive epidemiological literature is lacking, a recent review indicates that prevalence estimates for DLB range from 0.1% to 5.0% in the general population and from 1.7% and 30.5% in dementia cases [1]. In accordance with current consensus criteria, recurrent VH are among the core features indicative of DLB [2]. Approximately two-thirds of patients with DLB present with VH [3, 4]. Patients with DLB commonly present with hallucinations, and nearly half have hallucinations within 2 years after the first clinical symptom [5].

Factors Associated with VH in DLB

A recent community-based autopsy study found that cases with VH were more likely than cases without VH to have Lewy-related pathology (78% versus 45%) [6]. Overall cortical Lewy body (LB) burden is greater in cases with early VH (at onset or within the first 2 years of the disease course), which relates to more LBs in the inferior temporal cortices [5]. Additional neuropathological evidence indicates that VH are associated with more LB pathology in the parahippocampus and amygdala [5].

Neuroimaging technologies are also used to elucidate factors associated with VH. Although most effort focuses on identifying imaging markers that differentiate DLB from other dementing disorders, some investigations examine potential mechanisms related specifically to VH in DLB. ^{18}F-Fluorodeoxyglucose-positron emission tomography (^{18}F-FDG-PET) evaluations show that people living with DLB and VH have relative metabolic reductions in the right temporo-occipital junction and the right middle frontal gyrus compared to those with DLB without VH [7].

Certain clinical characteristics are also associated with VH in DLB. The Consortium on DLB [8] reports that VH may particularly present during periods of diminished consciousness. Visual impairment exacerbates VH; this is likely a consequence of selective sensory deprivation, and an increase in environmental stimulation may provide temporary relief [8]. People living with DLB and VH perform worse on overlapping figure identification compared to those without VH [9]. Additional evidence shows that DLB and demented PD patients with recurrent VH are significantly more impaired in visual discrimination, space-motion perception, and object-form perception than patients without VH [10].

Clinical Characteristics of VH in DLB

While people living with DLB have hallucinatory experiences that encompass a variety of modalities, VH are most common [4]. These VH are frequently complex, occur at least once a day, last for minutes, and consist of a single, colored, stationary object in the central visual field [11]. The experiences are often benign and not perceived as threatening. However, there are exceptions. These characteristics are largely similar to those evidenced in PD dementia. Specific phenomenological characteristics of VH in DLB include anonymous people/soldiers; body parts; animals; friends and family; children/babies; and machines [11]. VH in DLB tend to persist and are stable over time [12].

Clinical Impact and Treatment of VH in DLB

VH are considered one of the most important neuropsychiatric targets for intervention in DLB [13]. Several pharmacological intervention strategies show some success in the treatment of hallucinations in DLB. Deficits in cortical acetylcholine are associated with VH [14] and thus, unsurprisingly, VH are often responsive to pharmacotherapies with anticholinesterase properties. DLB patients with VH who are cognitive responders to acetylcholinesterase inhibitors such as donepezil, galantamine, and rivastigmine show greater improvement than responders without VH [15]. Furthermore, cognitive nonresponders with VH show less cognitive decline at follow-up than do cognitive nonresponders without VH [15]. Although these medications were originally created to treat AD, evidence shows a better response in the treatment of DLB than AD [16]. Because of the potential for severe adverse reactions to neuroleptics [2, 17], the use of antipsychotics in the treatment of DLB should only be initiated after careful consideration.

Parkinson's Disease

Epidemiology

Worldwide prevalence rates of Parkinson's disease (PD) tend to vary widely [18]. Estimates of the number of people living with PD in the world's ten most populous nations, along with Western Europe's five most populous nations, range between 4.1 and 4.6 million [19]. This number is expected to double to somewhere between 8.7 and 9.3 million by 2030. Annual incidence ranges between 4.9 and 26 per 100,000 [20]. Hallucinations occur in 20% to 40% of PD patients receiving symptomatic therapy [21], although as many as 75% of patients develop hallucinatory phenomena of a visual nature [22]. VH in PD are often considered treatment related because prevalence rates in the pre-levodopa era were as low as 5% [23, 24].

Factors Associated with the Presentation of Hallucinations in PD

Longer PD disease duration, higher unified PD rating scale (UPDRS) total score, and dementia show independent associations with the occurrence of medication-induced VH in PD [25]. All dopaminergic therapies (direct, through receptor stimulation, or indirect, through metabolic enzyme inhibition), and especially dopamine agonist therapy, can elicit hallucinations and psychosis [26]. Additionally, numerous studies find greater prevalence of hallucinations and other psychotic symptoms in demented versus nondemented patients with PD [27]. VH are present in 70% of PD patients with dementia [28]. Approximately 45% of nondemented PD patients with VH go on to develop dementia within a year [29]. Additional evidence suggests that deficient performance on cognitive tasks, such as verbal fluency, predicts the development of hallucinations in people living with PD [30]. Furthermore, REM (rapid eye movement) sleep behavior disorder comorbidity is associated with increased VH risk in PD.

Clinical Characteristics of VH in PD

The VH most often reported in PD are drug induced, complex, and consist of animate or inanimate objects or persons [31]. However, perceptual phenomena that are more transient and less clear can also occur [28]. VH typically appear several years after disease onset and usually contain five or fewer images, which are sometimes meaningful to the patient. The typical "hallucinator's experience" [32] occurs while alert and with eyes open, in dim surroundings. The hallucination is present for a few seconds and then suddenly vanishes. Initially, hallucinations are "friendly." Patients often see fragmented figures of beloved familiar persons or animals. As reality testing and insight further decrease, the content of the hallucinations may change to frightening images (e.g., insects, rats), inducing anxiety and panic attacks [33]. Hallucinations may become malignant, disabling, and intermingled with paranoid patterns, including suspiciousness, negativism, and sexual accusations. Ideas of persecution, fearfulness, agitation, aggression, confusion, and delirium become commonplace. It is at this point that the situation at home often becomes unbearable, and the patient is frequently placed in a nursing home [34]. Although VH are predominant, auditory hallucinations (mixed with visual) are reported to affect about 10% of patients [28].

Clinical Impact and Treatment of VH in PD

Without intervention, hallucinations with retained insight can evolve to malignant hallucinations without insight [35]. Presence of hallucinations can predict nursing home placement [36] and may predict mortality in PD [37]. When hallucinations first present, a systematic evaluation for potential causes should ensue. Once factors such as secondary illness or medication overdose are ruled out, the physician should revisit the diagnosis of PD to ensure premorbid psychosis or other neurodegenerative diseases do not explain the VH.

As a first-line treatment, visual, cognitive, and interactional coping strategies [38], along with appropriate sleep hygiene, should be encouraged. If these strategies do not effectively resolve the VH, removal or taper of medications with the lowest antiparkinsonian effect may be useful. Adjustment of dopaminergic therapy to balance the treatment of motor and nonmotor symptoms such as VH is perhaps the most effective treatment strategy. Although some evidence suggests that treatment with antipsychotics may delay psychiatric deterioration [39], the U.S. Food and Drug Administration (FDA) has determined that atypical antipsychotic use may contribute to increased mortality in elderly dementia patients [40]. Additional evidence linking antipsychotic use to increased risk of pneumonia is particularly relevant to treatment considerations, as pneumonia is the most commonly reported cause of death in PD [41]. Although clozapine is considered "probably effective" and quetiapine is considered "possibly effective" in the treatment of psychosis in PD [42], caution must be used when using antipsychotics "off-label" to treat hallucinations and other psychotic symptoms in PD. Pimavanserin tartrate, a selective 5-HT2A inverse agonist, has shown encouraging efficacy against psychotic symptoms in PD in phase II and is currently being tested in phase III pivotal trials [43]. Acetylcholinesterase inhibitors may also have potential utility in the treatment of VH in PD. A case report indicates donepezil may decrease VH in PD [44], and PD patients with VH may show greater benefit from rivastigmine than those without VH [45]. However, no large, controlled trials have been conducted to determine the efficacy of acetylcholinesterase inhibitors in the treatment of VH in PD.

Multiple System Atrophy

Multiple system atrophy (MSA) is a progressive neurodegenerative disorder with a diverse clinical presentation that can include parkinsonism, autonomic failure, urogenital dysfunction, cerebellar ataxia, and corticospinal disorders [46]. Prevalence estimates range from 1.9/100,000 to 4.9/100,000 per year, with an estimated incidence of 0.6/100,000 per year [47]. Nonmedication-induced hallucinations are considered nonsupportive of MSA diagnosis [46]. Nonetheless, evidence from case reports suggests that VH occur in up to 9.5% of pathologically confirmed MSA cases [48]. VH reported in a study by Papapetropoulos and colleagues consisted of small and friendly animals in one case not receiving dopaminergic therapy and fragmented friendly faces in dimly lit surroundings related to levodopa in another case. Neither case required treatment with antipsychotics [48].

VH in Tauopathies

Alzheimer's Disease

Epidemiology

AD is the most common degenerative dementia. There were 4.5 million people living with AD in the United States in 2000; this number is expected to nearly triple by 2050 [49]. A population-based European study estimates the age-standardized prevalence of AD to be 4.4%, with prevalence increasing with age [50]. Nearly 19% of patients with AD experience VH [51]. Data on persistence of psychotic symptoms, including VH, in AD are mixed, and methodological differences likely contribute to disparate findings.

Factors Associated with the Presentation of Hallucinations in AD

The severity of cognitive impairment in AD often relates to prevalence of hallucinations, with more impaired patients being at higher risk for hallucinations [51]. Several studies show that African Americans have a higher risk of developing hallucinations than Caucasians; however, this relationship appears to be more relevant in advanced disease stages. Data on other clinicodemographic factors are either mixed or equivocal and are discussed more fully by Ropacki and Jeste [51]. Additional evidence indicates that patients with dementia (including, but not limited to AD) and hallucinations are more likely to present with agitation, delusions, and apathy than those without hallucinations [6]. This cohort of hallucinators was also more likely to have Lewy-related pathology upon autopsy.

Clinical Characteristics of VH in AD

Assessing VH in people living with AD and other cognitive disorders is frequently challenging. Some studies rely on caregiver reports to identify patients experiencing VH, whereas others do not often report characteristics of the hallucinations other than prevalence or Neuropsychiatric Inventory score. Some work shows that VH in AD include images of familiar people, dead relatives, animals, and machinery [52]. Other work shows that 54% of AD patients with VH also experience an auditory component [53]. Because of the clinical presentation of AD, VH may not be adequately captured with common methodologies.

Clinical Impact and Treatment of VH in AD

Hallucinations in AD have been associated with aggressive behavior, verbal outbursts, asocial behavior, and falls; however, other studies have failed to show these relationships [54]. The presence of hallucinations predicts increased risk for cognitive/functional decline, institutionalization, and mortality in AD [55]. At present, regulatory authorities including the FDA have yet to approve any pharmacotherapeutic agent for the treatment of dementia-related psychosis. Consequently, as with previously mentioned disorders, nonpharmacological management is the recommended first-line treatment. Although some atypical antipsychotics may be modestly effective treatments for psychosis in AD, adverse event and mortality risk may significantly outweigh the treatment benefits in this population [17, 40, 56].

Progressive Supranuclear Palsy

Progressive supranuclear palsy (PSP) is a phenotypically heterogeneous, progressive neurodegenerative disorder consisting of parkinsonism, mild dementia, supranuclear gaze palsy, and postural instability [57]. Prevalence estimates range from 1.39/100,000 to 6.5/100,000 [58–60], and incidence is estimated to be 5.3 new cases per 100,000 person-years in people 50 to 99 years of age [61]. Estimates of VH prevalence in PSP range from 9.1% to 13.4% [62, 63]. Several studies report phenomenological characteristics of VH in PSP [62, 64–66]. VH are frequently whole people, animals, or fragmented faces. They are familiar sights and occur during twilight or nighttime more often than not. VH can present with an auditory component and may become frightening as complexity increases and disease progresses. The relationship between VH in PSP and antiparkinsonian treatment appears to be equivocal. Nonpharmacological interventions are the first-line treatment, and pharmacotherapy may be useful if the VH become threatening and severely impair quality of life. Antipsychotics show limited utility in treating VH in PSP. However, before implementation, the risk of severe adverse events must be strongly considered [62].

Frontotemporal Dementia

Frontotemporal dementia (FTD) is a term used to define a grouping of pathologically and clinically heterogeneous disorders that demonstrate degeneration of the frontal and temporal lobes. Prevalence estimates range from 4/100,000 to 15/100,000 for those aged 45 to 64 years [67, 68]. Incidence for the same age range is estimated to be 3.5 cases per 100,000 person-years [69]. Studies published after the initial frontotemporal lobar degeneration consensus diagnostic criteria [70] have examined hallucinations, without differentiating sensory types, and report prevalence of hallucinations ranging from 2% to 13% [71–73]. However, per recent review by the Committee on Research of the American Neuropsychiatric Association, there are several reports of psychotic symptoms in FTD with only one case [74] truly showing an association between possible FTD and bizarre VH [75]. Nonpharmacological interventions are the first-line treatment for hallucinations that may arise in people living with FTD. Pharmaceutical management decisions should be made on a case-by-case basis with particular caution given to potential neuroleptic hypersensitivity [76] and other adverse events.

VH in Heredodegenerative and Other Neurodegenerative Diseases

Huntington's disease (HD) is a progressive, heredodegenerative disorder that presents with neuropsychiatric, cognitive, and motor symptoms. Prevalence of psychosis in HD ranges from 3% to 11% [77], with approximately 2% presenting with hallucinations [78]. Studies of hallucinations in HD often group hallucinations with delusions and examine them collectively rather than individually. Psychiatric symptoms that occur in people living with HD are not related to cognitive or motor presentation [78, 79]. However, they may be related to mood disorders. Once mood disorders, intoxication, and delirium are taken into consideration, antipsychotics may be useful. Assuming neuroleptics are not needed for the control of involuntary movements, newer agents such as risperidone, olanzepine, or quetiapine may be best as these have less chance of extrapyramidal side effects [80]. Systematic review deems risperidone "possibly useful" for the treatment of psychosis in HD [81].

Creutzfeldt–Jakob disease (CJD), although quite rare, is the most common prion disease affecting humans. Several forms of the disease are currently recognized, including sporadic, familial, iatrogenic, and variant. Rapidly progressive dementia and myoclonus are the cardinal features of sporadic CJD (sCJD). One study describing VH in CJD reports patients hallucinate birds, people, and other visual phenomena [82]. Cases of sCJD are frequently referred to as the Heidenhain variant if visual disturbances, including VH, occur within the first week after onset [83]. VH are present in approximately 13% of Heidenhain variant cases and 2.3% of all sCJD cases [83]. However, other studies show hallucinations of unspecified modality occur in nearly 25% of cases [84].

Although VH occur in other neurodegenerative disorders, this review is unable to address them all. As the neuropsychiatric features of neurodegenerative disorders receive more attention in the literature, a more developed understanding of symptom presentation and treatment options will likely ensue.

Conclusions

Visual hallucinations (VH) are a common feature of neurodegenerative disease. Alpha-synuclein pathology may predispose individuals to develop VH. In PD, VH are frequently treatment related, and may lead to nursing home placement and increased mortality. In DLB, VH are very common, primary, and one of the core diagnostic features. Clinical treatment of VH in neurodegenerative disorders is complex. Neuroleptics should be considered with caution, particularly in disorders with dopamine deficit.

References

1. Zaccai J, McCracken C, Brayne C (2005) A systematic review of prevalence and incidence studies of dementia with Lewy bodies. Age Ageing 34(6):561–566
2. McKeith IG, Dickson DW, Lowe J et al (2005) Diagnosis and management of dementia with Lewy bodies: third report of the DLB Consortium. Neurology 65(12):1863–1872
3. Ballard C, Holmes C, McKeith I et al (1999) Psychiatric morbidity in dementia with Lewy bodies: a prospective clinical and neuropathological comparative study with Alzheimer's disease. Am J Psychiatry 156(7):1039–1045
4. Aarsland D, Ballard C, Larsen JP et al (2001) A comparative study of psychiatric symptoms in dementia with Lewy bodies and Parkinson's disease with and without dementia. Int J Geriatr Psychiatry 16(5):528–536
5. Harding AJ, Broe GA, Halliday GM (2002) Visual hallucinations in Lewy body disease relate to Lewy bodies in the temporal lobe. Brain 125(Pt 2):391–403

6. Tsuang D, Larson EB, Bolen E et al (2009) Visual hallucinations in dementia: a prospective community-based study with autopsy. Am J Geriatr Psychiatry 17(4):317–323
7. Perneczky R, Drzezga A, Boecker H et al (2008) Cerebral metabolic dysfunction in patients with dementia with Lewy bodies and visual hallucinations. Dement Geriatr Cogn Disord 25(6):531–538
8. McKeith IG, Galasko D, Kosaka K et al (1996) Consensus guidelines for the clinical and pathologic diagnosis of dementia with Lewy bodies (DLB): report of the consortium on DLB international workshop. Neurology 47(5):1113–1124
9. Mori E, Shimomura T, Fujimori M et al (2000) Visuoperceptual impairment in dementia with Lewy bodies. Arch Neurol 57(4):489–493
10. Mosimann UP, Mather G, Wesnes KA et al (2004) Visual perception in Parkinson disease dementia and dementia with Lewy bodies. Neurology 63(11):2091–2096
11. Mosimann UP, Rowan EN, Partington CE et al (2006) Characteristics of visual hallucinations in Parkinson disease dementia and dementia with Lewy bodies. Am J Geriatr Psychiatry 14(2):153–160
12. Ballard CG, O'Brien JT, Swann AG et al (2001) The natural history of psychosis and depression in dementia with Lewy bodies and Alzheimer's disease: persistence and new cases over 1 year of follow-up. J Clin Psychiatry 62(1):46–49
13. McKeith I, Mintzer J, Aarsland D et al (2004) Dementia with Lewy bodies. Lancet Neurol 3(1):19–28
14. Perry EK, McKeith I, Thompson P et al (1991) Topography, extent, and clinical relevance of neurochemical deficits in dementia of Lewy body type, Parkinson's disease, and Alzheimer's disease. Ann N Y Acad Sci 640:197–202
15. Pakrasi S, Mukaetova-Ladinska EB, McKeith IG et al (2003) Clinical predictors of response to Acetyl Cholinesterase Inhibitors: experience from routine clinical use in Newcastle. Int J Geriatr Psychiatry 18(10):879–886
16. Samuel W, Caligiuri M, Galasko D et al (2000) Better cognitive and psychopathologic response to donepezil in patients prospectively diagnosed as dementia with Lewy bodies: a preliminary study. Int J Geriatr Psychiatry 15(9):794–802
17. Schneider LS, Dagerman KS, Insel P (2005) Risk of death with atypical antipsychotic drug treatment for dementia: meta-analysis of randomized placebo-controlled trials. JAMA 294(15):1934–1943
18. Zhang ZX, Roman GC (1993) Worldwide occurrence of Parkinson's disease: an updated review. Neuroepidemiology 12(4):195–208
19. Dorsey ER, Constantinescu R, Thompson JP et al (2007) Projected number of people with Parkinson disease in the most populous nations, 2005 through 2030. Neurology 68(5):384–386
20. Schrag A (2007) Epidemiology of movement disorders. In: Jankovic J, Tolosa E (eds) Parkinson's disease and movement disorders. Lippincott Williams & Wilkins, Philadelphia
21. Papapetropoulos S, Mash DC (2005) Psychotic symptoms in Parkinson's disease. From description to etiology. J Neurol 252(7):753–764
22. Diederich NJ, Fenelon G, Stebbins G et al (2009) Hallucinations in Parkinson disease. Nat Rev Neurol 5(6):331–342
23. Lewy F (1923) Die Lehre vom Tonus und der Bewegung. Springer, Berlin
24. Schwab RS, Fabing HD, Prichard JS (1951) Psychiatric symptoms and syndromes in Parkinson's disease. Am J Psychiatry 107(12):901–907
25. Papapetropoulos S, Argyriou AA, Ellul J (2005) Factors associated with drug-induced visual hallucinations in Parkinson's disease. J Neurol 252(10):1223–1228
26. Tolosa E, Katzenschlager R (2007) Pharmacological management of Parkinson's disease. In: Jankovic J, Tolosa E (eds) Parkinson's disease and movement disorders. Lippincott Williams & Wilkins, Philadelphia
27. Papapetropoulos S, Gonzalez J, Lieberman A et al (2005) Dementia in Parkinson's disease: a post-mortem study in a population of brain donors. Int J Geriatr Psychiatry 20(5):418–422
28. Fenelon G, Mahieux F, Huon R et al (2000) Hallucinations in Parkinson's disease: prevalence, phenomenology and risk factors. Brain 123(Pt 4):733–745

29. Ramirez-Ruiz B, Junque C, Marti MJ et al (2007) Cognitive changes in Parkinson's disease patients with visual hallucinations. Dement Geriatr Cogn Disord 23(5):281–288
30. Santangelo G, Trojano L, Vitale C et al (2007) A neuropsychological longitudinal study in Parkinson's patients with and without hallucinations. Mov Disord 22(16):2418–2425
31. Haeske-Dewick HC (1995) Hallucinations in Parkinson's disease: characteristics and associated clinical features. Int J Geriatr Psychiatry 10(6):487–495
32. Barnes J, David AS (2001) Visual hallucinations in Parkinson's disease: a review and phenomenological survey. J Neurol Neurosurg Psychiatry 70(6):727–733
33. Wolters EC (2001) Intrinsic and extrinsic psychosis in Parkinson's disease. J Neurol 248(suppl 3):III22–III27
34. Baker MG (1999) Depression, psychosis and dementia in Parkinson's disease. Neurology 52(7 suppl 3):S1
35. Goetz CG, Fan W, Leurgans S et al (2006) The malignant course of "benign hallucinations" in Parkinson disease. Arch Neurol 63(5):713–716
36. Goetz CG, Stebbins GT (1993) Risk factors for nursing home placement in advanced Parkinson's disease. Neurology 43(11):2227–2229
37. Sinforiani E, Pacchetti C, Zangaglia R et al (2008) REM behavior disorder, hallucinations and cognitive impairment in Parkinson's disease: a two-year follow up. Mov Disord 23(10):1441–1445
38. Diederich NJ, Pieri V, Goetz CG (2003) Coping strategies for visual hallucinations in Parkinson's disease. Mov Disord 18(7):831–832
39. Goetz CG, Fan W, Leurgans S (2008) Antipsychotic medication treatment for mild hallucinations in Parkinson's disease: positive impact on long-term worsening. Mov Disord 23(11):1541–1545
40. U.S. Food and Drug Administration (2009) Deaths with antipsychotics in elderly patients with behavioral disturbances. http://www.fda.gov/Drugs/DrugSafety/PublicHealthAdvisories/ucm053171.htm. Accessed 15 Aug 2009
41. Knol W, van Marum RJ, Jansen PA et al (2008) Antipsychotic drug use and risk of pneumonia in elderly people. J Am Geriatr Soc 56(4):661–666
42. Miyasaki JM, Shannon K, Voon V et al (2006) Practice parameter: evaluation and treatment of depression, psychosis, and dementia in Parkinson disease (an evidence-based review). Report of the Quality Standards Subcommittee of the American Academy of Neurology. Neurology 66(7):996–1002
43. Abbas A, Roth BL (2008) Pimavanserin tartrate: a 5-HT2A inverse agonist with potential for treating various neuropsychiatric disorders. Expert Opin Pharmacother 9(18):3251–3259
44. Kurita A, Ochiai Y, Kono Y et al (2003) The beneficial effect of donepezil on visual hallucinations in three patients with Parkinson's disease. J Geriatr Psychiatry Neurol 16(3):184–188
45. Burn D, Emre M, McKeith I et al (2006) Effects of rivastigmine in patients with and without visual hallucinations in dementia associated with Parkinson's disease. Mov Disord 21(11):1899–1907
46. Gilman S, Wenning GK, Low PA et al (2008) Second consensus statement on the diagnosis of multiple system atrophy. Neurology 71(9):670–676
47. Wenning GK, Colosimo C, Geser F et al (2004) Multiple system atrophy. Lancet Neurol 3(2):93–103
48. Papapetropoulos S, Tuchman A, Laufer D et al (2007) Hallucinations in multiple system atrophy. Parkinsonism Relat Disord 13(3):193–194
49. Hebert LE, Scherr PA, Bienias JL et al (2003) Alzheimer disease in the US population: prevalence estimates using the 2000 census. Arch Neurol 60(8):1119–1122
50. Lobo A, Launer LJ, Fratiglioni L et al (2000) Prevalence of dementia and major subtypes in Europe: a collaborative study of population-based cohorts. Neurologic Diseases in the Elderly Research Group. Neurology 54(11 Suppl 5):S4–S9
51. Ropacki SA, Jeste DV (2005) Epidemiology of and risk factors for psychosis of Alzheimer's disease: a review of 55 studies published from 1990 to 2003. Am J Psychiatry 162(11):2022–2030

52. Lin SH, Yu CY, Pai MC (2006) The occipital white matter lesions in Alzheimer's disease patients with visual hallucinations. Clin Imaging 30(6):388–393
53. Wilson RS, Krueger KR, Kamenetsky JM et al (2005) Hallucinations and mortality in Alzheimer disease. Am J Geriatr Psychiatry 13(11):984–990
54. Bassiony MM, Lyketsos CG (2003) Delusions and hallucinations in Alzheimer's disease: review of the brain decade. Psychosomatics 44(5):388–401
55. Scarmeas N, Brandt J, Albert M et al (2005) Delusions and hallucinations are associated with worse outcome in Alzheimer disease. Arch Neurol 62(10):1601–1608
56. Ballard C, Waite J (2006) The effectiveness of atypical antipsychotics for the treatment of aggression and psychosis in Alzheimer's disease. Cochrane Database Syst Rev 1:CD003476
57. Williams DR, Lees AJ (2009) Progressive supranuclear palsy: clinicopathological concepts and diagnostic challenges. Lancet Neurol 8(3):270–279
58. Golbe LI, Davis PH, Schoenberg BS et al (1988) Prevalence and natural history of progressive supranuclear palsy. Neurology 38(7):1031–1034
59. Schrag A, Ben-Shlomo Y, Quinn NP (1999) Prevalence of progressive supranuclear palsy and multiple system atrophy: a cross-sectional study. Lancet 354(9192):1771–1775
60. Nath U, Ben-Shlomo Y, Thomson RG et al (2001) The prevalence of progressive supranuclear palsy (Steele-Richardson-Olszewski syndrome) in the UK. Brain 124(Pt 7):1438–1449
61. Bower JH, Maraganore DM, McDonnell SK et al (1997) Incidence of progressive supranuclear palsy and multiple system atrophy in Olmsted County, Minnesota, 1976 to 1990. Neurology 49(5):1284–1288
62. Papapetropoulos S, Mash DC (2005) Visual hallucinations in progressive supranuclear palsy. Eur Neurol 54(4):217–219
63. Williams DR, Warren JD, Lees AJ (2008) Using the presence of visual hallucinations to differentiate Parkinson's disease from atypical parkinsonism. J Neurol Neurosurg Psychiatry 79(6):652–655
64. Compta Y, Marti MJ, Rey MJ et al (2009) Parkinsonism, dysautonomia, REM behaviour disorder and visual hallucinations mimicking synucleinopathy in a patient with progressive supranuclear palsy. J Neurol Neurosurg Psychiatry 80(5):578–579
65. Cooper AD, Josephs KA (2009) Photophobia, visual hallucinations, and REM sleep behavior disorder in progressive supranuclear palsy and corticobasal degeneration: a prospective study. Parkinsonism Relat Disord 15(1):59–61
66. Diederich NJ, Leurgans S, Fan W et al (2008) Visual hallucinations and symptoms of REM sleep behavior disorder in Parkinsonian tauopathies. Int J Geriatr Psychiatry 23(6):598–603
67. Rosso SM, Donker Kaat L, Baks T et al (2003) Frontotemporal dementia in The Netherlands: patient characteristics and prevalence estimates from a population-based study. Brain 126(Pt 9):2016–2022
68. Ratnavalli E, Brayne C, Dawson K et al (2002) The prevalence of frontotemporal dementia. Neurology 58(11):1615–1621
69. Mercy L, Hodges JR, Dawson K et al (2008) Incidence of early-onset dementias in Cambridgeshire, United Kingdom. Neurology 71(19):1496–1499
70. Neary D, Snowden JS, Gustafson L et al (1998) Frontotemporal lobar degeneration: a consensus on clinical diagnostic criteria. Neurology 51(6):1546–1554
71. Le Ber I, Guedj E, Gabelle A et al (2006) Demographic, neurological and behavioural characteristics and brain perfusion SPECT in frontal variant of frontotemporal dementia. Brain 129(Pt 11):3051–3065
72. Mourik JC, Rosso SM, Niermeijer MF et al (2004) Frontotemporal dementia: behavioral symptoms and caregiver distress. Dement Geriatr Cogn Disord 18(3–4):299–306
73. Liu W, Miller BL, Kramer JH et al (2004) Behavioral disorders in the frontal and temporal variants of frontotemporal dementia. Neurology 62(5):742–748
74. Reischle E, Sturm K, Schuierer G et al (2003) A case of schizophreniform disorder in frontotemporal dementia (FTD). Psychiatr Prax 30(suppl 2):S78–S82

75. Mendez MF, Lauterbach EC, Sampson SM et al (2008) An evidence-based review of the psychopathology of frontotemporal dementia: a report of the ANPA Committee on Research. J Neuropsychiatry Clin Neurosci 20(2):130–149
76. Mendez MF, Lipton A (2001) Emergent neuroleptic hypersensitivity as a herald of presenile dementia. J Neuropsychiatry Clin Neurosci 13(3):347–356
77. van Duijn E, Kingma EM, van der Mast RC (2007) Psychopathology in verified Huntington's disease gene carriers. J Neuropsychiatry Clin Neurosci 19(4):441–448
78. Paulsen JS, Ready RE, Hamilton JM et al (2001) Neuropsychiatric aspects of Huntington's disease. J Neurol Neurosurg Psychiatry 71(3):310–314
79. Zappacosta B, Monza D, Meoni C et al (1996) Psychiatric symptoms do not correlate with cognitive decline, motor symptoms, or CAG repeat length in Huntington's disease. Arch Neurol 53(6):493–497
80. Rosenblatt A, Ranen N, Nance M, et al (1999) A physician's guide to the management of Huntington's disease. http://www.hdsa.org/images/content/1/1/11289.pdf. Accessed 1 Sept 2009
81. Bonelli RM, Wenning GK (2006) Pharmacological management of Huntington's disease: an evidence-based review. Curr Pharm Des 12(21):2701–2720
82. Proulx AA, Strong MJ, Nicolle DA (2008) Creutzfeldt-Jakob disease presenting with visual manifestations. Can J Ophthalmol 43(5):591–595
83. Appleby BS, Appleby KK, Crain BJ et al (2009) Characteristics of established and proposed sporadic Creutzfeldt-Jakob disease variants. Arch Neurol 66(2):208–215
84. Lundberg PO (1998) Creutzfeldt-Jakob disease in Sweden. J Neurol Neurosurg Psychiatry 65(6):836–841

Organic Delusional Syndrome: Tentative Neuropsychological Mechanism of Delusions

Yoshitaka Ohigashi and Makiko Yamada

Abstract Three organic delusions, namely, "persecutory delusions in psychotic disorder following traumatic brain injury (PDFTBI)," "Capgras syndrome, a major form of delusional misidentification syndrome," and "anosognosia for left hemiplegia or somatoparaphrenia," are discussed in this chapter. Concerning persecutory delusions in PDFTBI, we underscore the role of the temporal pole lesion that may segregate the function of the amygdala from visual information processed in the temporal lobe. The isolated function of the amygdala is speculated to cause an undiscerning oversensitive response to any incoming emotional stimuli. With regard to Capgras delusion, the most conventional neuropsychological account of "the mirror-image model of prosopagnosia" is reevaluated, and several important critiques are mentioned. Last, we have attempted to provide a novel explanation of anosognosia for left hemiplegia and somatoparaphrenia by refining definitions of "body consciousness" and "body schema" and by taking account of Edelman's reentry hypothesis for the genesis of consciousness. In the end, it is concluded that ingenious neuropsychological approaches are indispensable for the understanding of organic delusional syndromes.

Keywords Anosognosia • Capgras syndrome • Neuropsychology • Persecutory delusion • Somatoparaphrenia

---

Y. Ohigashi
International Center, Graduate School of Human and Environmental Studies,
Kyoto University, Kyoto, Japan
e-mail: ohigashi@mbox.kudpc.kyoto-u.ac.jp

M. Yamada (✉)
Molecular Imaging Center,
National Institute of Radiological Sciences, Chiba, Japan
e-mail: myamada@nirs.co.jp

K. Miyoshi et al. (eds.), *Neuropsychiatric Disorders*,
DOI 10.1007/978-4-431-53871-4_5, © Springer 2010

Introduction

Various types of organic delusions can be observed in neurological patients, yet their mechanisms are still to be determined. In this chapter, three major organic delusions are discussed, and we attempt to provide the neuropsychological mechanisms of each delusion. The first topic is the "persecutory delusion" that is observed in psychotic disorders following traumatic brain injury (PDFTBI). The second is the "delusional misidentification syndrome" (DMS), represented mainly by Capgras syndrome. The third is "anosognosia for left hemiplegia" [1] and "somatoparaphrenia" [2], both of which are generally observed following large right hemispheric lesions.

Given that the persecutory delusion and delusional misidentification can occur independently in neurological settings, these delusions are based on the distinct neurolopsychological mechanisms. Although the lesion in the temporal pole seems to be responsible for persecutory delusion in PDFTBI, abnormal functions in the limbic structures together with the right frontal lobe could be related to Capgras syndrome. The third type of delusion, anosognosia for left hemiplegia and somatoparaphrenia, is of special interest. Body schema and body consciousness are distinctive in nature. As the former is supposed to possess symbolic or semiotic features, it must be represented mainly in the left hemisphere. In contrast, the latter can be represented in the bilateral hemisphere in such a way that the right hemisphere represents whole-body consciousness while the left hemisphere supports only the contralateral, that is, the right side of body consciousness. As a consequence of a large right hemisphere lesion, a patient's bilateral body consciousness might be reduced, producing a residual consciousness of only the right side of his/her body. We consider that this is the fundamental feature of anosognosia for left hemiplegia and the phenomenon of somatoparaphrenia.

Persecutory Delusion and Delusional Perception in PDFTBI

Psychotic disorder following traumatic brain injury (PDFTBI), originally reported by Fujii and Ahmed [3, 4], is the psychotic state that consists predominantly of persecutory delusions and auditory hallucinations with an absence of negative symptoms. Abnormalities in the temporal and frontal areas are often associated with PDFTBI. The latency between traumatic brain injury and the onset of psychotic symptoms varies between patients, but the recent consensus falls around 4 to 5 years.

Our major interest here is whether delusional perception in PDFTBI is related to the patient's biased-emotion evaluations of others, which may provide insight regarding the neuropsychological mechanisms of persecutory delusion. In the following, we present two PDFTBI patients with temporal lobe lesions. Based on our examination of their ability to estimate emotion intensity from facial expressions, the critical role of the temporal pole for delusional perception is suggested.

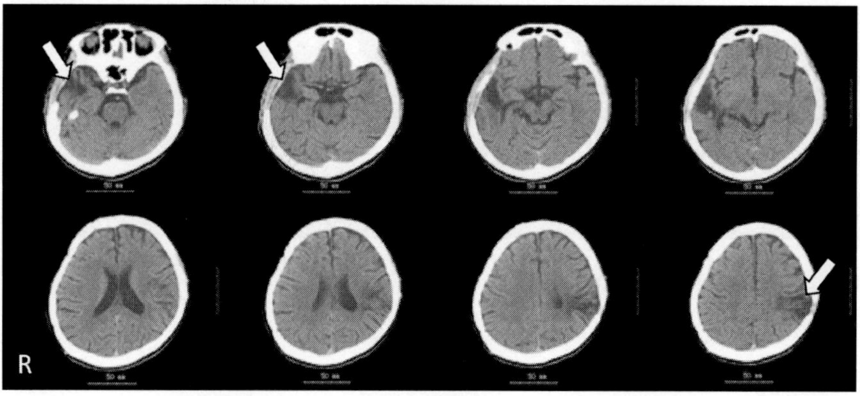

Fig. 1 Computed tomography (CT) findings of case SA

Case SA was a 23-year-old female ambidextrous college student. She had a traffic accident at age 16 years and had been unconscious for about 10 days. She received a craniotomy to remove a left parietal hematoma. Her lesions were detected in the right temporal pole and the left parietal lobe (Fig. 1). When she was discharged from hospital after 3 months, she showed mildly impaired memory retention, reduced calculation ability, articulation disorder, and mild right hemiparesis. After the accident, she was noticed by her family and friends to behave and talk like a child. She complained of her difficulty in memory retention and concentration; however, she had spent a quasi-normal daily life without many serious problems.

About 4 years later she began to experience hallucinations and delusions. She complained: "my father looks like a different person," "I feel as if TV is speaking of me," and "I'm very scared and always feel as if I'm chased by someone." She also experienced functional auditory hallucinations, such as "I hear the sound of typing computer keyboard as human voice."

Case DR was a 36-year-old right-handed woman. She received a college education. A traffic accident at age 14 resulted in skull fracture and intracranial hemorrhage with a loss of consciousness for 3 days. Her major complaint was headache, insomnia, and irritability. After 5 years after the accident, she began to develop persecutory delusion, such as "I hear some noise that speaks evil of me" and "my vulgar idea is detected by other people." She was first diagnosed as "schizophrenia" in a psychiatric department but was now rediagnosed as PDFTBI. Computed tomography (CT) and single-photon emission computerized tomography (SPECT) indicated apparent lesions in the left anterior temporal lobe and the left posterior frontal cortex (Fig. 2).

The ability of both patients to evaluate emotional intensity from others' faces was investigated using the Emotional Intensity Scale (EIS [5]) and compared with that of healthy subjects. In this task, subjects were asked to rate the perceived intensity of a given emotion word (six basic emotions in total) for each facial expression of six basic emotions (see [5] for detailed procedure). Results indicated that case SA perceived a sad facial expressions not only as "sadness" itself but also as high intensities of

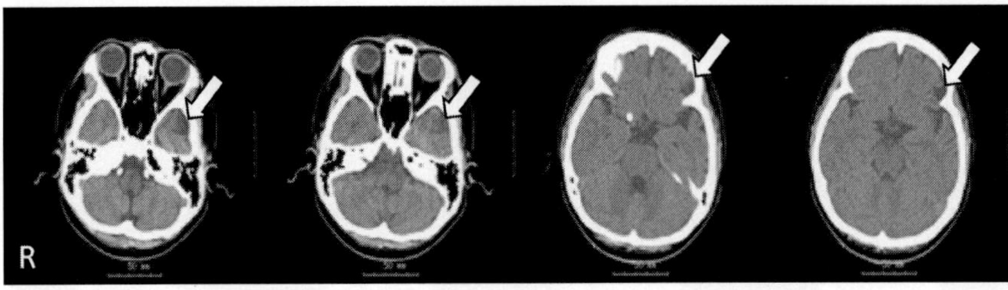

Fig. 2 CT findings of case DR

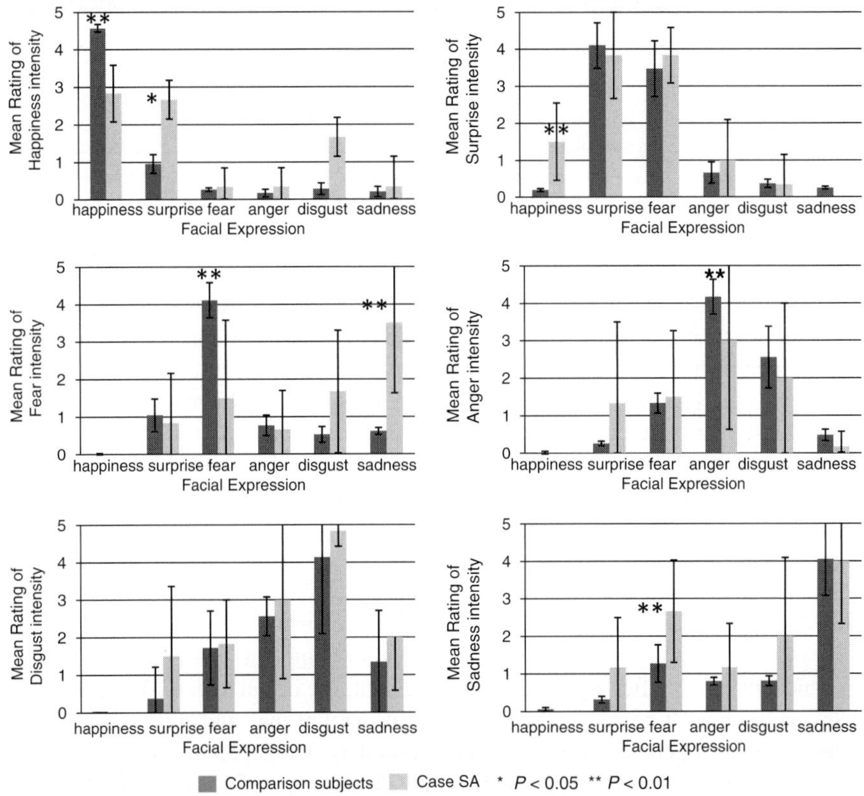

Fig. 3 Results of Emotional Intensity Scale in case SA. *Horizonta axis*, evaluated facial expressions; *vertical axis*, intensity of an emotion word

"surprise" and "fear" (Fig. 3). This patient showed a tendency to perceive facial expressions in heightened emotions of "surprise," "disgust," and "happiness" compared to normal subjects. Case DR perceived emotions of fear, anger, and sadness in almost all facial expressions except for happiness (Fig. 4).

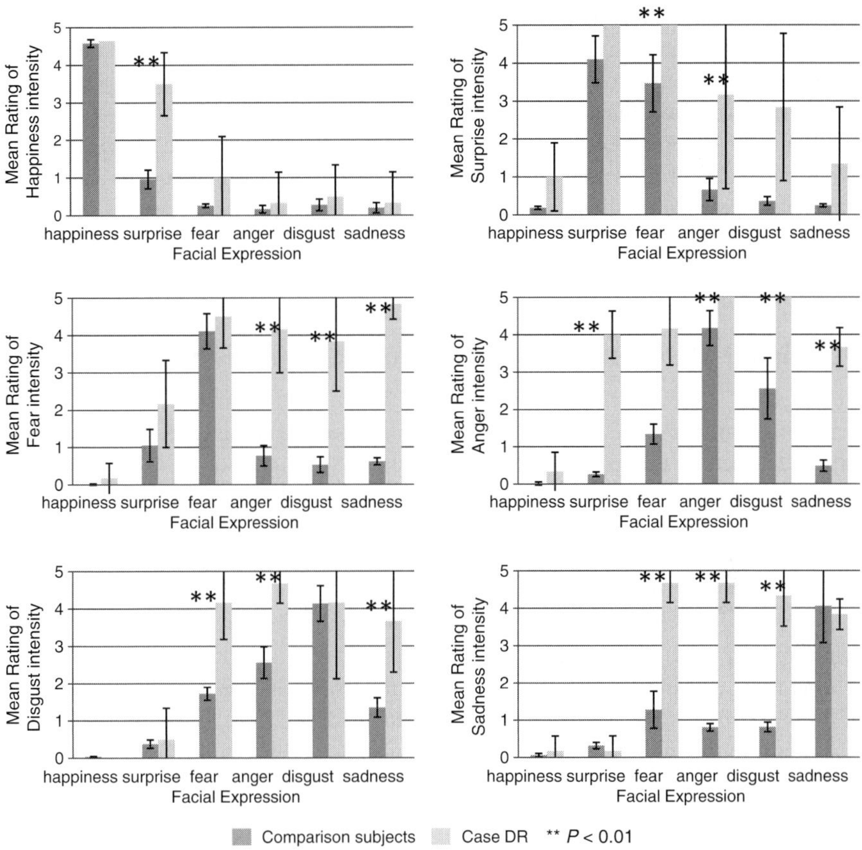

Fig. 4 Results of Emotional Intensity Scale (EIS) in case DR

Several common features between the two cases can be pointed out. (1) Their common lesion site was the temporal pole. (2) Psychotic states appeared 4 to 5 years after head injuries. (3) Persecutory delusion with hallucination was the predominant clinical picture in both cases. (4) Results of EIS suggested the confused judgments of facial expressions, characterized by a negatively biased-emotion estimation.

The temporal pole is known to play a crucial role in high-level recognition because it is anatomically located at the endpoint of the auditory and visual "what" stream. A general function of the temporal pole is supposed to be to couple emotional responses to highly processed sensory stimuli through a tight connection with the amygdala [6]. Thus, the temporal pole is regarded as a relay point that links the final "what" perception to emotional responses in the amygdala. The lesion sites in our cases suggest that the route from the temporal pole to the amygdala could be disrupted, and that the functions between these two sites might be isolated. As indicated by EIS results, the patients overestimated negative emotions regardless of the actual emotional signals of the facial expression. This overestimation of negative emotion has been observed in the case of ictal fear [7], which implied that the amygdala was not dysfunctional but rather hypersensitive. Consistent with this amygdala hypersensitivity account, a negatively biased perception in our cases could have persisted through limbic kindling, which might have created a trait-like misinterpretation of others' minds, or persecutory delusions.

In sum, the temporal pole lesions in patients with PDFTBI may segregate the function of the amygdala from visual information processing. This isolation may cause the amygdala to respond to emotional stimuli overly intensively and unselectively. We regard this as one possible cause of delusional perception and persecutory delusion in PDFTBI.

Delusional Misidentification Syndrome: Capgras Syndrome

Capgras syndrome is the most common form of delusional misidentification, originally described by Capgras and Reboul-Lachaux [8]. This disorder is characterized as the delusional belief that familiar persons have been replaced by identical impostors. This condition was once (or is still now) explained by the psychoanalytical view that posits this disorder as a defense mechanism against unconscious prohibited desires. However, accumulating neurological and neuropsychological evidence suggests that organic factors are important in the pathogenesis of Capgras syndrome [9].

One most conventional neuropsychological account is "the mirror-image model of prosopagnosia" [10], based on the dual-route theory of facial recognition (Fig. 5). According to this model, two anatomically independent routes to face recognition, namely, overt and covert recognition pathways (Fig. 5a, b, respectively), are damaged in a mirror-reversed manner between prosopagnosia and Capgras syndrome. As Fig. 5 illustrates, although the overt route interruption causes prosopagnosia, the covert route disconnection yields Capgras syndrome. This claim is derived exclusively from undifferentiated skin conductance responses (SCRs) toward known and unknown faces in Capgras patients, in contrast to normal SCRs toward unrecognized-yet-known faces in prosopagnostic patients. Disconnection between the face-processing areas and the amygdala has been considered to represent a lack of affection/familiar feeling toward known faces in Capgras syndrome. This disconnectionist account has been favored by several researchers ([12], etc.); however, it seems that quite a few serious objections impede upholding this idea.

Major criticisms include the following. (1) Although this model claims that the SCR is a measure of covert recognition, the relationship between SCRs and the true experience of patients is far less clear [13, 14]. (2) SCRs usually index a generalized arousal state following an unexpected external stimulus that is often threat- or fear related; this contradicts the assumption that SCRs signify a "familiar feeling" in the mirror-image model. (3) Correspondingly, although this model regards the amygdala functions as a "familiar feeling," the widely accepted view of this region is mainly to detect threat-related information. (4) The disconnection in the covert route is assumed in Capgras syndrome, but the actual anatomical disconnection has not

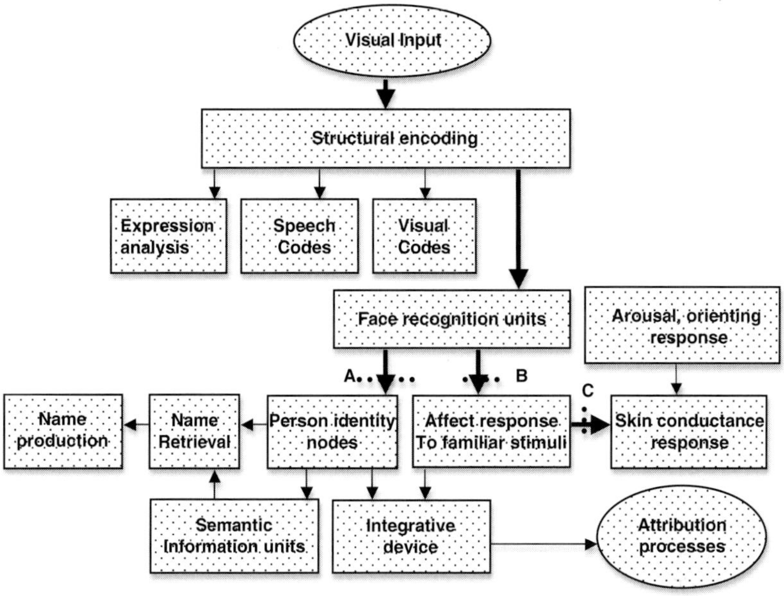

Fig. 5 Model of face recognition and Capgras delusion, formulated by Ellis and Young [10] (figure is a reprint from [11], modified for this publication). Disconnection in the overt recognition route (**a**) yields prosopagnosia, whereas that in the covert recognition route (**b**) produces Capgras syndrome

been identified. (5) The model explains the face recognition processing but ignores the occasional coexistence of misidentification of objects or places. (6) The model does not account for patients' resistance to modify their delusional belief in the presence of very strong evidence against it.

Among different explanations for DMS provided by other researchers, a two-factor model, proposed by Coltheart and his colleagues [15], takes into consideration the foregoing issue (see "6," above). In their model, although the first factor is composed of the failure of autonomic responsiveness to familiar faces, the second abnormal factor is the patient's resistance to revise the delusional belief, which is speculated to arise from a disrupted belief evaluation system associated with the right frontal cortex. In accord with their idea, neuroimaging studies revealed that the right prefrontal cortex was involved in mediating the ability to detect or resolve conflicts in thinking [16, 17]. In this sense, we also hypothesize that the delusion in Capgras syndrome as well as other DMSs might represent a dysfunction of the cognitive-conflict resolution mechanism, which is supported by the right frontal lobe. Further support for this view is observed from evidence that right frontotemporal lesions are predominant in patients with Capgras syndrome in the setting of focal brain damage [18–20]. The reduction in event-related potential (ERP) in the right frontal lobe was also reported in deluded patients [21].

Alghough Ellis &Young's original one-stage account was recently incorporated into two-factor model, called "an interactionist model" [11], the puzzle still remains as to what special mechanisms create the delusional misidentification. The examination of neurological patients suggests the involvement of the limbic structure, yet its functional relationship with the misidentification phenomenon must be determined in future research. Considering that the amygdala is an alarm system that deals with not only threat-related stimuli but also anything ambiguous for an organism, we dare advocate a new proposal of misidentification in Capgras syndrome. If the same argument that we made for delusional perception in PDFTBI can be applied to Capgras syndrome, we speculate that regardless of known or unknown persons (or objects), the maladaptive function of the hypersensitive amygdala creates a feeling too strongly suspicious to be rejected; that is, "a deluded misidentification in Capgras syndrome."

Anosognosia and Somatoparaphrenia

Anosognosia for left hemiplegia was first described by Babinski [1] as the denial of left hemiplegia. Somatoparaphrenia was reported by Gerstmann [2] as delusional beliefs concerning a contralesional side of body (the left side in most cases), which is characterized by a pathological alteration of the ownership of the limbs. In a famous monograph, *The Parietal Lobes* [23], Critchley classified the content of distortion of the body image as follows: (1) unilateral neglect, (2) lack of concern (anosodiaphoria), (3) unawareness of hemiparesis (anosognosia), (4) defective appreciation of the existence of hemiparesis, (5) denial of hemiparesis, (6) denial of hemiparesis with confabulation, (7) loss of awareness of one body-half (asomatognosia), (8) undue heaviness, deadness, or lifelessness of one half, (9) phantom third limb, (10) personification of paralyzed limb, and (11) misoplegia (the last two categories were included in 1955 and 1974, respectively). In his categorization, anosognosia and various somatoparaphrenia were not sharply demarcated but closely related. In 1972, Hécaen [24] distinguished hemi-somatognosic disorder into three categories: (1) anosognosia for the left hemiplegia, (2) hemi-asomatognosia raging from simple neglect to amnesia, unawareness of one side of the body, and (3) feeling of absence of one's body part or one side of the body, including disownership and phantom limbs. Apparently, these disorders still lie on a continuum.

Here we attempt to provide a neuropsychological mechanism of anosognosia (unawareness of left hemiparesis) and a feeling of disownership of the left side of the body, based on a novel framework of consciousness proposed by Edelman [25] and on our refined definitions of "body schema" and "body consciousness." Body schema represents a symbolic semiotic or linguistic body concept, possibly

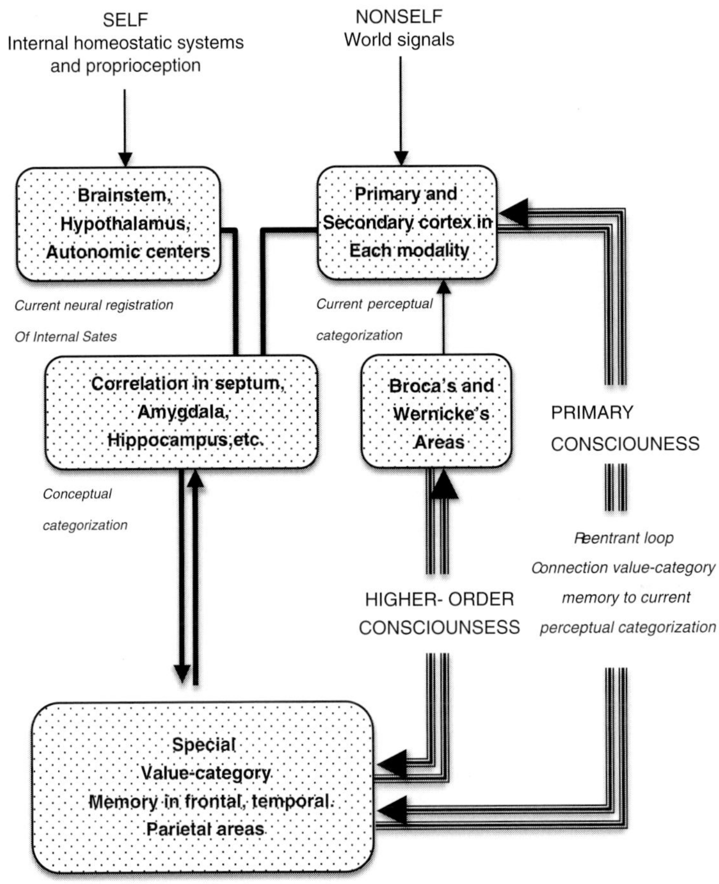

Fig. 6 Reentry genetic theory of consciousness by Edelman [25] (modified for this publication)

supported by the left parietal lobe. Phylogenetically, new "body schema," which would have coincided with the genesis of language, could be attributed to the higher-order consciousness within Edelman's reentry hypothesis for the genesis of consciousness [25] (Fig. 6). The close relationship between body schema and language is supported by the evidence that impaired body schema can provoke, for instance, bilateral finger agnosia or autotopagnosia. In contrast, body consciousness represents a basic and immediate body feeling that would be phylogenetically older than body schema. We would attribute body consciousness to the primary consciousness in Edelman's model, which may be supported predominantly by the right hemisphere.

We further speculate that body consciousness, which was originally distributed bilaterally and symmetrically, that is, the right body was in the left hemisphere and vice versa, gradually shifted to the right hemisphere as a consequent of a "body schema" lateralization in the left hemisphere. If so, it can be hypothesized that the right hemisphere represents the bilateral body consciousness, whereas the left hemisphere represents only a residual consciousness of the right side of the body. Recent lesion studies indicated that body consciousness would be represented by a neural circuitry of right hemisphere regions, including the temporo-parietal junction, posterior insula, and subcortical structures, such as basal ganglia [26–29]. Thus, damage to this neural circuitry in the right hemisphere may yield a loss of bilateral body consciousness whereas the right-body consciousness may survive without damage to the left hemisphere. Therefore, patients are aware of only the right side of the body, and the "anosognosia" and the "somatoparaphrenia" appear exclusively on the left side of the body.

In the patients' consciousness, the left body is no longer their own body. The conviction that they can move their own left arm would not work for them because the left arm no longer exists in their consciousness. In turn, they would say they can move it by showing their moving right arm, or would talk about their own left arm as if it did not belong to their body. These delusions are not false but quite real in their consciousness. We propose that this is the fundamental feature of "anosognosia for left hemiplegia" and the phenomenon of the "somatoparaphrenia."

Conclusion

In this chapter, we took a neuropsychological approach to understand organic delusional syndromes. One possible account for persecutory delusions in PDFTBI was the segregation of amygdala function caused by temporal pole lesions. The isolated amygdala may respond to any emotional stimuli because of inadequate visual information or rundown visual processing areas in the amygdala; this may create an overly reactive amygdala and shape the delusional perception in these patients. The pathogenesis of Capgras syndrome could be related to the abnormal functioning in the right hemisphere and the limbic areas; however, the most accepted neuropsychological account of "the mirror-image model of prosopagnosia" faces several critical problems, and the advanced theory warrants future research. Our novel explanation of anosognosia for left hemiplegia and somatoparaphrenia was provided within Edelman's reentry hypothesis for the genesis of consciousness, together with the refined definitions of "body consciousness" and "body schema."

References

1. Babinski MJ (1914) Contribution a l'értude des troubles mentaux dans l'hemiplegie organique cérébrale. Rev Neurol 1:845–848
2. Gerstmann J (1942) Problem of imperception of disease and of impaired body territories with organic lesions. Relation to body scheme and its disorders. Arch Neurol Psychiatry 48:890–913
3. Fujii DE, Ahmed I (2002) Psychotic disorder following traumatic brain injury: a conceptual framework. Cogn Neuropsychiatry 7:41–62
4. Fujii DE, Ahmed I, Hishimura E (2004) A neuropsychological comparison of psychotic disorder following traumatic brain injury, traumatic brain injury without psychotic disorder, and schizophrenia. J Neuropsychiatry Clin Neurosci 16:306–314
5. Adolphs R, Tranel D, Damasio H et al (1994) Impaired recognition of emotion in facial expressions following bilateral damage to the human amygdala. Nature (Lond) 372:669–672
6. Olson IR, Plotzker A, Ezzyatb Y (2007) The enigmatic temporal pole: a review of findings on social and emotional processing. Brain 130:1718–1731
7. Yamada M, Murai T, Sato W et al (2005) Emotion recognition from facial expressions in a temporal lobe epileptic patient with ictal fear. Neuropsychologia 43:434–441
8. Capgras J, Reboul-Lachaux J (1923) L'illusion des 'soises' dans un délire systématisé chronique. Bull Soc Clin Med Ment 11:6–16. In: Enoch MD, Trethowan WH (eds) Uncommon psychiatric syndromes. Wright and Sons, Bristol, 1979
9. Forstl H, Almeida OP, Owen AM et al (1991) Psychiatric, neurological and medical aspects of misidentification syndromes: a review of 260 cases. Psychol Med 21:905–910
10. Ellis HD, Young AW (1990) Accounting for delusional misidentification. Br J Psychiatry 157:239–248
11. Ellis HD (2007) Delusions: a suitable case for imaging? Int J Psychophysiol 62:146–151
12. Hirstein W, Ramachandran VS (1997) Capgras syndrome: a novel probe for understanding the neural representation of the identity and familiarity of persons. Proc Biol Sci 264:437–444
13. Breen N, Caine D, Coltheart M (2000) Models of face recognition and delusional misidentification: a critical review. Cogn Neuropsychol 17:55–71
14. Hohwy J (2004) Top-down and bottom-up in delusion formation. Philos Psychiatr Psychol 11:65–70
15. Coltheart M, Langdon R, McKay R (2007) Schizophrenia and monothematic delusions. Schizophr Bull 33:642–647
16. Fink GR, Marshall JC, Halligan PW et al (1999) The neural consequences of conflict between intention and the senses. Brain 122:497–512
17. Goel V, Buchel C, Frith C et al (2000) Dissociation of mechanisms underlying syllogistic reasoning. Neuroimage 12:504–514
18. Alexander MP, Stuss DT, Benson DF (1979) Capgras syndrome: a reduplicative phenomenon. Neurology 29:334–339
19. Staton RD, Brumback RA, Wilson H (1982) Reduplicative paramnesia: a disconnection syndrome of memory. Cortex 18:23–35
20. Moser DJ, Cohen RA, Malloy PF et al (1998) Reduplicative paramnesia: longitudinal neurobehavioral and neuroimaging analysis. J Geriatr Psychiatry Neurol 11:174–180
21. Papageorgiou P, Ventouras E, Lykouras L et al (2003) Psychophysiological evidence for altered information in delusional misidentification syndromes. Prog Neuropsychopharmacol Biol Psychiatry 27:365–372
22. Young G (2008) Capgras delusion: an interactionist model. Conscious Cogn 17:863–876
23. Critchley M (1953) The parietal lobes. Hafner, New York
24. Hécaen H (1972) Introduction à la neuropsychologie. Larousse, Paris
25. Edelman GM (2004) Wider than the sky: the phenomenal gift of consciousness. Yale University Press, New Haven

26. Cereda C, Ghika J, Maeder P et al (2002) Strokes restricted to the insular cortex. Neurology 59:1950–1955
27. Karnath HO, Baier B, Nagele T (2005) Awareness of the functioning of one's own limbs mediated by the insular cortex? J Neurosci 25:7134–7138
28. Baier B, Karnath H-O (2008) Tight link between our sense of limb ownership and self-awareness of actions. Stroke 39:486–488
29. Halligan PW, Marshall JC (1995) Supernumerary phantom limb after right hemispheric stroke. J Neurol Neurosurg Psychiatry 59:341–342

Neurological and Psychological Forms of Amnesia

Michael D. Kopelman

Abstract Amnesic disorders can be transient (a discrete episode of memory loss) or persisting. They can have a neurological or a psychological basis. Furthermore, neurological memory disorders can affect primarily episodic or semantic memory or both. Implicit (procedural) and working memory are commonly preserved. Psychogenic amnesia may be "global" or "situation specific." The global form affects the whole of a person's previous life and is commonly accompanied by a loss of the sense of personal identity. Situation-specific amnesia involves a discrete gap in a person's memory, usually related to a traumatic episode. Examples of these various forms of memory loss are given and discussed in relationship to our current concepts of memory and the underlying pathophysiology.

Keywords Amnesia • Anterograde • Neurological • Psychogenic • Retrograde

Introduction

Memory disorders have either a neurological or a psychological basis. Moreover, both these types may involve either a discrete (transient) episode of memory loss or a more persisting memory disorder. Figure 1 shows specific conditions giving rise to transient or persistent neurological or psychogenic memory disorders. Examples from each quadrant are discussed below. It should, of course, be acknowledged that admixtures of neurological and psychological factors are very common.

Anterograde amnesia (AA) consists of an impairment in new learning, that is, recall and recognition memory for episodes and facts that have arisen *after* the

M.D. Kopelman (✉)
Institute of Psychiatry, King's College London, London, UK
and
Academic Unit of Neuropsychiatry, 3rd Floor, Adamson Centre, South Wing, St. Thomas's Hospital, Westminster Bridge Road, London SE1 7EH, UK
e-mail: michael.kopelman@kcl.ac.uk

K. Miyoshi et al. (eds.), *Neuropsychiatric Disorders*,
DOI 10.1007/978-4-431-53871-4_6, © Springer 2010

onset of an illness or injury. Retrograde amnesia (RA) involves the loss of memory for episodes or facts that occurred *before* the onset of an illness or injury.

Primary or working memory ("short-term memory" in psychological parlance) consists of memories lasting a few seconds or as long as they are actively rehearsed and held in consciousness – what Williams James called the "specious present" [1]. This type of memory is characteristically preserved in the amnesic syndrome. Autobiographical memory involves a person's recollection of past incidents or events, which occurred at a specific time and place, such that the person can "travel back mentally in time." The term autobiographical memory is sometimes used interchangeably with "episodic memory," although the latter also includes a person's performance on standard learning tasks that may have a differing neurobiological basis [2]. By definition, autobiographical or episodic memory is severely impaired in amnesia. Semantic memory refers to a person's knowledge of language, concepts, and facts that do not have a specific location in time or place; this is variably affected in amnesia. Implicit memory refers to learning without awareness, and this incorporates both procedural (perceptuo-motor) skill learning and the response to priming. Implicit memory is characteristically spared in amnesia, as is discussed below. In principle, episodic, semantic, and implicit memory can each have an anterograde and a retrograde component. Figure 1 shows that they can be differentially affected in memory disorders: the amnesic syndrome principally affects episodic (autobiographical) memory, sometimes exclusively so; semantic dementia principally involves semantic

AMNESIC STATES

	Discrete Episode:	**Persistent:**
NEURO-	Toxic confusional state	Continuing drug toxicity
LOGICAL:	Head Injury	Amnesic syndrome - episodic
	Epilepsy	Semantic dementia -semantic
	Alcoholic 'black-out'	Alzheimer dementia - global
	Cerebral hypoxia	
	Transient Global Amnesia (TGA)	
	Post-ECT (electro-convulsive therapy)	
PSYCHOGENIC:	Situation – specific (e.g. offence, PTSD)	Depressive Pseudodementia
	Fugue states	'Focal retrograde amnesia'

Fig. 1 Specific conditions giving rise to transient or persistent, neurological or psychogenic memory disorders. *PTSD* posttraumatic stress disorder, *ECT*. (Modified from *British Journal of Psychiatry* (1987) 150:428–442)

memory; and Alzheimer dementia usually affects both the episodic and semantic components of memory, and eventually implicit skills may also be affected.

Transient Neurological Amnesias

Transient Global Amnesia

Transient global amnesia (TGA) occurs most commonly in the middle-aged or elderly, more frequently in men. It results in a period of amnesia usually lasting several hours.

TGA is characterized by repetitive questioning; there may be some confusion, but patients do not report any loss of the sense of personal identity; that is, they know who they are. Hodges and Ward found that in 114 cases of TGA the mean duration of amnesia was 4 h and that the maximum was 12 h [3]. Sometimes, the episode had been preceded by headache or nausea, a stressful life event, a medical procedure, or vigorous exercise. In 25% of their sample, there was a past history of migraine, which was considered to have a possible etiological role. In a further 7% of the sample, the patients subsequently developed epilepsy, usually complex partial seizures, although there had not been any past history of epilepsy or overt features of epilepsy evident during the original attack. In these latter cases, the memory loss was attributed in retrospect to epilepsy (see following). In this investigation, as in previous ones [4], TGA was not statistically associated with a past history of vascular disease, clinical signs suggestive of vascular pathology, or known risk factors for vascular disease. In particular, there was no specific association with transient ischemic attacks. Moreover, in 60–70% of this TGA sample, the underlying etiology was unclear.

More recently, Quinette et al. reviewed findings in 1,353 patients reported in the clinical literature since 1956 and their own data from 142 patients seen between 1994 and 2004 [5]. In general, the findings were consistent across the two sources. In these series, most of the attacks occurred between the ages of 50 and 80 (mean = 60.3), and they occurred equally among men and women. Most patients had a single attack, and the annual rate of recurrence ranged from 2.9% to 26.3% across different studies, being 6.3% in Quinette et al.'s own series. Moreover, in their own series, the duration of attacks ranged from 30 min to 16 h (mean = 5.6 h). These authors also investigated putative predisposing and precipitating factors in great detail, concluding that TGA may encompass at least three groups of patients: (1) younger patients with a history of migraine, in whom spreading neurochemical depression may be implicated; (2) women who have experienced acute emotional or physical stress, and who often have a history of anxiety or depression; and (3) men who, following physical exertion, develop venous congestion in the context of insufficient jugular vein valves and a precipitating Valsalva maneuver.

In those cases of TGA where neuropsychological tests have been administered to patients during the acute episode of memory loss [3, 6], the patients have shown a profound AA on tests of verbal and nonverbal memory, as would be expected. However, performance on tests of retrograde memory has been very variable, some patients showing no retrograde memory loss, others showing a brief retrograde loss, occasional others showing an extensive RA. Follow-up investigations have usually shown either complete or almost complete recovery of memories several weeks to months after the acute attack. In general, RA recovers before AA.

There is general agreement that the amnesic disorder in TGA results from transient dysfunction in limbic-hippocampal circuits, crucial to memory formation. Medial temporal abnormalities have been reported bilaterally on single-photon emission tomography (SPECT), positron emission tomography (PET), and diffusion-weighted imaging (DWI), and small hippocampal cavities have been seen on T_2 reversed magnetic resonance imaging (MRI) [7, 8]. Moreover, venous duplex sonography has shown jugular vein valve insufficiency in a proportion of cases [8].

Transient Epileptic Amnesia

Transient epileptic amnesia (TEA) refers to the minority of patients with TGA in whom epilepsy appears to be the underlying cause of the syndrome [3]. The term was originally coined by Kapur [9]. The main predictive factors for an underlying epileptic etiology in TGA are brief episodes of memory loss, lasting an hour or less, and a multiplicity of attacks [3]. It is important to note that standard electroencephalography (EEG) and computed tomography (CT) findings are often normal. However, an epileptic basis to the disorder may be revealed on a sleep-deprived EEG recording [3, 10].

TEA patients may show residual memory deficits between their attacks, presumably related to their underlying neuropathology. Kopelman et al. found a moderate degree of residual anterograde memory impairment, which was probably related to small foci of MRI signal alteration and bilateral medial temporal hypometabolism on PET in the medial temporal lobes bilaterally [10]. Such patients quite commonly also report "gaps" in their past personal memories [11]. Manes et al. and Butler and Zeman have reported abnormal long-term forgetting of newly learned material, which they attributed to hippocampal dysfunction [11, 12]. However, forgetting rates are extremely difficult to measure across long intervals, and these studies have been confounded by "ceiling" and "floor" effects, such that the apparently fast forgetting may have reflected impaired initial acquisition of the material. Similarly, disproportionate RA has been claimed, but whether a patient's reported gaps in past memories result from faulty initial encoding of those memories (because of subclinical ictal activity), impaired memory consolidation, or deficits in memory retrieval remains highly controversial and difficult to disentangle.

Epilepsy can, of course, give rise to automatisms or postictal confusional states. Such automatisms appear always to be associated with bilateral involvement of those medial temporal brain structures involved in memory formation. Hence, amnesia for the period of automatic behavior is always present and is usually complete; claims of automatism in the absence of significant amnesia should be rejected.

Persistent Neurological Memory Disorders

The amnesic syndrome can be defined as "an abnormal mental state in which memory and learning are affected out of all proportion to other cognitive functions in an otherwise alert and responsive patient" [13]. Please note that there is no reference to short-term memory in this definition and no reference to confabulation. Moreover, many patients may suffer from variable degrees of specific memory impairment (in the absence of generalized cognitive impairment), but not so severely as to constitute an amnesic syndrome; such patients are poorly categorized within the International Classification of Diseases.

The critical lesions that give rise to AA involve pathology in the medial temporal lobes (hippocampi, parahippocampal gyri), thalami, mammillary bodies, the mammillo-thalamic tract, the retrosplenium, and the fornix. Through their interconnections with these limbic circuits, pathology in the basal forebrain (particularly the septal nucleus) and elsewhere within the frontal lobes can also give rise to anterograde memory impairment. The neuropathological basis of RA is much more controversial, some theorists arguing that damage to the hippocampi (and their connections) is critical [14, 15], whereas others have argued that it is damage beyond the medial temporal lobes which is critical for RA [16, 17].

The diseases or disorders that give rise to an amnesic syndrome are those which implicate these critical brain structures. Hence, bilateral medial temporal lobectomy in the patient HM gave rise to profound amnesia [18], and bilateral damage is now a well-recognized reason for avoiding temporal lobe surgery in epilepsy. Herpes encephalitis or voltage-gated potassium channel pathology gives rise to structural damage in the medial temporal lobes and resulting memory disorder [19]; and profound hypoxia or hypoxic/ischemic insufficiency can also give rise to hippocampal damage and amnesia [20]. By contrast, thiamine deficiency (for example, in the alcoholic Korsakoff syndrome) particularly affects the thalami, the mammillary bodies, and the mammillo-thalamic tract. Vascular infarction in branches of the posterior cerebral artery can affect either the thalami, the hippocampi, or both, and subarachnoid hemorrhage sometimes produces profound amnesia by damage to the septal nucleus. Head injury, deep midline tumors, and TB meningitis can all produce amnesia by effects upon the medial temporal, diencephalic, or frontal structures of the brain.

The Korsakoff Syndrome

The term Korsakoff syndrome should nowadays be reserved for cases of the amnesic syndrome resulting from thiamine deficiency. These cases are almost invariably a consequence of alcohol misuse [21].

There is a profound AA, and a RA that extends back at least 20–25 years and involves autographical, personal semantic, and more general knowledge of public information [22]. Korsakoff noted these patients had severe disorientation in time, in particular, difficulty in remembering the temporal sequence of events [23]. He also noted his patients' preserved reasoning and other skills. Confabulation is not necessarily present, and it often consists of the inappropriate retrieval of fragments of real memory, jumbled up and confused in temporal context, as various others have also noted [13].

Many cases of the Korsakoff syndrome are diagnosed following an acute Wernicke encephalopathy, involving confusion, ataxia, nystagmus, and opthalmoplegia. Usually, not all these features are present, and the opthalmoplegia in particular responds rapidly to treatment with high-dose vitamins. These features are often also associated with a peripheral neuropathy. However, the Korsakoff syndrome can alternatively have an insidious onset, and such slower-onset cases are more likely to come to the attention of psychiatrists or clinical psychologists. In such cases, there may be either no known history of Wernicke features, or only a transient history of such signs. Moreover, reports from Scandinavia and Australia indicate that the characteristic Wernicke–Korsakoff neuropathology (see following) is found much more commonly at autopsy in alcoholics than the diagnosis is made in life, implying that many cases are missed [24, 25].

Victor et al. reported that 25% of patients with the Korsakoff's syndrome "recover," 50% show improvement through time, and 25% remain unchanged [13]. Although it is unlikely that any established patient shows complete recovery, the present author's experience is that a substantial improvement does occur over a matter of years if the patient remains abstinent. In such cases, it is probably correct to say that 75% of these patients show a variable degree of improvement while 25% show no change [21].

The characteristic neuropathology in the Wernicke–Korsakoff syndrome consists of neuronal loss, microhemorrhages, and gliosis in the paraventricular and the periaqueductal grey matter [13]. There has been considerable debate concerning which particular lesions are critical for the presence of chronic memory disorder (Korsakoff syndrome). Victor et al. argued that damage in the medial dorsal nucleus of the thalamus was critical in that patients who lacked pathology within this specific site showed only a transient Wernicke state [13]. However, Mair et al. and Mayes et al. argued that it was pathology within the mammillary bodies, the midline and anterior portions of the thalamus, but not the medial-dorsal nuclei, which was critical for memory disorder, and they based this observation on careful ante mortem neuropsychological and post mortem neuropathological assessments [26, 27]. More recently, Harding et al. compared eight patients who had suffered a persistent Korsakoff syndrome with five patients who experienced only a transient Wernicke episode: they argued that pathology in the anterior principal thalamic nuclei was the critical difference between these two groups of patients [28]. Taken together, these various findings suggest that the connections between the mammillary bodies, the mammillo-thalamic tract, and the anterior thalamus may be more important to memory dysfunction than pathology within the medial dorsal nucleus of the thalamus.

There are now a substantial number of neuroimaging studies in the Korsakoff syndrome, using CT, MRI, or PET. Atrophy of the thalami and mammillary bodies is found, but also a variable degree of accompanying cortical atrophy, particularly within the frontal lobes [29, 30]. Very commonly, there is also cerebellar atrophy with involvement of the vermis and pons, contributing to the ataxia. PET investigations show variable findings, but hypometabolism has been reported in the thalamic, orbital-medial frontal, and retrospleenial regions [31].

Herpes Encephalitis

Herpes encephalitis (HSE) can give rise to a particularly severe form of the amnesic syndrome as a result of devastating damage to the medial aspects of the temporal lobes [32, 33].

Many cases are said to be primary infections, although others may involve a reactivation of the virus after it has lain dormant in neural tissue. Characteristically, the disorder commences with a fairly abrupt onset of acute fever, headache, and nausea. There may be accompanying behavioral changes, and seizures can occur. Later, there is neck rigidity, vomiting, and motor and sensory deficits. However, some cases commence more insidiously with behavioral change or psychiatric phenomena, the confusion and neurological features becoming evident only much later. These latter cases are those most likely to be missed, which is now important because antiviral agents, such as acyclovir, are most effective when administered within the first 48 h of symptoms [34, 35]. Diagnosis is by polymerase chain reaction (PCR) test or a raised titer of antibodies in the cerebrospinal fluid (CSF), but a presumptive diagnosis sometimes has to be made on the basis of the clinical picture as well as severe signal alteration and subsequent atrophy in the medial temporal lobes on MRI.

Neuropathological and neuroimaging studies usually show extensive bilateral temporal lobe damage (signal alteration, volume loss, and hemorrhage), although occasionally the changes are surprisingly unilateral [29, 36]. There may be frontal changes, often in the orbitofrontal regions, and there may be focal changes elsewhere as well as a variable degree of general cortical atrophy. The medial temporal lobes are usually particularly severely affected, resulting in a profound AA, usually accompanied by an extensive retrograde memory loss. Autobiographical and episodic memory are particularly severely affected. Widespread damage to the left temporal lobes characteristically affects aspects of semantic memory, the patients often showing severe impairment in naming and word-finding, reading (a so-called surface dyslexia, in which the reading of irregularly spelled words is particularly affected), and impairments in comprehension. Right temporal lobe damage can result in particularly severe impairment in face recognition memory knowledge of people and/or remote autobiographical memory loss [37].

Wilson et al. have described a particularly severe case of amnesia following herpes encephalitis [33]. In this case, there was a long delay before the prescription of an antiviral agent, resulting in extensive left temporal lobe and right medial temporal lobe damage, evident on a quantified, structural MRI brain scan. An interesting feature of this patient was his relatively preserved skill as a musician (procedural/implicit memory). Despite this, he lacked any memory of having used his musical skills recently (episodic memory); when he was shown a video of himself playing the piano, he stated that he had not been "conscious" at the time that the video-clip was recorded. Indeed, for many years, he stated several times a day that he had "just woken up," and he also wrote this frequently in his diary.

Confabulation

Confabulation can be subdivided into "spontaneous" confabulation, in which there is a persistent, unprovoked outpouring of erroneous memories, and "momentary" or "provoked" confabulation, in which fleeting intrusion errors or distortions are seen in response to a challenge to memory, such as a memory test [37, 39].

Confabulation is widely believed to be particularly associated with the Korsakoff syndrome, but this is incorrect. Spontaneous confabulation arises in confusional states and in frontal lobe pathology, particularly where there is ventromedial or orbitofrontal damage [40–42]. Spontaneous confabulation is often seen in the confusional state of a Wernicke encephalopathy, but it is rare in the more chronic phases of the Korsakoff syndrome. On the other hand, fleeting intrusion errors or distortions ("momentary confabulation") do occur in the chronic phase of a Korsakoff syndrome, as well as other amnesic disorders or dementia, when a memory is challenged. However, such intrusion errors are also seen in healthy subjects when memory is "weak" for any reason, such as a prolonged delay until recall, and they are certainly not specific to the Korsakoff syndrome [39].

There has been considerable controversy concerning the underlying nature of spontaneous confabulation, which can extend across episodic, personal semantic, and more general semantic memories [43]. Korsakoff himself emphasized problems in the temporal ordering of memories, and the inappropriate retrieval of memory fragments, as discussed previously [23]. In a particularly elegant study, Schnider et al. found that spontaneous confabulators could be differentiated from other amnesic patients and healthy participants on the basis of their errors on a temporal context memory test, but not on other memory or executive tasks, and Schnider has more recently interpreted this as a failure in "reality monitoring" [39, 43]. By contrast, Gilboa et al. have argued that a failure in the strategic retrieval and postretrieval monitoring of memories, related to ventromedial and orbitofrontal pathology, is critical for confabulation to arise, and somewhat similar hypotheses have been proposed by others [41, 45, 46]. A third view, postulated by Fotopoulou and colleagues [46, 47], is that the content of confabulations is heavily influenced by motivational factors, and that confabulating patients tend to retrieve memories from a happier time or to manifest some degree of wish fulfilment [47, 48]. By contrast, Dalla Barba [48, 49] has argued that confabulating patients tend to retrieve the most stable elements from their long-term memories, often from earlier time periods [49, 50].

Transient Psychogenic Amnesia

Transient psychogenic amnesias ("dissociative amnesia") can be either global or situation specific. In global psychogenic amnesia, patients lose all memories of their earlier life, and this is often accompanied by a loss of the sense of personal identity or self: this occurs in a psychogenic fugue state. In situation-specific amnesia, there is a gap in memory for a particularly traumatic incident, which may be an accident or catastrophe, as in posttraumatic stress disorder; or being the victim of a crime, as in rape or child sexual abuse; and it also occurs in certain instances in the perpetrators of crime, particularly in violent offenses (see below).

Psychogenic Fugue

A fugue state is a syndrome consisting of the sudden loss of all autobiographical memories and knowledge of personal identity, usually associated with a period of wandering, for which there is a subsequent amnesic gap on recovery. Characteristically, fugue states last only a few hours or days – up to 3 or 4 weeks. If the state lasts longer than this, the question of simulation must always be considered, and if that is excluded, the diagnosis of "psychogenic focal RA" is probably the more appropriate (see following).

In clinical practice, fugue states can easily be differentiated from TGA or TEA, although these can also be precipitated by an emotional or traumatic event (see above) and may show no abnormalities on either brain imaging or a standard EEG. Although patients in TGA or TEA characteristically show repetitive questioning, this is not true of a fugue episode. Moreover, TGA/TEA patients virtually never lose their sense of personal identity, whereas this is characteristic in fugues. There are also differences in the pattern of retrograde memory loss: those with a neurological etiology characteristically show relative sparing of earlier memories, whereas those with a psychogenic etiology may show relative preservation of more recent memories [6, 10].

Fugue states are virtually always preceded by a severe precipitating stress, such as a marital crisis, financial crisis, or being charged with an offense, and they are more common in wartime (particularly in soldiers having to return to the front). Second, depressed mood is an extremely common antecedent to a psychogenic fugue state [51], and this may be associated with suicidal ideas evident just before the episode or following recovery from the fugue [52]. Various authors have noted that there is often a past history in such patients of a previous transient neurological amnesia, such as epilepsy, a head injury, or an alcoholic blackout, which may act as a kind of "learning experience" or "substrate" to the occurrence of the fugue at the time of depression and severe precipitating stress.

Schacter et al. described a patient who lost all his memories after attending the funeral of his grandfather [52]. He showed a severe amnesia for autobiographical memories with semantic memories and new learning relatively preserved. When constrained to recall memories from earlier time periods, he could do so mainly from just one particularly happy period of his life. This patient recovered his memories after watching a funeral on television a few days after the onset. Glisky et al. described a German who lost his memories in Tucson, Arizona, following offenses in Germany and being thrown out of accommodation in Tucson [53]. He appeared not to retain any memory of his past, or of the German language. However, he did show implicit knowledge of German on a paired-associate test, and he also manifested increased galvanic skin responses to personal information of which he denied "explicit" knowledge. A functional MRI (fMRI) task involving German words indicated relatively diminished frontal lobe activation.

Situation-Specific Amnesia

Situation-specific amnesia occurs in victims of crime such as rape [54] and, although controversial in some quarters, in cases of child sexual abuse [55, 56]. It can also occur in the perpetrators of crime, and it is claimed in 25–45% of offenders of homicide, approximately 8% of perpetrators of other violent crimes, and a small percentage of nonviolent offenders [57–59]. Although a few of these instances result from automatisms in epilepsy, parasomnias, hypoglycemia, or head injury, and many cases result from severe intoxication with alcohol or substances, more purely psychogenic cases of amnesia occur in so-called crimes of passion.

In these "crimes of passion," there has commonly been extreme emotional arousal and pretraumatic depression, the offense is unplanned and unpremeditated, and the victim is usually a lover, wife, or family member. Such amnesias remain controversial [60], but it should be noted that many offenders claiming amnesia report their own offense or, at least, fail to take measures to avoid capture. There are consistencies across their reports that are striking, and their descriptions do indeed bear resemblances to other patients' accounts of psychological forms of amnesia in other clinical circumstances. Moreover, victims sometimes report similar amnesias, and memory errors are common in eye-witnesses: nobody disputes the motives of these parties. In addition, amnesia itself only rarely has legal implications (as in automatisms), and it may actually be damaging to the conduct of a person's defense.

Gudjonsson and MacKeith described a 67-year-old man who had apparently battered his wife to death without any obvious motive [60]. He then telephoned the police and gave himself up. On their arrival, he reported that he had no memory of the actual attack, but that he recalled standing over the body, realizing that he had been responsible for his wife's death. His amnesia persisted until trial. (Other cases are described by Kopelman [57].)

Pyszora et al. examined the psychiatric reports of all offenders given a life sentence in England and Wales in 1994 [58]. They found that 29% of these offenders claimed amnesia and 31% of the homicide offenders reported amnesia. Detailed follow-up reports were available 3 years after conviction, and these were also examined. At this follow-up, only about 2% of the cases were thought to have been malingering their amnesia. Of the other cases who had claimed amnesia, 33% reported complete return of their memories at 3 years post conviction, 26% had partial recovery of their memories, and 41% reported no change in their amnesia.

Persistent Psychogenic Amnesia

Persistent psychogenic amnesia occurs in so-called psychogenic focal RA (FRA). Again, this is a controversial topic [61, 62]. Kapur coined the term focal RA (FRA) to describe patients who appeared to show their RA in the absence of any anterograde memory loss [63]. There have been various reports of such cases in the neuropsychological literature. Sometimes these cases have been initially accompanied by loss of the sense of personal identity, but this is usually transient and not characteristically accompanied by a period of wandering. Moreover, unlike a fugue state, the memory disorder persists. Often (but not always) the amnesia follows a mild concussion or other minor cerebral event that is insufficient to account for the severity or disproportionate nature of the retrograde memory loss. Moreover, brain imaging is almost invariably normal. In a detailed critique of such cases, Kopelman argued that many, if not all, such cases have a psychogenic basis [61].

Kopelman described a 55-year-old man who collapsed at work during early 1998 with a transient left-sided weakness and complete loss of autobiographical memory and personal identity [61]. At initial admission, this patient was disorientated in time and place as well as person, and there was a mild loss of power in the left arm and left leg with an equivocal left plantar response. A CT scan was normal, but an MRI brain scan showed evidence of a few pinpoint regions of altered signal bilaterally, consistent with a history of previously diagnosed hypercholesteremia and diabetes. However, the physicians attending this man felt confident that his memory loss was entirely disproportionate to his neurological signs, which resolved rapidly. The man did not recognize his wife, and he could not remember the names and ages of his wife or children. He claimed to have “relearned” language and mental calculation, and stated that each day he remembered more about the day before. On formal tests, he showed severe and extensive autobiographical and remote memory loss with intact anterograde memory. When first seen, he and his family were extremely angry at any suggestion that there might be a psychological component to his memory loss. However, during the succeeding weeks, his wife informed the clinical team about an emotionally deprived childhood and subsequent psychological problems. The initial onset had occurred following dismissal from two jobs that he had been carrying out simultaneously. After being seen on a regular basis for several weeks, the patient was more willing to accept a psychological contribution to his RA. At that point, following an interview under sedation, virtually all of this man’s memories were recovered.

There are now psychological models for such amnesias. For example, Anderson and Green have demonstrated that the deliberate suppression of associative memories can result in subsequent forgetting [64]. Moreover, in a functional MRI investigation [65], they demonstrated that this suppression of memories is associated with bilateral dorsolateral prefrontal activation as well as with frontopolar and bilateral hippocampal deactivation [65]. However, there have also been a number of neuroimaging studies of patients reporting psychogenic amnesias, usually of FRA type; these have produced rather conflicting findings, and the neurophysiological correlates of psychogenic amnesia remain to be fully elucidated.

Conclusions

In summary, memory disorders can be either neurological or psychogenic, and sometimes there is a complex admixture of contributory factors. In this chapter, I have focused on severe disorders of autobiographical or episodic memory, but there are other disorders in which either semantic memory or procedural memory can be particularly severely affected. There is now good understanding of the brain circuits that are critical for memory formation, damage to which gives rise to AA. The nature of neurological RA is more controversial. Similarly, we now have a fairly good understanding of the precipitating factors that can give rise to a psychogenic amnesia, which may often particularly affect aspects of retrograde memory. However, the neurophysiological correlates of psychologically induced amnesias remain to be properly elucidated.

References

1. James W (1890) The principles of psychology, vol 1. Holt, New York
2. Gilboa A (2004) Autobiographical and episodic memory – one and the same? Neuropsychologia 42:1336–1349
3. Hodges JR, Ward CD (1989) Observations during transient global amnesia: a behavioural and neuropsychological study of five cases. Brain 112:595–620
4. Miller JW, Petersen RC, Metter EJ et al (1987) Transient global amnesia: clinical characteristics and prognosis. Neurology 1987:733–737
5. Quinette P, Guillery-Girard B, Dayan V et al (2006) What does transient global amnesia really mean? Review of the literature and thorough study of 142 cases. Brain 129:1640–1658
6. Kritchevsky M, Squire LR, Zouzounis JA (1988) Transient global amnesia: characterization of anterograde and retrograde amnesia. Neurology 38:213–219
7. Nakada T, Kwee IL, Fujii Y et al (2005) High-field, T_2 reversed MRI of the hippocampus in transient global amnesia. Neurology 64:1170–1174
8. Sander K, Sander D (2005) New insights into transient global amnesia: recent imaging and clinical findings. Lancet Neurol 4:437–444
9. Kapur N (1990) Transient epileptic amnesia: a clinically distinct form of neurological memory disorder. In: Markowitsch H (ed) Transient global amnesia and related disorders. Hogrefe and Huber, New York, pp 140–151
10. Kopelman MD, Panayiotopoulos CP, Lewis P (1994) Transient epileptic amnesia differentiated from psychogenic 'fugue': neuropsychological, EEG and PET findings. J Neurol Neurosurg Psychiatry 57:1002–1004

11. Butler CR, Zeman A (2008) Recent insights into the impairment of memory in epilepsy: a systematic review of transient epileptic amnesia, accelerated long-term forgetting and remote memory impairment. Brain 131:2243–2263
12. Manes F, Graham KS, Zeman A et al (2005) Autobiographical amnesia and accelerated forgetting in transient epileptic amnesia. J Neurol Neurosurg Psychiatry 76:1387–1391
13. Victor M, Adams RD, Collins GH (1971) The Wernicke-Korsakoff syndrome. Davis, Philadelphia
14. Nadel L, Moscovitch M (1997) Memory consolidation, retrograde amnesia and the hippocampal complex. Curr Opin Neurobiol 7:217–227
15. Moscovitch M, Nadel L, Winocur G et al (2006) The cognitive neuroscience of remote episodic, semantic and spatial memory. Curr Opin Neurobiol 16:179–190
16. Bayley PJ, Gold JJ, Hopkins RO et al (2005) The neuroanatomy of remote memory. Neuron 46:799–810
17. Bright P, Buckman J, Fradera A et al (2006) Retrograde amnesia in patients with hippocampal, medial temporal, temporal lobe, or frontal pathology. Learn Mem 13:545–557
18. Scoville WB, Milner B (1957) Loss of recent memory after bilateral hippocampal lesions. J Neurol Neurosurg Psychiatry 20:11–21
19. Vincent A, Buckley C, Schott JM et al (2004) Potassium channel antibody-associated encephalopathy: a potentially immunotherapy-responsive form of limbic encephalitis. Brain 127:701–712
20. Caine D, Watson JD (2000) Neuropsychological and neuropathological sequelae of cerebral anoxia: a critical review. J Int Neuropsychol Soc 6:86–99
21. Kopelman MD, Thomson A, Guerrini I et al (2009) The Korsakoff syndrome: clinical aspects, psychology and treatment. Alcohol Alcohol 44:148–154
22. Kopelman MD (1989) Remote and autobiographical memory, temporal context memory, and frontal atrophy in Korsakoff and Alzheimer patients. Neuropsychologia 27:437–460
23. Korsakoff SS (1889) Psychic disorder in conjunction with peripheral neuritis (translated and republished: Victor M, Yakovlev PI (1955)) Neurology 5:394–406
24. Harper C (2009) The neuropathology of alcohol-related brain damage. Alcohol Alcohol 44:136–140
25. Torvik A, Lindboe C, Rogde S (1982) Brain lesions in alcoholics: a neuropathological study. J Neurol Sci 56:233–248
26. Mair WGP, Warrington EK, Weiskrantz L (1979) Memory disorder in Korsakoff's psychosis; a neuropathological and neuropsychological investigation of two cases. Brain 102:749–783
27. Mayes AR, Meudell PR, Mann D et al (1988) Location of lesions in Korsakoff's syndrome: neuropsychological and neuropathological data on two patients. Cortex 24:367–388
28. Harding A, Halliday G, Caine D et al (2000) Degeneration of anterior thalamic nuclei differentiates alcoholics with amnesia. Brain 123:141–154
29. Colchester A, Kingsley D, Lasserson D et al (2001) Structural MRI volumetric analysis in patients with organic amnesia: 1. Methods and comparative findings across diagnostic groups. J Neurol Neurosurg Psychiatry 71:13–22
30. Sullivan EV, Pfefferbaum A (2009) Neuroimaging of the Wernicke–Korsakoff syndrome. Alcohol Alcohol 44:155–165
31. Reed LJ, Lasserson D, Marsden P et al (2003) ^{18}FDG–PET findings in the Wernicke–Korsakoff syndrome. Cortex 39:1027–1045
32. Hokkanen L, Launes J (2007) Neuropsychological sequelae of acute-onset sporadic viral encephalitis. Neuropsychol Rehabil 17:429–449
33. Wilson BA, Kopelman M, Kapur N (2008) Prominent and persistent loss of past awareness in amnesia: delusion, impaired consciousness or coping strategy? Neuropsychol Rehabil 18:527–540
34. McGrath N, Anderson NE, Croxson MC et al (1997) Herpes simplex encephalitis treated with acyclovir: diagnosis and long term outcome. J Neurol Neurosurg Psychiatry 63:321–326
35. Raschilas F, Wolff M, Delatour F et al (2002) Outcome of and prognostic factors for herpes simplex encephalitis in adult patients: results of a multicenter study. Clin Infect Dis 35:254–260

36. Reed LJ, Lasserson D, Marsden P et al (2005) Correlations of regional cerebral metabolism with memory performance and executive function in patients with herpes encephalitis or frontal lobe lesions. Neuropsychology 19:555–565
37. Kopelman MD (2002) Disorders of memory. Brain 125:2152–2190
38. Kopelman MD (1987) Two types of confabulation. J Neurol Neurosurg Psychiatry 50:1482–1487
39. Schnider A (2003) Spontaneous confabulation and the adaptation of thought to ongoing reality. Nat Rev Neurosci 4:662–671
40. Gilboa A, Alain C, Stuss DT et al (2006) Mechanisms of spontaneous confabulations: a strategic retrieval account. Brain 129:1399–1414
41. Turner MS, Cipolotti T, Yousry TA et al (2008) Confabulation: damage to a specific interior medial prefrontal system. Cortex 44:637–648
42. Kopelman MD, Ng N, Van den Brouke O (1997) Confabulation extending across episodic memory, personal and general semantic memory. Cognit Neuropsychol 14:683–712
43. Schnider A, von Däniken C, Gutbrod K (1996) The mechanisms of spontaneous and provoked confabulations. Brain 119:1365–1375
44. Burgess PW, Shallice T (1996) Confabulation and the control of recollection. Memory 4:359–411
45. Schacter DL, Norman KA, Koustaal W (1998) The cognitive neuroscience of constructive memory. Annu Rev Psychol 49:289–318
46. Fotopoulou A, Solms M, Turnbull O (2004) Wishful reality distortions in confabulations: a case study. Neuropsychologia 42:727–744
47. Fotopoulou A, Conway MA, Solms M et al (2008) Self-serving confabulation in prose recall. Neuropsychologia 46:1429–1441
48. Dalla Barba G (1993) Confabulation: knowledge and recollective experience. Cognit Neuropsychol 10:1–20
49. Dalla Barba G, Cappelletti YJ, Signorini M et al (1997) Confabulation: remembering "another" past, planning "another" future. Neurocase 3:425–436
50. Berrington WP, Liddell DW, Foulds GA (1956) A re-evaluation of the fugue. J Ment Sci 102:280–286
51. Stengel E (1941) On the aetiology of the fugue states. J Ment Sci 87:572–599
52. Schacter DL, Wang PL, Tulving E et al (1982) Functional retrograde amnesia: a quantitative case study. Neuropsychologia 5:523–532
53. Glisky EL, Ryan L, Reminger S et al (2004) A case of psychogenic fugue: I understand, aber ich verstehe nichts. Neuropsychologia 42:1132–1147
54. Mechanic M, Resick PA, Griffin MG (1998) A comparison of normal forgetting, psychopathology, and information-processing models of reported amnesia of recent sexual trauma. J Consult Clin Psychol 66:948–957
55. Andrews B, Brewin CR, Rose S et al (2000) Predicting PTSD symptoms in victims of violent crime: the role of shame, anger, and childhood abuse. J Abnorm Psychol 109:69–73
56. Taylor PJ, Kopelman MD (1984) Amnesia for criminal offences. Psychol Med 14:581–588
57. Kopelman MD (2002) Psychogenic amnesia. In: Baddeley AD, Kopelman MD, Wilson BA (eds) The handbook of memory disorders, 2nd edn. Wiley, Chichester
58. Pyszora NM, Barker AF, Kopelman MD (2003) Amnesia for criminal offences: a study of life sentence prisoners. J Forens Psychiatry Psychol 14:475–490
59. Christianson SA, Merckelbach H, Kopelman MD (2006) Crime-related amnesia. In: Heaton-Armstrong A, Shepherd E, Gudjonsson G et al (eds) Witness testimony: psychological, investigative and evidential perspectives. Oxford University Press, Oxford, pp 105–126
60. Gudjonsson GH, MacKeith JAC (1983) A specific recognition deficit in case of homicide. Med Sci Law 23:37–40
61. Kopelman MD (2000) Focal retrograde amnesia and the attribution of causality: an exceptionally critical review. Cognit Neuropsychol 17:585–621

62. Kapur N (2000) Focal retrograde amnesia and the attribution of causality: an exceptionally benign commentary. Cognit Neuropsychol 17:623–637
63. Kapur N (1993) Focal retrograde amnesia in neurological disease: a critical review. Cortex 29:217–234
64. Anderson MC, Green C (2001) Suppressing unwanted memories by executive control. Nature (Lond) 410:366–369
65. Anderson MC, Ochsner KN, Kuhl B et al (2004) Neural systems underlying the suppression of unwanted memories. Science 303:232–235

Part III
Seizure Disorders

Part III
[illegible]

The Neuropsychological Aspect of Epilepsy

Yoshio Morita

Abstract A supplementary relationship is observed between clinical epileptology and clinical neuropsychology with regard to the method of studying higher brain functions in the human cortex. For example, ictal illusions and hallucinations associated with localization-related epilepsy can contribute to the phenomenological works dealing with both epilepsy and neuropsychology. We evaluated the content and type of aura-sensations and determined the laterality of epileptic focus using scalp EEG. Epigastric and visual auras ware the most frequently observed sensations. However, the laterality of the aura-sensations was not clarified in the EEG recordings.

Keywords Aura-sensations • Epilepsy • Ictal illusions and hallucinations • Lateralization • Neuropsychology

Introduction

In studies of higher brain function, clinical neuropsychology and clinical epileptology are closely related. Both sciences aim at the elucidation of local brain functions: clinical neuropsychology presents syndromes of functional loss and stimulation associated with local injuries of the human brain, whereas various syndromes of human epileptic seizures are observed in clinical epileptology.

Studies attempt to elucidate the association between changes in brain function induced in the cerebral disease process and the psychological process employing methods supplementing each other. Clinical brain wave measurement including evoked responses and psychological measurement are employed in this study. Paroxysmal neuropsychological symptoms; visuo-spatial disorders and body-scheme

Y. Morita (✉)
Department of Neuropsychiatry, Hyogo College of Medicine,
1-1, Mukogawa-cho, Nishinomiya, 663-8501, Hyogo, Japan
e-mail: npsy@hyo-med.ac.jp

K. Miyoshi et al. (eds.), *Neuropsychiatric Disorders*,
DOI 10.1007/978-4-431-53871-4_7, © Springer 2010

disorders (heautoscopy) in temporal lobe epilepsy will be mentioned in this chapter for understanding the close relations between neuropsychology and epileptology.

Neuropsychological Symptoms in Epilepsy

According to W.G. Lennox, epilepsy is defined as recurrent self-sustained paroxysmal disorders of brain function.

Epilepsy encompasses paroxysmal disorders, and the international classification categorizes epileptic seizures as follows [1]:

1. Localization-related (focal, local, and partial) epilepsies and syndromes
   (a) Idiopathic (with age-related onset)
   (b) Symptomatic
   (c) Cryptogenic
2. Generalized epilepsies and syndromes
3. Epilepsies and syndromes undetermined as to whether focal or generalized
4. Special syndromes

Temporal lobe epilepsy, one of the types of complex partial seizures, is classified as symptomatic epilepsy in this classification [1]. The paroxysmal symptoms of this type of epilepsy are closely related to anatomical localization of the lesion in the temporal lobe.

In addition to paroxysmal symptoms, accompanying signs and symptoms at onset are important indices of the origin of paroxysmal discharge. On the other hand, classical clinical neuropsychology searches for associations between functional changes in brain disorders and psychological processes.

Neurological symptoms; essential sensation and movement disorders, as well as neuropsychological symptoms; aphasia, apraxia, and agnosia, are common symptoms in epileptic patients. On the other hand, neuropsychiatric symptoms, such as hallucination, disturbance of memory, spontaneity disorder, personality disorder are less frequently noted in epilepsy.

Paroxysmal Visuo-Spatial Disorders

Fifty-seven episodes of aura sensations in 18 patients with temporal lobe epilepsy are tabulated in Table 1 and 2.

The main symptoms of temporal lobe syndrome in temporal lobe epilepsies (TLEs) are simple and complex partial seizures, secondarily generalized seizures, or a combination of these symptoms.

Complex partial seizure can be categorized into P0–P4 based on the phasal development of seizures; P0 aura-sensations, P1 represents the tonic-lapse phase, P2 oral automatism, P3 behavioral automatism, and P4 secondarily generalized tonic-clonic seizures. Aura-sensations of visuo-spatial distortions were noted in the P0 stage of 18 patients with temporal lobe epilepsy.

Table 1 Classification of aura-sensations

	n	Percent
Cephalic	11	19.3
Visceral	8	14.0
Autonomic	3	5.3
Somatosensory	2	3.5
Emotional	7	12.3
Illusional	17	29.8
Hallucinatory	7	12.3
Ideational	2	3.5
	57	100

(a) On interictal scalp-recorded EEG, paroxysmal abnormality was detected in right anterotemporal lobe (15 patients), left anterotemporal lobe (29 patients) and bilateral anterotemporal lobe (7 patients).
(b) Fifty-seven episodes of aura sensation occurred in the 18 patients, and 24 (about 42%) showed visuo-spatial distortion.

The anterotemporal spikes during the interictal period on scalp-recorded EEG in the 18 patients was detected in right anterotemporal lobe (7 patients), left anterotemporal lobe (7 patients) and bilateral anterotemporal lobe (7 patients).

The 57 episodes of aura-sensations are tabulated in Table 2.

When foci of aT spikes on the left and right sides were counted on interictal scalp-recorded EEG, no distinct difference of laterality was noted in the cases of aura-sensations.

Visuo-spatial distortions are usually complaint by the patients with temporal lobe epilepsy as distortion of the size, shape, distance and dimension of objects, disorientation, experiences of déjà vu and/or jamais vu, distortion of scene and body schema [2–4].

Visceral auras, like epigastric distress, and changes of feeling of familiarity are the common aura symptoms in the patients with temporal lobe epilepsy.

Aphasia is also reported as one of the symptoms of an aura-sensation [2] (Table 3).

Taylor and Lochery [4] reported the idiosyncratic auras in temporal lobe epilepsy. Déjà vu with micropsia, sense of being enveloped by a "monster", feeling of inferiority, rerealization, and other peculiar feelings are reported in this category. Illusions of recognition and illusional emotions, caused by experimental stimulation of the brain, appeared to be similar to the illusions in visuo-spatial aura in temporal lobe epilepsy [5] (Table 5).

Body Scheme Disorders (Heautoscopy)

Paroxysmal heautoscopy accompanied by visuo-spatial disorder occurred in 2 of the 51 patients with temporal lobe epilepsy. Paroxysmal heautoscopy is rare in epilepsy, but it well known in psychopathology. Penfield and Perot reported four electrical stimulation-induced human cases of heautoscopy in an epilepsy study in

Table 2 Ictal visual spatial distortions and lateralization

	RaT	LaT	Bil
Size	2	0	2
Shape	2	0	2
Distance	2	1	2
Dimension	3	4	2
Orientation	1	4	1
Deja ve/jamais vu	2	1	1
Scene	1	1	1
Body schema	2	1	0
n=38 (19 patients)			

Table 3 Frequency of different aura-sensations in our patients (from Kanemoto and Janz [2])

	n	Percent
Epigastric	50	35
Familiarity	45	31
(Déjà vu)	28	19
Aphasia	24	17
Anxiety	23	16
Thought-disorder	19	13
"Es"	16	10
Visual	12	8
Somatosensory	12	8
Gustatory	12	6
Porropia-porracousia	8	5
Olfactory	7	5
Auditory	7	3
Dysarthria	4	4
Others	5	22
No aura	31	
Total N	143	

which 69 patients underwent electric stimulation during brain surgery. It showed another characteristic in that it concomitantly occurred with other visuo-spatial distortions [4].

Penfield and Perot [5] reported the case of patient with heautoscopy. Their case was a 37-year-old housewife, who began to have seizures at the age of 20, consisting of the following pattern: (1) thoracic sensation and palpitation, (2) experiential hallucination, visual type, and (3) occasional major seizures, mainly right sided. At the beginning of an attack, she would mentally visualize scenes that she sometimes had difficulty recognizing or remembering, but they were often from her own past. Frequently, the scene consisted of herself during childbirth and also in a picture. Often, as soon as she recognized the scene it would disappear. On surgery, the left temporal lobe was exposed, and an area of gliosis identified. Stimulation at point N (Brodmann 21) caused the patient to say that she suddenly

Table 4 Interpretive responses and illusions (from Penfield and Perot [5])

Auditory illusions: Sounds heard seemed louder or clearer, fainter or more distinct, nearer or farther
Visual illusions: Things seen seemed clearer or blurred; nearer or farther; larger or smaller; fatter or thinner
Illusions of recognition: Present experience seemed familiar (déjà vu), strange, altered, or unreal
Illusional emotions: Feelings of fear, loneliness, sorrow, or disgust

Table 5 Ictal autoscopy hallucination [6]

	Author		Focus
1	Nouet	1923	r. temporal
2	Ehrenwald	1931	r. central
3	Lunn	1948	r. central
4	Lunn	1948	l. central
5	Hecaen and Ajuriaguerra	1952	l. centro-parieto occipital
6	Ionasescu	1960	l. temporal-occipital
7	Ionasescu	1960	r. temporal
8	Ohashi	1965	r. temporal
9	Hamanaka	1974	bil. diffuse
10	Morita	1978	r. temporal
11	Sengoku	1981	r. temporal
12	Kamiya and Okamoto	1982	r. temporal
13	Kamiya and Okamoto	1982	l. temporal
14	Kamiya and Okamoto	1982	r. temporal

saw herself in childbirth and she felt as if she were reliving the experience [5] (Table 4).

Here the brief history of our patient with heautoscopy is presented.

The female patient of 26 years old who suffered with aura-sensation of complex partial seizure of temporal lobe epilepsy complaint the frequent episodes of heautoscopic experiences and inverted vision. Inter-ictal scalp-record electroencephalogram showed the spike and slow wave complex at left anterior temporal lobe of this patient [6] (Table 5).

Ictal autoscopy hallucination is observed frequently in the patients with temporal lobe epilepsy. This peculiar experience is considered one of the feeling of alteration of body scheme and asomatognosia.

Discussion and Conclusion

Visuo-spatial and body-schema cognitions are firmly established brain functions in humans and are rarely impaired. However, paroxysmal distortions of visuo-space and body image frequently occur simultaneously in the patients with temporal lobe

Table 6 Paroxysmal disorders of body image (from Ohhashi et al. [8])

1. Sentiment dábsence dune partie du corps
2. Illusion de transformation corporalle
3. Illusion de deplacement cofporel
4. Membre fantome
5. Héautoscopie

epilepsy [2,3]. And, occasionally the symptoms are accompanied by the state of double consciousness [7]. Neuropsychological symptoms, like aphasia, heautoscopy [8], and inverted vision, distortion of the time sense [9] are also encountered in the complex partial seizures.

Heautoscopy is regarded as one of the disorder of body scheme (asomatognosia) [8] (Table 6). Paroxysmal episodes of the peculiar experience of seeing one's self or "double" self (heautoscopy) may occur in the patients with temporal lobe epilepsy. In the brain stimulation study reported by Penfield and Perot [5], heautoscopy was reproduced in 4 of 69 cases, and the foci of the seizures were present in the temporal lobe, similarly to our patients.

As we see in the present chapter, neuropsychological symptoms commonly occur in paroxysmal seizures of the complex partial epilepsy, especially temporal lobe epilepsy. Therefore, collaborative studies in the fields of epileptology and neuropsychology are important to understand the complexity of the psychiatric symptoms in temporal lobe epilepsy.

Although the complete understanding of human brain function might not be possible at this moment, it should be a goal of the clinical neurosciences in the future. There is no doubt, however, neuropsychological studies of epileptic patients contribute to understand the brain function, as the encourage words of Penfield and Jackson: "He who is faithfully analyzing many different cases of epilepsy is doing far more than studying epilepsy" (Wilder Penfield and Hughlinge Jackson).

References

1. Commission on classification and terminology of the international league against epilepsy (1981) Proposal for revised clinical and electroencephalographic classification of epileptic seizures. Epilepsia 22:489–501
2. Kanemoto K, Janz D (1989) The temporal sequence of aurasensations in patients with complex focal seizures with particular attention to ictal aphasia. J Neurol Neurosurg Psychiatry 52:52–56
3. Ionasescu V (1960) Paroxymal disorders of the body image in temporal lobe epilepsy. Acta Psychiatr Scand 35:171–181
4. Taylor D, Lochery M (1987) Temporal lobe epilepsy: origin and significance of simple and complex auras. J Neurol Neurosurg Psychiatry 50:673–681
5. Penfield W, Perot P (1963) The brain's record of auditory and visual experience. Brain 86:39–696
6. Morita Y (1978) Paroxysmal disorders of body image, 2 cases. Clin Electroencephalogr 20:223–224

7. Kamiya S, Okamoto S (1982) Double consciousness in epileptics: a clinical picture and minor hemispheric specialization. Advances in epileptology. Raven, New York
8. Ohhashi H, Kawai I, Hamanaka T (1969) A clinical and electroencephalographic study on the paroxysmal disorders of body image. Psychiatr Neurol Jpn 71:435–449
9. Kawai I, Kawagoe T, Hatada K et al (1983) Ictal distortion of time sense in epileptic patients. J Jpn Epilepsy Soc 1:17–22

The Interictal Dysphoric Disorder of Epilepsy

Marco Mula

Abstract Depression represents a common psychiatric comorbidity in patients with epilepsy, particularly among those with partial seizures of temporal lobe origin, ranging between 24% and 74% according to the population investigated. However, a number of authors have pointed out that the phenomenology of depression, especially among patients with refractory epilepsy, frequently fails to meet widely standardized criteria for psychiatric disorders such as DSM-IV. In this regard, it has been suggested that, within the overall presentations of depression in epilepsy, a subgroup of patients may develop an affective-somatoform syndrome also known as the interictal dysphoric disorder of epilepsy. This chapter is aimed at reviewing, with historical reference, the psychopathological and clinical features of such a controversial entity in the light of recent studies pointing out the commonalities with a specific subset of cyclothymic subjects in which depressive periods and labile–angry–irritable moods dominate the clinical picture. It is, therefore, tempting to speculate that the interictal dysphoric disorder may represent an interesting biological model to further clarify a number of issues on the neurobiology of mood regulation.

Keywords Antiepileptic drugs • Bipolar disorder • Depression • Epilepsy • Interictal dysphoric disorder

Epilepsy and Depression: An Overview

It has been known for a long time that there are some associations between epilepsy and depression. The Greek physician Hippocrates, around 400 B.C., observed that "*melancholics ordinarily become epileptics, and epileptics, melancholics: what*

M. Mula (✉)
Division of Neurology, Maggiore Hospital, Amedeo Avogadro University, C.so Mazzini 18, 28100, Novara, Italy
e-mail: marco.mula@med.unipmn.it

K. Miyoshi et al. (eds.), *Neuropsychiatric Disorders*,
DOI 10.1007/978-4-431-53871-4_8, © Springer 2010

determines the preference is the direction the malady takes; if it bears upon the body, epilepsy, if upon the intelligence, melancholy" [1].

There are several reasons why these two conditions may be closely linked, and such reasons are both biological and psychosocial. Epilepsy is a chronic disorder, which still brings about much social discrimination, and as with any chronic disorder, epilepsy might be expected to be linked to demoralization and a negative perspective toward life. On the other hand, the biological contribution to the association, based on neuroanatomical and neurochemical principles, needs to be taken into account. Epilepsy is frequently associated with damages in the limbic system, which plays a key role in the processing of emotions. Also, patients with epilepsy are chronically exposed to antiepileptic drugs that are potent psychoactive compounds with a number of effects on mood and behavior. For all these reasons it is expected that depression is more frequent among patients with epilepsy when compared to the general population, and data coming from community studies support such an impression. The General Practice UK study reported a 22% prevalence of depression in unselected samples of patients with epilepsy [2]. A Canadian Community Health Survey noted very similar lifetime prevalence rates for depression (around 22%), much higher than those reported in the general population (around 12%) [3]. A U.S. survey pointed out that depression is more frequent in epilepsy (36.5%) in comparison to people with asthma (27.8%) and healthy controls [4], suggesting that depression is more frequently reported in epilepsy than in other chronic medical conditions. Another relevant point relates to seizure control being such comorbidity greater in those patients with higher seizure frequencies and with continuing seizures compared to seizure-free patients. In fact, several authors have noted a correlation with seizure frequency that most likely reflects in a large part on the intractability of the seizure disorders. Jacoby et al. [5] reported depression in 4% of seizure-free patients, 10% in patients with less than one seizure per month, and 21% in patients with higher seizure frequency. O'Donoghue et al. [6] pointed out that patients with epilepsy with continuing seizures are significantly more likely to suffer from depression than those in remission (33% vs. 6%).

The association between depression and epilepsy has relevant implications in terms of prognosis and treatment; in fact, it seems quite established that depressive symptoms are the most important predictor of quality of life of patients with epilepsy, an even more powerful predictor than the actual seizure frequency [7–9].

An important finding that has been replicated by several studies is that the link between depression and epilepsy is not necessarily unidirectional; that is, patients with such a comorbidity always present with the seizure disorder before the emergence of the depression, but it has been noted that having a prior mood disorder can be associated with an increased risk of epilepsy [10, 11]. Although it is reasonable to hypothesize that the development of the epilepsy may be related to suicidal attempts, or to drug abuse, or follow some other kinds of trauma such as head trauma, it tempting to speculate that such a finding may reflect an underlying common pathogenesis, which may relate to some as yet unknown genetic factor, or some link with neurotransmitter function (for example, related to transmitters that are known to play a role in both epilepsy and depression such as serotonin or GABA) [12, 13].

Is Depression Associated with Any Specific Epilepsy Syndrome?

There has been considerable debate, which is unresolved, as to the association between depression and any particular epilepsy syndrome. It is well known that people with lesional mesial temporal lobe epilepsy are likely to have intractable seizures, and they are also likely to be on a polytherapy regimen. It has been suggested that such patients are more prone to develop depression than other groups, and this association seems to be strictly related to the degree of involvement of the limbic structures [14]. However, other authors failed to show any difference between temporal lobe and extratemporal lobe epilepsy in terms of mood disorders [15]. In this regard, it is interesting to note that there are a number of studies outside the field of epilepsy suggesting that hippocampal volume loss is associated with depression [16, 17]. Thus, although further research in this area is needed, neuroimaging studies are revealing an underlying brain network of depression in psychiatric patients without a neurological disorder, which includes the hippocampus, nicely in keeping with the findings in epilepsy patients.

Current literature on neurobiology of depression in epilepsy has also focused on frontal lobe dysfunction, the latter having emerged from investigations using brain imaging techniques [positron emission tomography (PET) or single-photon emission computed tomography (SPECT)] and neuropsychological testing. It has been shown that patients with left-sided temporal lobe epilepsy and depression were more likely to perform poorly on frontal lobe tasks [18]. Similar results have been reported by neuroimaging studies [19, 20]. Although these findings, of necessity, were derived from a limited number of patients, the concordance between the conclusions does support an anatomical association between temporal lobe epilepsy, especially left-sided epileptic activity, depression, and frontal lobe dysfunction.

Is There a Mood Disorder Specific of Epilepsy? The Interictal Dysphoric Disorder

The issue of phenomenology of depression in epilepsy has been and still is very much a matter of debate. Some authors have emphasized the endogenous features [21] while others commented on the reactive nature of depression [22]. In general terms, the spectrum of manifestations is likely to be large, and it is reasonable to hypothesize that patients with epilepsy can experience forms of mood disorders identical to those of patients without epilepsy. However, it is equally reasonable to assume that the underlying brain pathology may influence the final phenomenology of mood disorder symptoms, emphasizing some aspects or attenuating others.

Data favoring the existence of an epilepsy-specific mood disorder come from the clinical observation that the psychopathology of patients with epilepsy often has unique manifestations that are poorly reflected by conventional classification systems such as Diagnostic and Statistical Manual of Mental Disorders (DSM)-IV and International Classification of Diseases (ICD)-10 [23]. Some authors observed that up to 22% of patients consecutively assessed for the phenomenology of depression could be classified as having atypical features [24]. In fact, it is a common observation that classic endogenous-type depressive symptoms, such as feelings of guilt, lack of emotions or "*Gefühl der Gefühllosigkeit*," and a circadian pattern of symptom severity are rarely reported by patients with epilepsy. Kanner et al. [25] reported that such atypical symptoms are much more frequent among subjects with refractory epilepsy with percentages as high as 71%; moreover, it is important to point out that 64% fail to meet any DSM-IV criteria using two structured clinical interviews, namely, the Structured Clinical Interview for DSM-IV Axis I (SCID-I) and the Mini International Neuropsychiatric Interview (MINI) [26]. Among different potential causes for the atypical features of mood disorders in epilepsy, the periictal cluster of symptoms, to some degree, may account for such an atypicality [27], but the possibility that the mood disorders of epilepsy may have unique characteristics has plausibility.

In classic psychiatric writings, especially the German literature [28, 29], patients with epilepsy were described as having a pleomorphic pattern of symptoms, including affective symptoms with prominent irritability intermixed with euphoric moods, fear, anxiety as well as anergia, pain, and insomnia. Such observations have been confirmed by Gastaut [30], and later Blumer coined the term interictal dysphoric disorder to refer to this type of depressive disorder seen in patients with epilepsy [31]. Blumer used the term "dysphoria" to emphasize the periodicity of mood changes and the presence of outbursts of irritability and aggressive behavior as key symptoms. Other authors [25, 32, 33] highlighted the chronic course of this state of moderate neurotic depression with symptom-free intervals typical of epilepsy, referring to a dimension very close to dysthymia. It is obvious that the interictal dysphoric disorder may present in our time with features that are different from those described by premodern psychiatry. For example, depressed mood and anergia may be much more evident than previously because modern antiepileptic medications may attenuate the dysphoric symptoms.

The phenomenology of this somatoform-affective disorder, as reported by Blumer, is particularly intriguing [31, 34]. He described eight key symptoms grouped in three major categories: labile depressive symptoms (depressive mood, anergia, pain, and insomnia), labile affective symptoms (fear, anxiety), and supposedly "specific" symptoms (paroxysmal irritability, and euphoric moods; Table 1). The dysphoric episodes are described as occurring without external triggers and without clouding of consciousness; beginning and ending rapidly and recurring fairly regularly in a uniform manner (every few days to every few months and lasting for a few hours up to 2 days). The concept of the interictal dysphoric disorder theorized by Blumer goes beyond the mood disorder itself to encompass a spectrum of conditions with transient psychotic features, to an even more debilitating disorder with prolonged psychotic states. In fact, according to Blumer's view, the schizophrenia-like psychoses of epilepsy can be considered as a severe interictal dysphoric disorder with psychotic features or better a schizoaffective interictal dysphoric disorder [31, 34]. Such a hypothesis is deeply influenced by classic German psychiatric

Table 1 Principal symptom groups of the interictal dysphoric disorder of epilepsy according to Blumer's definition

Labile depressive symptoms	Anergia
	Depressed mood
	Insomnia
	Pain
Labile affective symptoms	Anxiety
	Fear
Specific symptoms	Euphoric moods
	Paroxysmal irritability

literature, especially Kraepelin's view of the relationship between manic-depressive illness and schizophrenia [28].

Recent studies from my group specifically investigated the clinical and psychopathological features of the interictal dysphoric disorder [35, 36]. We observed that such a syndrome represents a homogeneous construct with specific clinical features and affects a relevant proportion of patients with epilepsy (about 17%). However, it seems not to be specifically associated to the epilepsy itself, being diagnosed also in subjects with migraine (about 18%) [35]. Therefore, it needs to be clarified whether the so-called interictal dysphoric disorder is an organic affective syndrome that occurs in patients with brain disturbances or whether it can be diagnosed also in subjects with chronic medical conditions not affecting primarily the central nervous system. Theoretically, this issue was partly addressed by Blumer himself, stating that such a syndrome can occasionally occur in the absence of clinical seizures, in patients with brain lesions (with or without an abnormal EEG) [37]. From a psychopathological point of view, we speculated that some features of the interictal dysphoric disorder, especially the co-occurrence of mood instability and irritability, belong to the bipolar spectrum rather than to unipolar depression [38, 39]. This concept seems to be further supported by the use of standardized clinical instruments for manic and depressive symptoms. In fact, the Mood Disorder Questionnaire came out to be more specific for a diagnosis of interictal dysphoric disorder (86.0%) then the Beck Depression Inventory (65.9%) [35], the former being highly specific for manic symptoms [40]. From a clinical point of view, patients with the interictal dysphoric disorder have several features in common with a subset of cyclothymic subjects where depressive periods and labile–angry–irritable moods dominate the clinical picture, representing the more unstable form of bipolar II disorder [41]. In this regard, it interesting to note that Blumer reported a combined therapy of antiepileptic and antidepressant drugs as effective [34], a combination extensively used in bipolar depression. In another study from my group, we looked at the prevalence and clinical features of manic symptoms in patients with epilepsy observing that although they are highly present (12–14%), in a large proportion of cases these symptoms are related to the interictal dysphoric disorder and can be misleadingly interpreted as bipolar symptoms [36], whereas the prevalence of a true manic-depressive illness in epilepsy showed to be in line with that reported in the general population (about 2%) [42].

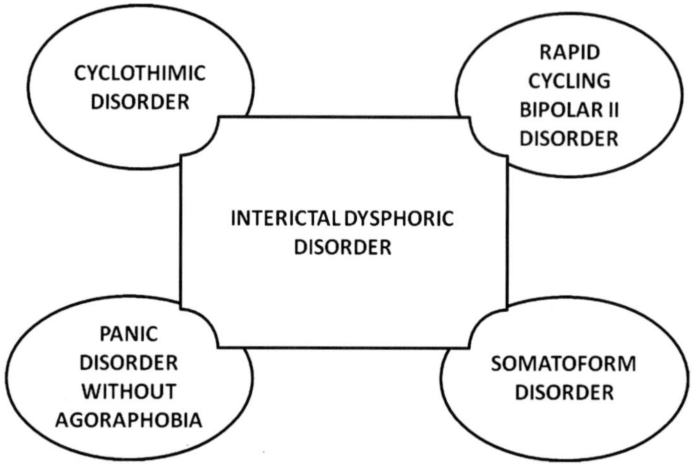

Fig. 1 Major DSM-IV Axis I diagnoses overlapping with the interictal dysphoric disorder

The features of the so-called interictal dysphoric disorder overlap with a variety of affective disorders seen in clinical psychiatric practice (Fig. 1); however, data presented suggest that such a syndrome represents a frequent comorbidity in patients with epilepsy and its diagnosis can be challenging even for expert clinicians because of the pleomorphic phenomenology of the syndrome.

Diagnosing Mood Disorders in Patients with Epilepsy

As already discussed, a diagnosis of depression can be challenging in patients with epilepsy because of the atypicality and pleomorphic nature of symptoms. Moreover, a number of manifestations, which are recognized as diagnostic criteria for a depressive episode by the ICD-10 and DSM-IV (e.g., loss of energy, insomnia or hypersomnia, increase or decrease in appetite, loss of libido, psychomotor retardation, diminished ability to think or concentrate), may occur in epilepsy secondary to seizure activity or the antiepileptic drug treatment. For all these reasons, clinicians need to fully explore the mental state of their patients, trying to identify key symptoms that cannot be influenced by epilepsy-related variables. For example, anhedonia has been suggested to be an excellent indicator of the presence of depression [13]. This issue is strictly related to that of available clinical instruments specifically validated in patients with epilepsy. In this regard, Krishnamoorthy pointed out that the vast majority of studies use measures or cutoff scores that may not be valid in the epilepsy population [43].

Mintzer and Lopez [44] proposed the Epilepsy Addendum for Psychiatric Assessment (EAPA), an instrument expressly designed for use with the MINI, and a version of the SCID-I adapted for patients with epilepsy, named SCID-E, has been proposed [45]. However, the relative benefits of these various instruments, in the assessment of generic psychopathology in community-based studies, are the subject of considerable debate. Among well-known screening instruments, the psychometric properties of the Beck Depression Inventory have been investigated in epilepsy, showing a good sensitivity (0.93), an acceptable specificity (0.81), and an excellent negative predictive value (0.98), but a very low positive predictive value (0.47) [46]. A six-item, self-report, screening instrument, the Neurological Disorders Depression Inventory for Epilepsy (NDDI-E), was validated to screen for major depressive episodes in epilepsy [47]. It has the advantage of being constructed specifically to minimize confounding factors, such as adverse events related to AEDs or cognitive problems associated with epilepsy, and showed an internal consistency of 0.85 and a test–retest reliability of 0.78. A score of 15 or higher has a specificity of 0.90 and a sensitivity of 0.81 for a diagnosis of major depressive episode. However, all these instruments relate to a diagnosis of a mood disorder characterized by symptoms identical to those referred by psychiatric populations without epilepsy. Therefore, a number of atypical manifestations that can be seen in the epilepsy setting may remain undetected. The Seizure Questionnaire developed by Blumer and collaborators contains questions for the eight key symptoms of the interictal dysphoric disorder [48]. Patient and caregiver answer them jointly, and the examiner then reviews all answers for completeness and accuracy. We have developed a specific instrument, named the Interictal Dysphoric Disorder Inventory (IDDI), a 38-item, self-report questionnaire, to evaluate all symptoms of the interictal dysphoric disorder in terms of presence, frequency, severity, and global impairment [35]. This questionnaire explores a time interval of 12 months. The diagnosis of interictal dysphoric disorder follows Blumer's criteria [34], namely, the presence of at least three symptoms of "moderate" or "severe" severity and causing "moderate" or "severe" distress. It is possible to obtain a total score and three subscale scores that mirror the three major symptom categories described by Blumer: labile depressive symptoms, labile affective symptoms, and specific symptoms. Furthermore, the IDDI allocates also "*severeness*" (IDDIsev) total and partial scores that reflect the degree of interference or distress caused by symptoms. The IDDI total and subscale scores showed strong or very strong correlations among themselves (0.68–0.85), and the instrument displayed an acceptable sensitivity and an excellent specificity when compared to a validated questionnaire for the screening of major depression or bipolar disorder (i.e., Beck Depression Inventory and Mood Disorder Questionnaire) [35]. Finally, in the appendix to the questionnaire, six questions investigate the time course of the disorder, duration of dysphoric symptoms, and their associations with seizures or antiepileptic drug therapy. The entire questionnaire has been published and it is fully available [49].

It seems clear that the correct diagnosis of mood disorders in epilepsy is still affected by unmet needs. However, some screening instruments shown to be valid in depression (i.e., BDI and NDDI-E) and others are available for specific syndromes (i.e., IDDI). Nevertheless, clinical observation through a careful assessment of the mental state of the patient still remains the gold standard.

Conclusions

Depression in epilepsy represents a frequently encountered psychiatric comorbidity that is likely to be related to a number of variables which are both biological and psychosocial. The arguments for whether the majority of the clinical presentations could be explained by psychosocial factors have been variably prominent across authors. However, whatever way one views this, the literature suggests that the link between depression and epilepsy may not be unidirectional, further supporting the hypothesis of common underlying biological mechanisms.

It does seem generally agreed that the clinical picture of depression in epilepsy is not typical in all cases for a DSM categorization, and a number of authors have noted the atypical nature of the clinical picture. Within the overall presentations of depression in epilepsy, it appears that a subgroup of patients may have an affective syndrome, which some have referred to as the interictal dysphoric disorder. Such a condition seems to have overlapping features with the bipolar spectrum, with possible consequences in terms of prognosis and therapeutic strategies. It is, therefore, essential that clinicians assess for these varied forms as well.

References

1. Temkin O (1971) The falling sickness. John Hopkins, Baltimore
2. Edeh J, Toone B (1987) Relationship between interictal psychopathology and type of epilepsy. Results of a survey in general practice. Br J Psychiatry 151:95–101
3. Tellez-Zenteno JF, Patten SB, Jetté N et al (2007) Psychiatric comorbidity in epilepsy: a population-based analysis. Epilepsia 48:2336–2344
4. Ettinger A, Reed M, Cramer J et al (2004) Depression and comorbidity in community-based patients with epilepsy or asthma. Neurology 63:1008–1014
5. Jacoby A, Baker GA, Steen N et al (1996) The clinical course of epilepsy and its psychosocial correlates: findings from a UK community study. Epilepsia 37:148–161
6. O'Donoghue MF, Goodridge DM, Redhead K et al (1999) Assessing the psychosocial consequences of epilepsy: a community-based study. Br J Gen Pract 49:211–214
7. Perrine K, Hermann BP, Meador KJ et al (1995) The relationship of neuropsychological functioning to quality of life in epilepsy. Arch Neurol 52:997–1003
8. Gilliam F, Kuzniecky R, Faught E et al (1997) Patient validated content of epilepsy specific quality of life measurement. Epilepsia 38:233–236
9. Boylan LS, Flint LA, Labovitz DL et al (2004) Depression but not seizure frequency predicts quality of life in treatment-resistant epilepsy. Neurology 62:258–261
10. Forsgren L, Nystrom L (1990) An incident case-referent study of epileptic seizures in adults. Epilepsy Res 6:66–81
11. Hesdorffer DC, Hauser WA, Annegers JF et al (2000) Major depression is a risk factor for seizures in older patients. Ann Neurol 47:246–249
12. Kanner AM, Balabanov A (2002) Depression and epilepsy: how closely related are they? Neurology 58(8 suppl 5):S27–S39
13. Kanner AM (2006) Depression and epilepsy: a new perspective on two closely related disorders. Epilepsy Curr 6:141–146
14. Quiske A, Helmstaedter C, Lux S et al (2000) Depression in patients with temporal lobe epilepsy is related to mesial temporal sclerosis. Epilepsy Res 39:121–125

15. Swinkels WA, van Emde BW, Kuyk J et al (2006) Interictal depression, anxiety, personality traits, and psychological dissociation in patients with temporal lobe epilepsy (TLE) and extra-TLE. Epilepsia 47:2092–2103
16. Bremner JD, Narayan M, Anderson ER et al (2000) Hippocampal volume reduction in major depression. Am J Psychiatry 157:115–118
17. Frodl T, Meisenzahl EM, Zetzsche T et al (2002) Hippocampal changes in patients with a first episode of major depression. Am J Psychiatry 159:1112–1118
18. Hermann BP, Seidenberg M, Haltiner A et al (1991) Mood state in unilateral temporal lobe epilepsy. Biol Psychiatry 30:1205–1218
19. Schmitz EB, Moriarty J, Costa DC et al (1997) Psychiatric profiles and patterns of cerebral blood flow in focal epilepsy: interactions between depression, obsessionality, and perfusion related to the laterality of the epilepsy. J Neurol Neurosurg Psychiatry 62:458–463
20. Bromfield E, Altschuler L, Leiderman D (1990) Cerebral metabolism and depression in patients with complex partial seizures. Epilepsia 31:625
21. Betts TA (1974) A follow up study of a cohort of patients with epilepsy admitted to psychiatric care in an English city. In: Harris P, Mawdsley C (eds) Epilepsy: Proceedings of the Hans Berger Centenary Symposium. Churchill Livingstone, Edinburgh, pp 326–338
22. Mulder DW, Daly D (1952) Psychiatric symptoms associated with lesions of the temporal lobe. JAMA 141:173–176
23. Krishnamoorthy ES, Trimble MR, Blumer D (2007) The classification of neuropsychiatric disorders in epilepsy: a proposal by the ILAE Commission on Psychobiology of Epilepsy. Epilepsy Behav 10:349–353
24. Mendez MF, Cummings JL, Benson DF (1986) Depression in epilepsy. Significance and phenomenology. Arch Neurol 43:766–770
25. Kanner AM, Kozac AM, Frey M (2000) The use of sertraline in patients with epilepsy: is it safe? Epilepsy Behav 1:100–105
26. Kanner AM, Soto A, Gross-Kanner H (2004) Prevalence and clinical characteristics of postictal psychiatric symptoms in partial epilepsy. Neurology 62:708–713
27. Kanner AM (2008) Do peri-ictal psychiatric symptoms account for the differences between depressive disorders in patients with and without epilepsy? In: Kanner AM, Schachter S (eds) Psychiatric controversies in epilepsy. Elsevier, New York, pp 201–209
28. Kraepelin E (1923) Psychiatrie. Band 3. Johann Ambrosius Barth, Leipzig
29. Bleuler E (1949) Lehrbuch der Psychiatrie, 8th edn. Springer-Verlag, Berlin
30. Gastaut H, Morin G, Lesevre N (1955) Etude du comportement des epileptiques psychomoteurs dans l'intervalle de leurs crises: les troubles de l'activitè globale et de la sociabilitè. Ann Med Psychol (Paris) 113:1–27
31. Blumer D (2000) Dysphoric disorders and paroxysmal affects: recognition and treatment of epilepsy-related psychiatric disorders. Harv Rev Psychiatry 8:8–17
32. Himmelhoch JM (1984) Major mood disorders related to epileptic changes. In: Blumer D (ed) Psychiatric aspects of epilepsy. American Psychiatric, Washington, DC, pp 271–94
33. Kanner AM (2003) Depression in epilepsy: a frequently neglected multifaceted disorder. Epilepsy Behav 4:S11–S19
34. Blumer D, Montouris G, Davies K (2004) The interictal dysphoric disorder: recognition, pathogenesis, and treatment of the major psychiatric disorder of epilepsy. Epilepsy Behav 5:826–840
35. Mula M, Jauch R, Cavanna A et al (2008) Clinical and psychopathological definition of the interictal dysphoric disorder of epilepsy. Epilepsia 49:650–656
36. Mula M, Schmitz B, Jauch R et al (2008) On the prevalence of bipolar disorder in epilepsy. Epilepsy Behav 13:658–61
37. Blumer D, Heilbronn M, Himmelhoch J (1988) Indications for carbamazepine in mental illness: atypical psychiatric disorder or temporal lobe syndrome? Compr Psychiatry 29:108–122
38. Möller HJ, Curtis VA (2004) The bipolar spectrum: diagnostic and pharmacologic considerations. Expert Rev Neurother 4(6 suppl 2):S3–8

39. Benazzi F (2007) Is there a continuity between bipolar and depressive disorders? Psychother Psychosom 76:70–6
40. Hirschfeld RM, Holzer C, Calabrese JR et al (2003) Validity of the mood disorder questionnaire: a general population study. Am J Psychiatry 160:178–180
41. Akiskal HS, Pinto O (1999) The evolving bipolar spectrum. Prototypes I, II, III, and IV. Psychiatr Clin North Am 22:517–34
42. Judd L, Akiskal HS (2003) The prevalence and disability of bipolar spectrum disorders in the U.S. population: re-analysis of the ECA database taking into account subthreshold cases. J Affect Disord 73:123–131
43. Krishnamoorthy ES (2006) The evaluation of behavioral disturbances in epilepsy. Epilepsia 47(suppl 2):3–8
44. Mintzer S, Lopez F (2002) Comorbidity of ictal fear and panic disorder. Epilepsy Behav 3:330–337
45. Krishnamoorthy ES (2005). Epidemiology and assessment of psychiatric disorders of epilepsy. Ph.D. thesis, University College London
46. Jones JE, Hermann BP, Woodard JL et al (2005) Screening for major depression in epilepsy with common self-report depression inventories. Epilepsia 46:731–735
47. Gilliam FG, Barry JJ, Hermann BP et al (2006) Rapid detection of major depression in epilepsy: a multicentre study. Lancet Neurol 5:399–405
48. Blumer D, Montouris G, Davies K et al (2002) Suicide in epilepsy: psychopathology, pathogenesis, and prevention. Epilepsy Behav 3:232–241
49. Mula M, Trimble MR (2008) What do we know about mood disorders in epilepsy? In: Kanner AM, Schachter S (eds) Psychiatric controversies in epilepsy. Elsevier, New York, pp 49–66

Neuropsychiatric Symptoms of Seizure Disorders with Special Reference to the Amygdala

Michael Trimble

Abstract In this chapter, the anatomy and function of the amygdala in relationship to emotional processing are explored. It is now known that the amygdala can be activated by certain emotional stimuli, and the fearful faces paradigm has been well tested experimentally. Studies with epilepsy reveal that amygdala sclerosis often accompanies hippocampal sclerosis. Studies of patients with amygdala sclerosis show that this affects the activity to emotional stimuli of the amygdala but also the fusiform and related cortical areas distant from the amygdala. Studies of patients who have undergone temporal lobectomy show the influence of the amygdala in relation to both preoperative and postoperative affective states, especially of the nondominant hemisphere. It is concluded that further studies of the amygdala in epilepsy and other neurological disorders are valuable in studying the functions of the limbic system.

Keywords Amygdala • Psychiatry • Epilepsy • Fusiform area

Introduction

The clinical associations between epilepsy and psychiatric syndromes have now been widely accepted, and the term comorbidity is often used to express such a relationship. In the past, psychological and psychosocial explanations were widely used to explain links between such syndromes as anxiety and depression in epilepsy, although the more severe syndromes such as psychoses or the controversial personality disorders were less likely to be accounted for without considering the underlying biology of the epilepsy [1].

Part of this confusion was the result of the almost exclusive psychological approach to neuropsychiatric disorders taken by psychiatrists, and the relative neglect by neurologists of behavior problems that could be associated with

M. Trimble (✉)
Institute of Neurology, Queen Square, London, WC1N3BG, UK
e-mail: mtrimble@ion.ucl.ac.uk

K. Miyoshi et al. (eds.), *Neuropsychiatric Disorders*,
DOI 10.1007/978-4-431-53871-4_9, © Springer 2010

neurological disorders. Further, in the field of epilepsy there was confusion over the distinction between seizures and epilepsy. Many people equated the two, but seizures as signs and causing symptoms are quite distinct from the underlying pathological processes of the epilepsy. The ongoing interictal electrophysiological disturbances, which presumably reflect underlying electrochemical aberrations within the brain, which are easily identifiable by various imaging techniques, may be expected to lead to continuing interictal disturbances of cerebral function, and if these occur in areas of the central nervous system that have an impact on emotion and behavior, then psychiatric disturbances may be the expected outcome for at least some people with epilepsy, depending upon the site and type of the underlying epileptic discharge.

There has been a growing literature that emphasizes not only the possible neurological underpinnings of psychiatric disorders generally, but also the psychiatric complications of neurological disorders, including epilepsy. From a purely anatomical point of view, the unravelling of the concept of the limbic system, from the earlier circuitry proposed by Papez, to the later more sophisticated elaborations of people such as MacLean, has emphasized that within the brain there were neuronal structures and circuits which have specifically to do with modulation of emotion. This was a new idea, as before the development of the limbic system concept there was no clear cerebral framework for an understanding of how the brain felt and expressed emotion. It was crucial to elaborating on the link between epilepsy and emotion to realize that two key limbic structures, the hippocampus and the amygdala, were frequently involved in the underlying pathology of epilepsy, particularly in the localization-related epilepsies, and newly developed techniques of recording from sites within the brain revealed that between seizures, interictal abnormalities were recorded from such structures. More recently, the uncovering and elaboration of the direct associations between medial temporal structures and limbic forebrain structures, and the unraveling of the neuroanatomy of the limbic forebrain by authors such as Heimer and colleagues, have given clear neurological underpinnings for an understanding of the behavioral consequences of neurological disorders, epilepsy being no exception [2].

The Amygdala

That the amygdala plays a central role in animal behaviour has been known for many years, although its precise role, and its relative importance across different species, have yet to be fully determined. Until recently several lines of evidence have pointed to the role of the amygdala in human behavior, and there is considerable evidence that this structure is closely involved with emotional responsivity in humans. Using functional magnetic resonance imaging (fMRI), it has become commonplace to image the amygdala in vivo, and there are case histories of patients who have had either damage to the amygdala or degeneration of the amygdala, revealing behavioral problems [3].

The amygdala is located at the anterior part of the temporal lobes, in front of and above the temporal horn of the lateral ventricle. It abuts the rostral part of the hippocampus and is a composite of several neuronal aggregates. There are two main components, a larger basolateral complex, which has extensive connections with the neocortex and from which it receives polysensory information, and a central-medial division, extending medially and establishing continuity with the bed nucleus of the stria terminalis (extended amygdala; see following). The laterobasal complex is cortical, whereas the centromedial nucleus is striato-pallidal like.

The main afferent and efferent pathways traverse the stria terminalis and the ventral amygdalofugal pathway. The latter is a longitudinal association bundle linking to the ventral striatum and the medial frontal cortex. There is also a caudal part going to the lateral hypothalamus and, via the medial forebrain bundle, to the brainstem. The uncinate fasciculus that projects to the frontal cortex. The connections to the brainstem come almost exclusively from the central nucleus, the fibers ending in structures that serve autonomic and visceral functions: these include the hypothalamus, the catecholamine and serotonin brainstem nuclei, the ventral tegmental area (VTA) and the substantia nigra, the central grey matter, the dorsal motor nucleus of the vagus, and the nucleus of the solitary tract (NTS). There are also connections to the midbrain and medullary tegmentum. Those to the hypothalamus may influence the control of pituitary hormone release, especially the projections to the ventromedial nucleus, which itself projects to the arcuate nucleus. In the cortex, amygdaloid fibers are found in the orbital and medial frontal lobe, the rostral cingulate gyrus, and most of the temporal lobe [3].

It is further appreciated that the amygdala has extensive distributions to sensory cortical areas, especially the visual cortex, which presumably modify early sensory inputs [4]. The connections of the amygdala to the hippocampus are primarily via the entorhinal cortex, which is a major source of hippocampal afferents. There are direct connections to the subiculum part of the hippocampus.

Some of the widespread connections of the amygdala are shown diagrammatically in Fig. 1. Thus, the amygdala has extensive afferent and efferent connections, and when the amygdala speaks, the rest of the brain listens. The amygdala provides affective valence to sensory representations and is crucial for the emotional tone of memories. The reciprocal connections with the same cortical structures from which it receives information, including even the primary sensory cortical areas, allow for an influence of emotional tone directly on cortical sensory impressions.

Thus the structures of the limbic system, but especially the amygdala, are of great importance for the interpretation of sensory stimuli, and its efferents directly influence motor output. A reliable finding from fMRI studies is that emotional stimuli, notably emotional facial expression, enhance amygdala activity, and there is accumulating evidence that it is also associated with decision making, guiding and driving human behavior [5]. The latter may include the social appraisal of the emotional state of others and the making of value judgements in complex social situations.

The Amygdala in Epilepsy

One of the main pathologies of treatment-resistant epilepsy is mesial temporal sclerosis; this is usually linked with hippocampal lesions, of varying severity, but in some 10% of cases isolated amygdala damage can be seen, and amygdala sclerosis often accompanies hippocampal sclerosis [6]. MRI technology has now been widely

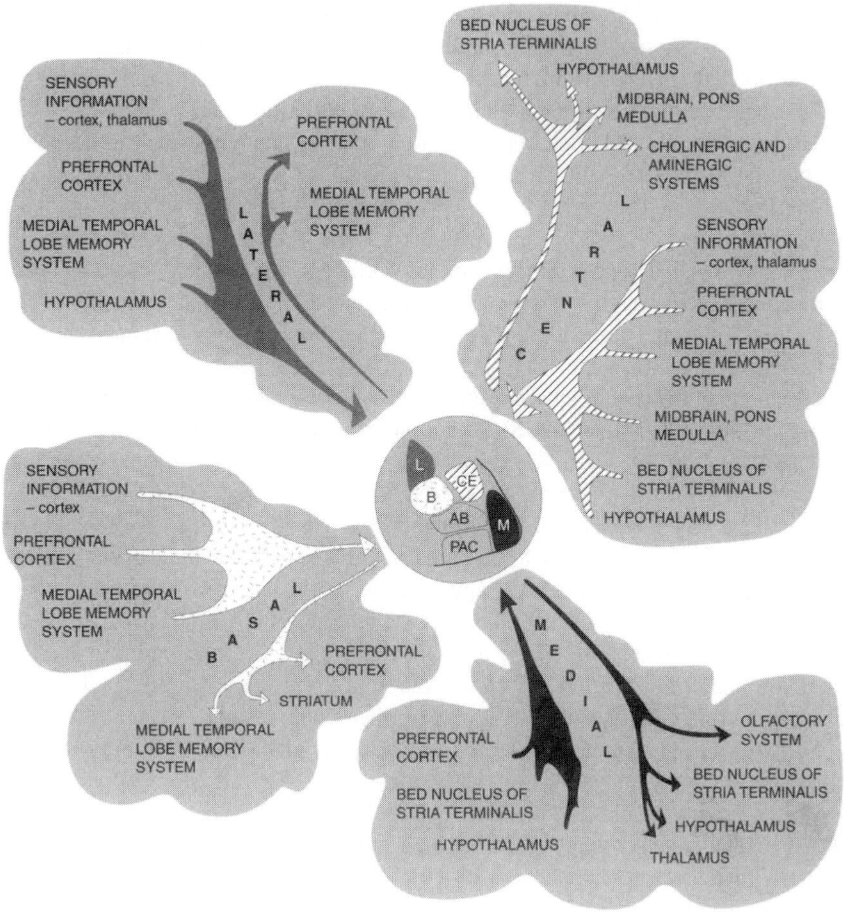

Fig. 1 The amygdala has widespread influence on cortical and subcortical structures. *L* lateral; *CE* central; *M* medial; *B* basal; *AB* accesory basal nucleus; *PAC* periamygdaloid cortex. (Reproduced with permission from Asla Pitkanen)

used to explore the brains of patients with epilepsy, and data from both structural volumetric analyses and functional data using fMRI have drawn attention to the importance of the amygdala for regulating behavior in patients with epilepsy.

Structural Changes

van Elst et al. 2000 [7, 8] carried out a series of studies examining the volume of the amydala in different groups of patients with epilepsy. In the first investigation, they examined a group of patients with intermittent explosive disorder (DSM4) associated with epilepsy, comparing their data to patients with epilepsy without such behaviors. They reported that the aggression group contained a subgroup of patients with very small amygdala, and there was a higher prevalence of amygdala sclerosis in the aggressive patients. Twenty percent of their sample had severe amygdala atrophy in the context of a history of encephalitis. Left-sided lesions were overrepresented.

In further studies, they looked at the volumes of the amygdala in patients with epilepsy and psychosis. Two patient groups were examined: the first were patients with epilepsy and interictal psychosis ($n=11$), and the second had post-ictal psychosis ($n=15$). Two control groups consisted of 20 healthy volunteers and 20 randomly selected cases of temporal lobe epilepsy who had not displayed any psychopathology; these were matched for age, sex, duration of epilepsy, and anti-epileptic medication to the study group. The psychotic episodes were defined according to ICD10 criteria for the paranoid subtype of schizophrenia; the minimum requirement for the diagnosis of psychosis was the presence of delusions or hallucinations. The relationship of the psychopathology to the seizures was also determined, and the groups therefore divided into those with post-ictal and those with interictal psychoses. Further, patients with other first-axis psychiatric disorders were excluded from the study except for those with minor affective symptoms that are common in patients with temporal lobe epilepsy.

The results from the study are shown in Fig. 2. When adjusted for cerebral size (patients with psychoses of epilepsy had significantly smaller total brain volumes

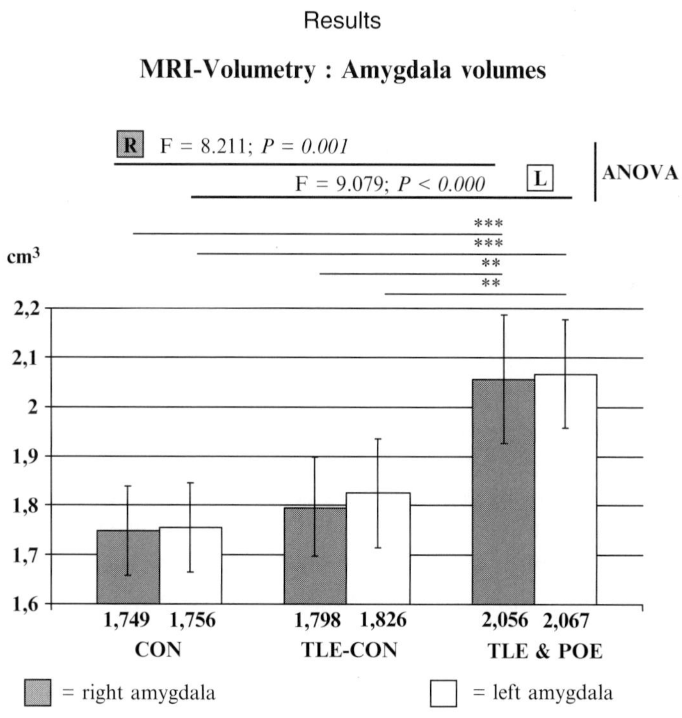

Fig. 2 Results of amygdala volumetry in epileptic psychoses. *MRI* magnetic resonance imaging; *CON* control; *TLE* temporal lobe epilepsy; *POE* psychoses of epilepsy. (From van Elst et al. [8])

compared with both healthy controls and patients without psychopathology), a highly significant (16–18%) enlargement of both the right and left amygdala volumes was found in the patients with the psychoses of epilepsy. Neither gender or age contributed to this variance, and post hoc subgroup analysis revealed that the bilateral enlargement of the psychotic patients was responsible for the overall significant findings in a factorial analysis of variance (ANOVA). When the data from the patients with post-ictal psychoses were compared with those of the interictal psychoses, no significant volumetric differences emerged. Interestingly, no significant differences in hippocampal volumes were noted.

Functional Studies

Maier et al. [9] examined patients with schizophrenia-like psychoses of epilepsy, and schizophrenia in the absence of epilepsy, using magnetic resonance spectroscopy. The hippocampus and amygdala complex were examined, and differences were noted from healthy controls. In particular, they noted a decrease of NAA in the left-sided medial temporal structures in the psychotic patients, which was maximal in the patients with psychoses and epilepsy. However, in this study the amygdala were not well defined or examined separately from the hippocampus.

More recent data have been published using fMRI. Richardson et al. [10] examined patients with epilepsy who had varying degrees of hippocampal and amygdala pathology. They gave patients a task of emotional memory encoding, comparing amygdala responses to neutral emotional stimuli. All their patients had left hippocampal sclerosis, and the responses were compared with normal controls. The extent of the medial temporal damage, in particular the severity of amygdala pathology, was reported. They showed that the encoding-related hippocampal activity for successfully remembered emotional items correlated with a degree of amygdala pathology, and the amygdala-evoked activity to remembered emotional items correlated with the degree of left hippocampal pathology. There were no correlations between measures of pathology between the examined hippocampus and amygdala. They considered that the influence of the amygdala on hippocampal encoding was expressed through effects on the hippocampus because the pathology in the left amygdala (assessed by T2 measurements) predicted reduced activity in the adjacent hippocampus for emotional stimuli, but not for neutral items.

In a subsequent investigation, the same group [11] examined the influence of viewing fearful faces on areas of cortex distant from the amygdala, again comparing patients with hippocampal as opposed to hippocampal plus amygdala pathology. Thus, seeing fearful faces not only produces a greater activation of the amygdala in healthy volunteers, but it also produces a greater activation in the face-responsive areas of the fusiform gyrus than does seeing faces with neutral expressions.

In these studies, healthy volunteers were shown to have higher bilateral activity in the fusiform and extra striate cortex in response to the fearful as opposed to the neutral faces. In the epilepsy patients, when they examined the amygdala T2 values they found a significant relationship between the amount of sclerosis and reduced emotional activation, especially in the posterior fusiform and left occipital areas. These data reveal that the visual responsiveness of the occipital cortical areas was intact, but the enhanced emotional responses did not occur.

These data are complemented by neurophysiological studies, and also studies of patients who have had a temporal lobe removed to treat intractable epilepsy. Vuilleumier and Driver [12], using a similar experimental paradigm, reported that amygdala damage reduced or completely eliminated the enhancement of the P1 component of the visual evoked potential for fearful faces, relative to neutral faces. These findings supported the view of the distance effects of amygdala lesions on emotional processing.

Bonelli et al. [13] examined patients with anterior temporal lobe resections having assessed the preoperative amygdala activation of these patients using the fearful face paradigm. The responses of patients with refractory epilepsy were compared with healthy controls, and measures of anxiety and depression were taken preoperatively and 4 months postoperatively, being assessed with standardized anxiety and depression rating scales.

Preoperatively, the patients with left temporal lobe epilepsy had significantly reduced activation of the amygdala bilaterally, whereas patients with right temporal lobe epilepsy showed bilateral amygdala activation. Patients with right temporal lobe epilepsy revealed left and right amygdala activation that was correlated to the preoperative anxiety and depression levels, and the preoperative right amygdala activation was correlated significantly with the postoperative increases of both anxiety and depression scores. Similar correlations were not found for patients with left-sided temporal lobe epilepsy.

These data, in accordance with the other findings reported above, not only support the view that the amygdala is of considerable importance in relationship to the affective state of patients with epilepsy, but they also contributed to the studies of laterality. Thus, these data suggest that the right amygdala is of more importance in relationship to affective disorders, in keeping with the known role of the nondominant hemisphere in relationship to control of affect, and predict that resection of the right amygdala with patients who have surgery for epilepsy is more likely to lead to emotional disturbances.

Conclusions

Studies of temporal lobe epilepsy have until recently concentrated much more on the hippocampus than on the amygdala. However, particularly since the advent of modern brain imaging, with the ability to examine not only the structure, but also the function, of the amygdala, the role of the amygdala in emotional processing in a variety of settings has become clear. Further, there are studies that show that alteration of the function of the amygdala, either from structural lesions or from epilepsy, have an influence on the processing of emotional stimuli in patients with such pathologies.

In the studies reviewed in this chapter, the influence of amygdala pathology on emotional processing is revealed to be not only related to the pathology at the amygdala, but distant in its effect, influencing areas of cortex connected with the amygdala that are normally activated to a greater degree when emotional processing is required. The findings from the temporal lobe surgery studies suggest that more attention should be paid to the amygdala preoperatively in assessing patients who are more likely to develop psychiatric disturbances following surgery, postoperative depression being a particularly problematic clinical problem [14].

In contrast to the direct link shown between emotional processing and emotional responsivity in patients with epilepsy, the study with epileptic psychoses is particularly revealing. In the past there has been much discussion on the relationship between the schizophreniform psychoses of epilepsy and schizophrenia in the absence of epilepsy. In the studies of Slater and in subsequent work there has remained the suggestion that the main differences are related to the lack of the long-term deterioration of people with the schizophrenia-like psychoses of epilepsy and the maintenance of affective warmth and responsiveness. The increased size of the amygdala as reported by van Elst et al. may reflect on these phenomenological differences. Thus, outside the studies of epilepsy, an increased size of the amygdala has been noted in a number of studies of affective disorder and particularly in bipolar disorder (for review [15]). Whether the findings of increased volumes and also activity of the amygdala [with positron emission tomography (PET) studies] reflect on state or trait factors is unknown, but the findings in the psychoses of epilepsy are quite distinct from the findings in schizophrenia without epilepsy, where the consensus of studies is that the amygdala are reduced as opposed as being increased in size [15].

These studies reveal the importance of further evaluation of the amygdala in relationship not only to the psychiatric syndromes encountered outside epilepsy, but also to the importance of epilepsy as a potential model for studying links between the brain and behavior, particularly those structures intimately related to the limbic system.

References

1. Trimble MR (1991) The psychoses of epilepsy. Raven, New York
2. Heimer L, Van Hoesen GW, Trimble MR et al (2008) Anatomy of neuropsychiatry. Academic, Amsterdam
3. Adolphs RD, Tranel D, Hamann S et al (1999) Recognition of facial emotion in nine subjects with bilateral amygdala damage. Neuropsychologia 37:111–117
4. Amaral DJ, Avendano C, Benoit R (1989) Distribution of somatostatin-like immunoreactivity in the monkey amygdala. J Comp Neurol 284:284–313
5. Dolan R (2007) The human amygdala and orbital prefrontal cortex in behavioural regulation. Philos Trans R Soc Lond B Biol Sci 362:787–799
6. Van Paesschen W, Connelly A, Johnson CL et al (1996) The amygdala and intractable temporal lobe epilepsy: a quantitative magnetic resonance imaging study. Neurology 47:1021–1031
7. van Elst LT, Woermann FG, Lemieux L et al (2000) Affective aggression in patients with temporal lobe epilepsy: a quantitative MRI study of the amygdala. Brain 123:234–243

8. van Elst L, Baeumer D, Lemeiux L et al (2002) Amygdala pathology in psychosis of epilepsy: a magnetic resonance imaging study in patients with temporal lobe epilepsy. Brain 125:140–149
9. Maier M, Mellers J, Toone B et al (2000) Schizophrenia, temporal lobe epilepsy and psychosis: an in vivo MRS and imaging study of the hippocampus/amygdala complex. Psychol Med 30:571–581
10. Richardson MP, Stange BA, Dolan RJ (2004) Encoding of emotional memories depends on amygdala and hippocampus and their interactions. Nat Neurosci 7:278–285
11. Vuilleumier P, Richardson MP, Armorny JL et al (2004) Distant influences of amygdala lesion on visual cortical activation during emotional face processing. Nat Neurosci 7:1271–1278
12. Vuilleumier P, Driver J (2007) Modulation of visual processing by attention and emotion: windows on causal interactions between human brain regions. Philos Trans R Soc Lond B Biol Sci 362:837–855
13. Bonelli B, Powell R, Yogarjah M et al (2009) Preoperative amygdala fMRI in temporal lobe epilepsy. Epilepsia 50:217–227
14. Ring HA, Moriarty J, Trimble MR (1988) A prospective study of the early postsurgical psychiatric associations of epilepsy surgery. J Neurosurg Psychiatry 64:601–604
15. Trimble MR, George M (2010) Biological psychiatry, 3rd edn. Wiley-Liss, Chichester

Part IV
Traumatic Brain Injury

Neuropsychiatric Assessment of Traumatic Brain Injury During Acute Neurorehabilitation*

David B. Arciniegas

Abstract Traumatic brain injury (TBI) is a common and costly problem worldwide. In the United States, 1.5 million people sustain TBI each year, and approximately 230,000 of these require hospitalization for management of their injury. The majority of TBI resulting in hospitalization are moderate to severe in nature and produce significant mortality and morbidity. Among those surviving their injuries, most will develop cognitive, emotional, and behavioral (collectively referred to here as neuropsychiatric) disturbances in the acute postinjury period and will require acute rehabilitation management. These posttraumatic neuropsychiatric sequelae present substantial clinical management challenges that the consulting neuropsychiatrist is well suited to evaluate and manage. In the service of offering the consulting neuropsychiatrist with information that may be of use in the care of persons with TBI receiving care in the acute neurorehabilitation setting, this chapter first defines and describes TBI and reviews the neuroanatomical and neurobehavioral consequences of TBI relevant to understanding posttraumatic neuropsychiatric disturbances. These disturbances are organized under the framework of posttraumatic encephalopathy, and the characteristic forms and stages of recovery of this condition are discussed. Finally, a neuropsychiatric approach to the evaluation of persons with TBI in the acute inpatient neurorehabilitation setting is described.

Keywords Cognitive impairment • Encephalophathy • Frontal assessment battery (FAB) • Mini-mental state exam (MMSE) • Traumatic brain injury (TBI)

---

*This work was supported in part by HealthONE Spalding Rehabilitation Hospital

D.B. Arciniegas (✉)
Brain Injury Rehabilitation Unit, HealthONE Spalding Rehabilitation Hospital,
Aurora, CO, USA
and
Neurobehavioral Disorders Program, Department of Psychiatry,
School of Medicine, University of Colorado Denver, 13001 East 17th Place,
Campus Box F546, Aurora, CO, 80045, USA
e-mail: David.Arciniegas@UCDenver.edu

K. Miyoshi et al. (eds.), *Neuropsychiatric Disorders*,
DOI 10.1007/978-4-431-53871-4_10, © Springer 2010

Introduction

Neuropsychiatrists and behavioral neurologists are increasingly involved in the early postinjury and neurorehabilitation management of persons hospitalized after traumatic brain injury (TBI). In the United States, approximately 230,000 persons annually are hospitalized in the acute injury period [1, 2]. Most of these individuals sustain TBI as a result of road traffic accidents, transportation, falls, or assaults, including incidents involving firearms. Among those whose injuries require hospitalization, adolescents, young adults, and older persons are overrepresented, and most of these sustained TBI of moderate or greater severity [1, 2]. Between the early 1980s and late 1990s, the overall annual rate of hospitalization following TBI declined by 51% [1, 2]. This decline is generally attributed to 61% and 19% reduction in hospital-based care of persons with mild and moderate TBI, respectively. At the same time, annual hospitalization rates following severe TBI increased 90%, from 10 to 19 per 100,000 persons. Additionally, in-hospital mortality following TBI declined by 17% as a result of advances in pre-hospital and in-hospital trauma care [1, 2]. As a result of these changes in the epidemiology of TBI, individuals admitted to hospital following TBI are more likely than in past decades to have sustained a relatively severe injury and to survive it.

More than 40% of persons hospitalized following moderate-to-severe TBI (or about 125,000 persons in the United States annually) are expected to develop permanent disability as a result of that injury [3]. Posttraumatic neuropsychiatric disturbances – a term used here to denote the broad spectrum of impairments in cognition, emotional regulation, behavior, and elementary neurological function produced by mechanical trauma to the brain – are particularly common among persons with moderate or severe TBI [4–8]. Neuropsychiatric disturbances are substantial contributors to postinjury disability [9–11] and reduced quality of life for patients and their families during and after the early postinjury period [10, 12–14].

The care provided to persons with TBI in acute inpatient rehabilitation settings is intrinsically neuropsychiatric. The neurorehabilitation of persons with moderate-to-severe TBI requires identification and management of cognitive impairments (e.g., disturbances of arousal, attention, processing speed, memory, and executive function, among others), emotional disturbances (e.g., irritability, liability, depression, anxiety), behavior (e.g., restlessness, agitation, disinhibition, aggression, apathy), and elementary neurological functions (e.g., sleep–wake cycle disturbances, seizures, motor impairments, sensory impairments). Identifying and treating neuropsychiatric disturbances as early as possible during the course of postinjury care as well as avoiding interventions with the potential for acute and/or long-term neuropsychiatric complications will reduce long-term posttraumatic neuropsychiatric morbidity. Accordingly, developing further the consulting neuropsychiatrists' expertise in the neuropsychiatric assessment and management of persons with TBI is an important objective.

With these goals in mind, this chapter begins by defining TBI and reviewing the commonly used methods of identifying TBI and characterizing its severity. The neurobiology of TBI is reviewed briefly, including the neuroanatomy, neurochemistry, and brain–behavior relationships relevant to the management of acute and subacute posttraumatic neuropsychiatric disturbances. Finally, a neuropsychiatric approach to the evaluation of persons with TBI in the acute neurorehabilitation setting is described.

Defining TBI

TBI is defined as a functionally significant disruption of brain function produced by blunt or penetrating trauma or rapid acceleration/deceleration forces that results in immediately apparent cognitive or physical impairments [15]. Although the CDC clinical case definition permits skull fracture to serve as a proxy marker for TBI, in this chapter we exclude from consideration those injuries that produce only skull fracture: although the association between skull fracture and TBI is well described [16–18], this association is neither invariate nor a sufficiently reliable predictor of TBI to permit skull fracture to serve as the sole clinical finding upon which to predicate a TBI diagnosis [19]. Additionally, brain injuries from other causes such as birth trauma, hypoxic-ischemic (anoxic), inflammatory, toxic, or metabolic encephalopathies, primary ischemic or hemorrhagic strokes, seizure disorders, intracranial surgery, and cerebral neoplasms, although these are all causes of acquired brain injury, are excluded from this definition of TBI (Table 1).

Table 1 Clinical case definition of traumatic brain injury (adapted from the Center for Disease Control *Guidelines for the Surveillance of Central Nervous System Injury*, 2002)

Clinical phenomena	Description
Objective neurological abnormality	Focal motor, sensory, or reflex abnormalities Seizures (focal or generalized)
Alteration of consciousness	Loss of consciousness (LOC) Impairment of wakefulness (arousal) and/or awareness
Amnesia	Loss or impairment of peri-event memory Retrograde amnesia (RGA): impaired memory for events immediately preceding the injury Anterograde amnesia (AGA): impaired memory for the injury or the events that follow it Posttraumatic amnesia (PTA): the period of dense impairment in new learning following TBI; inclusive of both AGA and RGA
Objective neuropsychological abnormality	Standardized neuropsychological examination (in the immediate postinjury period) reveals impairment of cognition (e.g., disorientation, confusion), disturbances of behavior (e.g., agitation), or other abnormalities in neuropsychiatric status (e.g., personality change)
Diagnosed intracranial lesion	On computed tomography (CT), magnetic resonance imaging (MRI), or another neurodiagnostic (i.e., neuroimaging) study, there is evidence of diffuse axonal injury, and/or epidural, subdural, subarachnoid, or intracerebral hematoma, and/or cerebral contusion or laceration, and/or penetration of brain by foreign body (e.g., gunshot wound)

With respect to the cognitive manifestations of brain dysfunction at the time of injury, no single symptom or sign is pathognomic of TBI. Instead, any one (or more) of several features, including loss of consciousness (LOC), dense impairment in declarative new learning (posttraumatic amnesia, PTA), and alteration in higher cognitive functions (e.g., feeling "dazed and confused" without LOC or PTA), is sufficient evidence of brain dysfunction to merit assignment of this diagnosis, regardless of the duration of these disturbances. With regard to elementary neurological impairments, the intended referents of this term are focal neurological signs (e.g., hemiparesis, hemianopia), focal neurological symptoms (e.g., hemisensory loss), or seizure. Nonlocalizing or generalized neurological symptoms such as headache, fatigue, dizziness, blurred vision, and so forth, although common post-concussive symptoms, are frequently produced by peripheral nervous system injury, musculoskeletal (i.e., cervicospinal) injury, and facial/head (without brain) trauma. Accordingly, these are less useful as indicators of brain injury and therefore not used as evidence of TBI in the standard definition of this condition [15].

Characterizing TBI Severity

TBI severity is generally divided into three categories: mild, moderate, and severe. Among hospitalized patients, the Glasgow Coma Scale (GCS) [20] is the most commonly used metric for determining TBI severity. Mild, moderate, and severe TBI are defined by GCS scores of 13–15, 9–12, and 3–8, respectively, reflecting performance on three relatively elementary assessments of verbal, eye opening, and motor responses. While the GCS is an excellent research and clinical measure when administered in a consistent and timely manner [6, 21, 22], its use in many hospitals is inconsistent, at best, and the data it yields are frequently confounded by other non-TBI factors [23].

In the absence of GCS scores, or as a supplement or complement to them, determination of the duration of PTA is also a useful gauge of TBI severity [24]. PTA describes the period of dense impairment in the ability to learn new information (with or without some degree of retrograde amnesia). Although PTA is most accurately understood as one of the later stages within the larger condition of posttraumatic encephalopathy (PTE; discussed later in this chapter) [25], the conventional assessment of PTA duration encompasses the entire period between injury and the recovery of reasonably continuous and accurate memory for daily events. There are several measures with which to formally assess PTA severity and duration, the most commonly used of which are the Galveston Orientation and Amnesia Test (GOAT) [26] and the Orientation Log (O-Log) [27, 28]; among these, we prefer the O-Log given its ease of administration and interpretation and its excellent statistical comparison to the GOAT [29].

When neither GCS nor prospective PTA data are available, TBI severity may be characterized retrospectively using the American Congress of Rehabilitation Medicine (ACRM) definition of mild TBI [30, 31]. These criteria define TBI as a physiological disruption in brain function resulting from the application of an external physical (including acceleration/deceleration) force, as evidenced by any one (or more) of the following: LOC, PTA, altered mental state ("dazed and confused"), and/or a focal neurological deficit that may or may not be transient. To remain in the mild category, LOC must be less than 30 min, after which GCS scores are in the 13–15 range, and/or PTA duration is no longer than 24 h. Injuries that produce LOC of 30 or more min, GCS scores less than 13 at 30 min (or later) post injury, and/or PTA longer than 24 h are classified as moderate to severe. McMillan and colleagues in 1996 [31] demonstrated that retrospective interview-based estimates PTA of duration among hospitalized individuals with TBI correlate highly with prospective, GOAT-determined duration of PTA. Among patients whose PTA duration is longer than 24 h, practical classification of injuries as moderate or severe may be made according to PTA duration (whether prospectively or retrospectively determined) of 1–7 days and more than 7 days, respectively.

For the consulting neuropsychiatrist, the usefulness of measured or estimated PTA duration and PTA-based severity classifications lies in the prognostic utility of this value: PTA duration (as a continuous variable) is a robust predictor of functional independence [29, 34] and disability [34] at the end of acute inpatient rehabilitation, Glasgow Outcome Scale [35] scores at 6 and 12 months post injury [36, 37], long-term cognitive recovery [38–40], productivity [41], employment [42], and community reintegration [43]. As with the GCS, noninjury factors (e.g., sedating medications, severe communication impairments) must be considered when estimating PTA duration, particularly among subjects with more severe general physical injuries and complications. Nonetheless, in our clinical experience time between injury and emergence from PTA – regardless of the TBI and concurrent factors contributing to the duration of that period – define usefully the severity of injury and offer valuable prognostic information that the consulting neuropsychiatrist can use when communicating with patients and their families as well as other healthcare providers about the patient's prognosis and likely posthospital treatment and resource needs.

An important qualifier on ACRM-based TBI severity classification of which the consulting neuropsychiatrist should be aware is "complicated mild TBI" [32, 33]. This subtype of mild TBI is used to denote individuals who meet ACRM criteria for mild TBI but whose computed tomography (CT) or magnetic resonance imaging (MRI) of the brain demonstrates abnormalities consistent with TBI. The importance of noting this subtype is that the outcome of subjects with complicated mild TBI more closely resembles that of persons with moderate TBI than those with uncomplicated (i.e., "simple") mild TBI; awareness of this issue will allow the consulting neuropsychiatrist to interpret the patient's clinical presentation more accurately and to offer more fully informed education, counseling, and prognostic information to patients and their families.

Neurobiology of TBI

In addition to understanding the diagnosis and implications of TBI severity, the consulting neuropsychiatrist needs also to be familiar with the neuroanatomy, neurochemistry, and typical brain–behavior relationships that inform on neuropsychiatric outcome following TBI.

The injurious biomechanical effects of TBI consist primarily of two general types: contact and inertial. Contact injuries refer to those resulting from the penetration of the brain by material (e.g., projectiles, bone fragments) entering the intracranial space, as well as those injuries produced by movement of the brain within the intracranial space that results in the brain striking or being abraded by the inner surface of skull. The movement of the brain against the various ridges and bony protuberances of the anterior (frontal) and middle (temporal) fossae is especially injurious to the temporal and frontal poles as well as the ventral anterior, medial, and lateral temporal and frontal cortices (see Bigler [44] for a review of this subject). In case of penetrating injuries, tissue displacement/destruction by a projectile, fragmentation and deposition of bone or a projectile within brain tissue, and contamination of the intracranial space by potential infectious material on a projectile or the tissues through which it passes may all contribute to brain injury. The damage sustained in penetrating injuries is relatively focal, involving most brain tissue in the linear path of the material penetrating the intracranial space. In non-penetrating and penetrating contact injuries types of injuries, subarachnoid, subdural, and/or epidural hematomas may complicate this type of injury.

Inertial forces include linear translation and rotation, which in combination produce angular acceleration/deceleration forces. These forces strain, shear, and/or compress brain tissue [45–50]. Although all these forces are potentially injurious, strain and shear forces are tolerated particularly poorly by brain tissue and are major contributors to TBI at all levels of severity. These forces are maximal in brain areas experiencing high angular acceleration/deceleration forces (superficial > deep tissues, anterior > posterior regions of the brain); at the junctions between tissues of different densities and elasticities (i.e., gray–white junctions); and at the intracranial rotational center of mass (i.e., rostral brainstem). High-speed, long-duration acceleration/deceleration injuries exert their greatest effect on axonal projections and small blood vessels within and projecting from the brainstem, on parasagittal cerebral white matter, on the corpus callosum, and at the superficial cortical gray–white junctions [51], particularly in the ventral and anterior frontal and temporal lobes (see Bigler [44] for review). In light of these patterns of neuropathology, "diffuse axonal injury" (DAI) is probably a misnomer and is more accurately understood as "multifocal," rather than diffuse, axonal injury [51]. Although inertial forces may play a role in the pathophysiology of penetrating TBI [52], this type of TBI tends to be relatively stroke-like with respect to the pattern of tissue involvement (focal vs. multifocal/diffuse), the neuropsychiatric problems it produces, and long-term functional outcomes.

As reviewed in Povlishock and Katz [53], Bigler [54], and Meythaler et al. [51], injurious cytotoxic processes are initiated by biomechanical injury; these processes both add to and also complicate biomechanical injury in TBI. Injury-induced calcium and magnesium dysregulation, free radical formation, and excitatory amino acid and neurotransmitter disturbances are the principal contributors from this cytotoxic cascade to neuronal injury and cell death. Excitatory amino acid excesses facilitate calcium influx into neurons, resulting in neuronal depolarization, initiation of oxidative processes, activation of proteolytic enzymes, and eventually injury to or destruction of neurons and/or their axonal termini. Excitatory amino acid excesses also overdrive glucose utilization, and oxidative metabolism, and produce potentially toxic accumulations of lactate. Concurrent excess of acetylcholine also appear to be excitotoxic and may amplify the destructive effects of excitatory amino acid excesses and be particularly injurious to brain areas where these neurotransmitters are densely colocated (i.e., hippocampus, frontal cortices; see Phillips and Reeves [55], Arciniegas [56], and Arciniegas and Silver [57] for review). The effects, benign or malignant, of acute cerebral monoaminergic (i.e., dopamine, norepinephrine, and serotonin) excesses that are part of the cytotoxic cascade remain uncertain. All these neurotransmitter excesses appear to wane over the first several weeks following TBI [58, 59], although the exact time course over which these excesses abate is not characterized fully. It is clear, however, that by several weeks post-TBI there is a relative cholinergic deficit resulting from injury to ventral forebrain cholinergic nuclei and their cortical projections [56, 57]. It is possible that TBI also results in primary or secondary disturbances in cerebral monoaminergic, and particularly noradrenergic and dopaminergic, systems [60], the effects of which may be modified by genetically mediated variations in catecholamine metabolism. These issues are particularly important for the consulting neuropsychiatrist, as the types and timings of posttraumatic neurotransmitter disturbances carry implications for pharmacotherapies directed at cognitive, emotional, and behavioral problems during the acute rehabilitation period and thereafter.

In addition to biomechanical and cytotoxic injury processes, persons with TBI who require hospitalization often experience other secondary neurological and systemic problems, whether as a consequence of TBI or as a comorbid process, that may complicate or exacerbate TBI. Such problems include traumatic intracerebral hematomas, focal or diffuse cerebral edema, elevated intracranial pressure (ICP), obstructive hydrocephalus, hypoxic-ischemic injury, intracranial/intracerebral infection, and subfalcine or transtentorial herniation. These latter problems may be fatal or, if not fatal, may compromise vascular supply in the areas of brain compression and thereby superimpose acute ischemic stroke on TBI. Additionally, systemic medical complications such as volume depletion/blood loss, hypoperfusion, hypothermia or hyperthermia, hypoxia, infection, and related problems may further complicate TBI. Aggressive treatment directed at these problems during acute care and, when necessary, in the acute rehabilitation period, therefore is essential.

Brain–Behavior Relationships and TBI

As noted in the prior section of this chapter, TBI disproportionately affects the anterior and ventral aspects of the frontal and temporal lobes, medial frontal and temporal areas, ventral forebrain, the diencephalon (thalamus, hypothalamus), the rostral and ventral areas of the upper brainstem, and the white matter within and between these areas [44, 53, 54, 61, 62]. Injury to these neuropsychiatrically salient areas produces typical, but not invariate, patterns of posttraumatic neuropsychiatric

Table 2 Brain–behavior relationships relevant to understanding the neurobehavioral sequelae of TBI commonly encountered in the acute rehabilitation setting

Structure injured	Neuropsychiatric consequence
Upper brainstem	
Reticulothalamic systems	Loss or impairment of consciousness caused by rotational strain/shear on ascending reticular activating system (ARAS) and ↑ ACh
Reticulocortical system	Acute and functionally disruptive ↑ GLU, ACh, DA, NE, 5HT
Ventral forebrain (cholinergic nuclei 1–4)	Acute and functionally disruptive ↑ AChChronic and functionally impairing ↓ ACh
Cerebral white matter	Slowed and inefficient information processing
Medial temporal areas	
Entrorhinal-hippocampal complex	Impaired sensory gating, attention, working memory, and declarative memory
Amygdala	Affective placidity, Klüver–Bucy-like syndromes
Anterior temporal cortices	Impaired sensory-limbic integration (cortical), declarative memory (uncinate fasciculus)
Ventral (orbital) prefrontal cortices	Behavioral dyscontrol (e.g., impulsivity, disinhibition, irritability, agitation, aggression)
Medial prefrontal (cingulate) cortex	Decreased goal-directed cognition, emotion, and behavior (apathy)
Inferior (inferolateral) prefrontal cortex	Impaired working memory
Dorsolateral prefrontal cortex	Impaired executive function, including executive control of other basic cognitive functions

disturbances in the acute and subacute postinjury periods (Table 2). These patterns of neuropsychiatric disturbances evolve in the days to weeks following TBI and are subsumed under the heading of PTE [25].

Posttraumatic Encephalopathy

Posttraumatic encephalopathy (PTE) is characterized by five stages: posttraumatic coma, posttraumatic delirium, PTA, posttraumatic dysexecutive syndrome, and recovery (Fig. 1). These stages are named according to the most salient (although clearly not the only) neurobehavioral feature of the clinical presentation. During posttraumatic coma, the most salient feature of the patient's presentation is complete impairment of arousal. The transition from posttraumatic coma to posttraumatic delirium is marked by the return of wakefulness (arousal), albeit sometimes in a fluctuating manner, and marked impairments in selective, sustained, and other aspects of attention; in the parlance of the American Psychiatric Association's Diagnostic and Statistic Manual, Fourth Edition, Text Revised [63], "reduced clarity of awareness of the environment." Although posttraumatic delirium also entails other disturbances in cognition, emotion, and behavior, profound inattention is the most salient and characteristic feature of this stage of PTE.

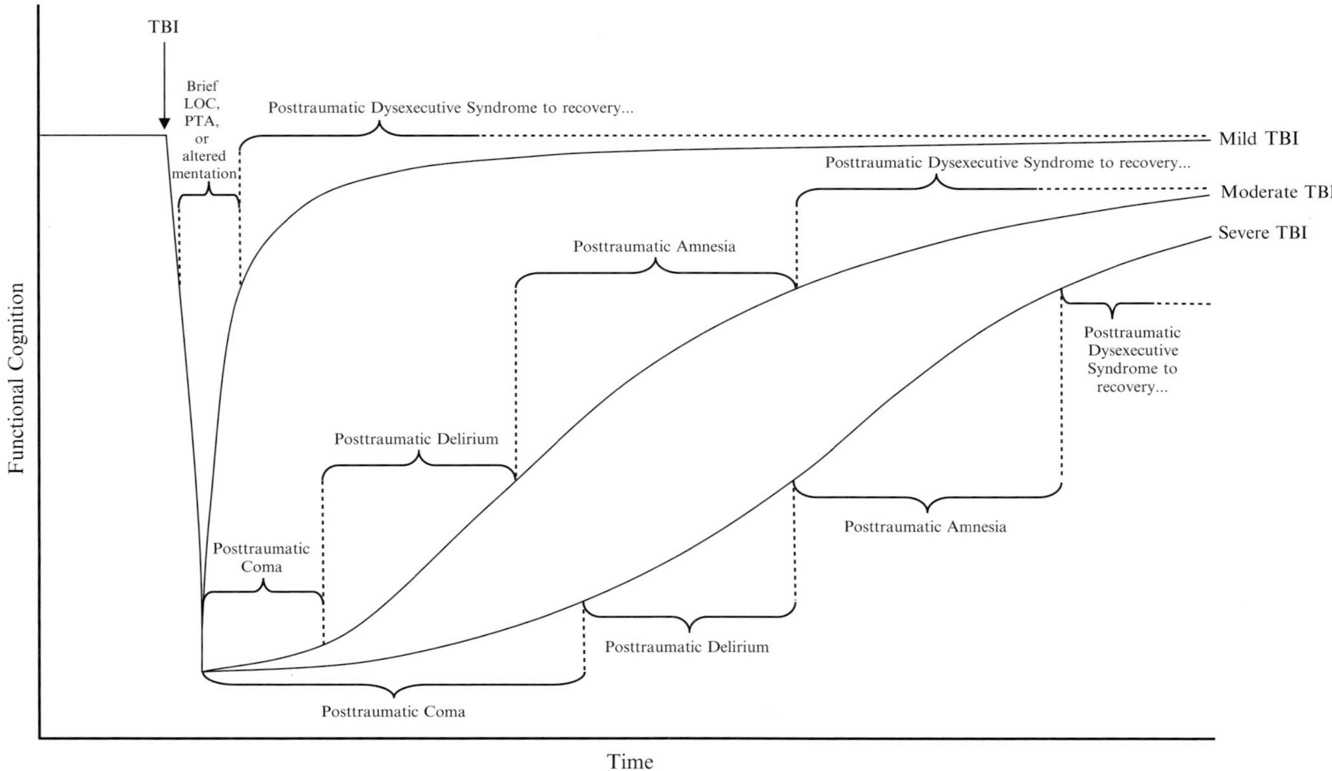

Fig. 1 Typical course of recovery through the stages of posttraumatic encephalopathy (PTE) following mild, moderate, and severe traumatic brain injury. *TBI* traumatic brain injury; *LOC* loss of consciousness; *PTA* posttraumatic amnesia

As the patient emerges from this stage, basic selective and sustained attention improve markedly; as a consequence, the patient's striking and dense impairment in declarative new learning becomes the most salient feature of the clinical presentation, and marks the patient's transition into PTA. As with posttraumatic delirium, the period of PTA also entails impairments in other aspects of cognition, especially executive function and executive control of attention, language, memory, and praxis. The patient is regarded as "in PTA" until his or her declarative new learning improves to the point that he or she is able to construct a reasonably continuous narrative of daily events from that point forward (formal criteria for emergence from PTA using the GOAT or O-Log are described in the next section of this chapter). The interval between onset of injury and subsequent recovery of declarative new learning defines the duration of PTA.

Unfortunately, the measured period of PTA duration is sometimes misunderstood as suggesting that the entire period measured is first and foremost characterized by impaired declarative new learning (i.e., amnesia); this clearly is not the case. It is important to be clear that although the formally measured duration of PTA necessarily encompasses posttraumatic coma, posttraumatic delirium, and (by some accounts) any preinjury period of retrograde amnesia, neither the concept of PTA nor its clinical manifestations are synonymous with posttraumatic delirium or, more obviously, posttraumatic coma. It is true that declarative new learning is impaired in these earlier stages of PTE; however, each of these entails other, and more salient, cognitive impairments. Nonetheless, duration of PTA as defined and used in the TBI literature is useful for both TBI severity characterization as well as a predictor of TBI outcomes and is, in this author's view, the most useful of the early stages of PTE to measure assiduously when offering prognoses to patients, their families, and other rehabilitation clinicians.

Upon emergence from PTA, impairments of executive function are the most salient feature of the clinical presentation; accordingly, this stage of PTE is referred to as the posttraumatic dysexecutive syndrome. Common clinical features of this syndrome include impairments of intrinsic executive function (e.g., abstraction, problem solving, the ability to generate, shift, and alter cognitive sets independent of environmental contingencies, judgment, and insight) as well as impaired executive control of other, more basic, cognitive functions. As illustrated in Fig. 1, some patients emerge from this stage of PTE into complete cognitive recovery whereas for others this becomes a chronic posttraumatic neurocognitive disorder.

The impairments that comprise each stage of PTE occur on a continuum clinically and temporally: patients at the transition between stages of PTE may vacillate for days (or longer) between those stages. Nonetheless, identifying the stage of PTE that best describes that patient is useful in that it facilitates the development of a treatment plan which is appropriate to the patient's current clinical status and also allows clinicians and the patient's family members to anticipate the course of continued recovery. By extension, this approach to PTE also helps clinicians to identify deviations from the expected course of recovery after TBI and therefore the need to evaluate the patient for conditions that explain such deviations.

Neuropsychiatric Evaluation of TBI in the Acute Rehabilitation Setting

The neuropsychiatric assessment of patients with TBI begins with corroboration of the diagnosis of TBI and entails characterization of its type and severity in the manner described in the preceding sections of this chapter. Next, identifying the stage of PTE using the framework described above is essential. It then is important to contextualize TBI and PTE by comprehensively assessing the patient's preinjury medical, neurological, psychiatric, and substance histories. It is particularly important to obtain collateral history on these issues from reliable informants (family, close friends, employers, etc.) because patients in the midst of PTE are frequently unable to provide this information themselves. Concurrently, assessment of the patient's social history (e.g., level of education, developmental history, legal history, military experience) and social supports should be obtained. This information often identifies strengths and limitations in the patient's personal and social contexts that may influence long-term outcomes and community reintegration, as well as the financial resources (or lack thereof) available to support the rehabilitation process. The assessment then moves from history-taking to examinations, including general physical, neurological, and neurobehavioral status examinations, as well as review of neuroimaging and other neurodiagnostic studies.

Bedside Assessment Methods

Standardized assessments appropriate to the phase of PTE in which the patient presents facilitate accurate diagnosis and guide prognostic and therapeutic formulations. Data derived from these measures may be used to gauge not only the extent and rate of recovery but also responses to treatment.

Although it is uncommon in the United States for patients to present to rehabilitation settings in posttraumatic coma, presentation of patients in this and other states of impaired arousal and awareness (i.e., with disorders of consciousness) is not uncommon in other parts of the world. The Coma/Near-Coma Scale [64] is particularly useful as an assessment of coma severity and recovery.

Upon emergence from posttraumatic coma, patients enter the period of posttraumatic delirium; at this point, it is very common for patients to be admitted to an acute inpatient rehabilitation hospital. The Delirium Rating Scale-Revised-98 (DRS-R-98) [65] or the Confusion Assessment Protocol (CAP) [66] are appropriate and useful measures for the consulting neuropsychiatrist to apply to the evaluation and monitoring of patients in posttraumatic delirium. The period of posttraumatic delirium corresponds to levels II–V of the Rancho Los Amigos Scale (RLAS) [67]. This scale and the descriptors of these lower levels of recovery after TBI are used frequently by rehabilitation physicians and therapists; the consulting neuropsychiatrist will be well served to be familiar with this scale to ensure proper interdisciplinary communication when discussing patients in posttraumatic delirium.

Consistent with the description of RLAS levels II–V, posttraumatic delirium generally begins as a state of impaired arousal and profound inattention (RLAS level II). As arousal improves, inattention and behavioral disturbances (agitation) become prominent features of the clinical presentation (RLAS levels III–IV). As agitation remits and attentional disturbances become less problematic (RLAS level V), patients transition into a state in which impaired declarative new learning is the most salient clinical problem, or PTA. Identifying the point of transition between these states may be facilitated by the use of appropriate cutoff scores from delirium on the DRS-R-98 or the CAP and continued impairment on measures of PTA such as the O-Log or the GOAT [26].

With this in mind, it is useful to begin the assessment of PTA using the O-Log or the GOAT early during the course of posttraumatic delirium. Assessment using the O-Log of the GOAT continues until the patient meets criteria for emergence from PTA (on two consecutive days, O-Log scores ≥25 or GOAT scores ≥76). Although the validity of assessing orientation and memory function in the severely delirious patient is dubious, early and daily assessment with these measures ensures that the end of PTA will be captured accurately; as noted earlier, and as demonstrated by our own work [29], duration of PTA offers short- and long-term prognostic information that is useful to clinicians and also to patients and their families.

Neuropsychiatric assessment is most often undertaken when patients are in posttraumatic delirium or PTA. Our service, which provides Behavioral Neurology and Neuropsychiatry consultations on an acute inpatient neurorehabilitation unit, integrates neurological and neuropsychiatric assessments to offer diagnostic and treatment recommendations as well as guidance on rehabilitation prognosis and the types of support and caregiving resources that are likely to be needed during these periods of PTE as well as during and after subsequent rehabilitation care. In addition to elementary neurological and general mental status examinations, our consultations include detailed examination for subtle neurological signs (SNS) and a thorough bedside cognitive examination.

The assessment for SNS focuses on paratonia (*mitgehen* and/or *gegenhalten*) and also several primitive reflexes (also known as “frontal release signs”): glabellar response, snout response, suck reflex, palmomental response (left and right), grasp response (left and right), and rooting response. These simple additions to the neurological examination, from which we have developed a preliminary metric referred to as the SNS score [68], yield important information regarding neurobehavioral status and rehabilitation outcome: SNS score predicts raw and Z-transformed mini-mental state examination (MMSE) and frontal assessment battery (FAB) scores (all $P<0.003$), FIM scores at consultation (all $P<0.04$), and rehabilitation discharge (all $P<0.03$), and RLOS ($P<0.0002$). Accordingly, inclusion of these items in the neuropsychiatric assessment of persons with TBI during the acute rehabilitation period is recommended.

The bedside cognitive examination used on our service includes, among other items, the MMSE [69] and FAB [70]. Because performance on these measures is influenced strongly by the effects of age and education, our interpretation of a patient's performance on them is normatively adjusted (for the MMSE, we use norms developed by Crum et al. [71], and for the FAB we use norms developed by Appollonio et al. [72]). After Z-transforming these data, the MMSE and, particularly, the FAB predict functional status and rehabilitation length of stay [73]. While other measures such as the Neurobehavioural Rating Scale – Revised [74, 75] may also be useful, the combination of the MMSE and FAB is time efficient and unlikely to overlap substantially with the assessments performed by neuropsychologists and rehabilitation therapists concurrently assessing these patients. For these reasons, this brief bedside battery of cognitive assessments is used in our clinical practice.

After patients emerge from PTA, neuropsychiatric assessment is most usefully directed toward disturbances in frontally mediated cognition, emotion, and behavior; in other words, at the posttraumatic dysexecutive syndrome. As noted previously, we have found the FAB particularly valuable for the evaluation of the cognitive components of this syndrome [73] but have employed other measures such as the Executive Interview (EXIT) [76] and the Behavioral Dyscontrol Scale (BDS) [77, 78] as well.

Assessment of other neuropsychiatric disturbances such as depression, mania, pathological laughing and crying, anxiety disorders, psychosis, and nondelirium-related impulse control problems and aggression also require neuropsychiatric assessment and treatment during PTE – and may require more specific assessment during PTA and posttraumatic dysexecutive syndrome in light of the fact that emotional and behavioral disturbances that occur during these stages of PTE cannot be dismissed as features of posttraumatic delirium. The Neurobehavioural Rating Scale – Revised [74, 75] is particularly well suited to the identification of such problems among patients able to participate in direct interview and examination. Among patients too impaired (neurologically or neuropsychiatrically) to engage effectively in interview and examination, assessment of posttraumatic emotional and behavioral disturbances may be performed productively by using the Neuropsychiatric Inventory (NPI) [79] as a guide to interviews of nursing and rehabilitation staff familiar with the patient. Our group at HealthONE Spalding Rehabilitation Hospital in Aurora, Colorado, is presently engaged in the development of an assessment instrument modeled after the NPI and adapted specifically for the assessment of persons with TBI in the acute neurorehabilitation setting; we expect to publish findings pertaining to this project in the near future.

Neurodiagnostic Methods

There is considerable debate regarding the timing of formal neuropsychological testing after TBI [80]. This debate generally centers around the validity of testing before the resolution of PTA and the potential bias of premature testing (due to test exposure) on later assessments. Recent studies [80, 81] suggest that a brief battery composed of the GOAT, California Verbal Learning Test-II, Trail Making Test,

Symbol Digit Modalities Test, grooved pegboard, phonemic and categorical word generation tasks, Wechsler Test of Adult Reading, and Wisconsin Card Sorting Test-64 may be a useful and practical brief neuropsychological assessment battery in the inpatient neurorehabilitation setting. Additionally, this battery – and, more specifically, its Weschler Test of Adult Reading and Trail Making Test-Part B components – are significant predictors of 1-year outcome after TBI as measured by the Disability Rating Scale, Supervision Rating Scale, and Glasgow Outcome Scale-Extended [81]. When it is feasible to obtain neuropsychological testing of this type in the acute neurorehabilitation setting, it is advisable to do so as a complement to other data obtained during the neuropsychiatric assessment.

Structural neuroimaging is an integral component of the neuropsychiatric assessment of patients receiving acute neurorehabilitation after TBI. In many (perhaps most) cases, CT of the brain will be performed in the acute care setting; unfortunately, CT is sensitive to gross abnormalities (i.e., skull fracture, acute hemorrhage or hemorrhagic contusion, severe DAI) but its value is generally limited to cases in which very severe injuries were sustained. MRI of the brain is frequently more useful as a neuroimaging guide to the severity of TBI; as a tool with which to determine the correspondence between bedside examination-identified neurological/neuropsychiatric problems and neuroimaging abnormalities; and as a guide to prognosis and treatment planning. For example, ventral prefrontal cortical and white matter injury is a relatively common consequence of severe TBI (see Table 2) and frequently is associated with impulsive, disinhibited, and/or aggressive behavior. MR evidence of overtly destructive damage (i.e., traumatic ablation) to these structures influences the selection of pharmacologic agents directed at these behaviors: selective serotonin reuptake inhibitors, anticonvulsants, or atypical antipsychotics suppressing brain (limbic) areas driving these behaviors is likely to be more useful than are agents (e.g., stimulants or cholinesterase inhibitors) intended to augment the function of the ventral prefrontal-subcortical circuit. Accordingly, we recommend obtaining (or reviewing one previously obtained) an MRI of the brain in all neurorehabilitation inpatients receiving neuropsychiatric assessment after TBI. When MRI is performed, T_1, fluid-attenuated inversion recovery (FLAIR), T_2* gradient echo, susceptibility-weighted, and diffusion-weighted sequences are the most useful sequences to obtain [82].

Electroencephalography (EEG), including evoked potentials, event-related potentials, and quantitative EEG (qEEG), does not usually contribute usefully to the neuropsychiatric assessment of patients undergoing acute neurorehabilitation after TBI [83]. When clinical history suggests the possibility of seizures (particularly complex partial seizures with post-ictal confusion or behavioral disturbances), then it is appropriate to obtain EEG to identify potentially epileptiform abnormalities. However, it is important to remain mindful that interictal EEG is relatively insensitive to epileptiform abnormalities and that the decision to treat patients for post-traumatic seizures rests on the event semiology and not on the presence or absence of electroencephalographic abnormalities.

The literature guiding the selection of laboratory assessments relevant to the neuropsychiatric assessment in the acute neurorehabilitation setting is underdeveloped. It is reasonable and appropriate to review and/or obtain laboratory data (including serum and urine studies) that may inform on contributors to, or alternate explanations for, delirium and cognitive impairments experienced by persons with TBI. Recent reviews suggest that neuroendocrine disturbances are common and underdiagnosed in this population [84]; other than assessment of thyroid-stimulating hormone and thyroid hormone levels, however, the optimal methods for assessing and treating other posttraumatic neuroendocrine disturbances remains uncertain.

Review of Concurrently Prescribed Treatments

An essential component of the neuropsychiatric assessment of persons with TBI receiving acute neurorehabilitation services is a review of pharmacologic treatments that may be causing or contributing to neurological and neuropsychiatric problems identified during that assessment.

Treatment with anticonvulsant medications is common in this population, but this requires careful consideration with respect to both benefits and adverse effects on posttraumatic neurological and neuropsychiatric status. Persons with TBI are at risk for the development of posttraumatic seizures [85], and these are generally divided into two types according to the timing of their onset post injury: early (within 1 week of injury) and late (after the first week post injury). Administration of anticonvulsant medications (so-called seizure prophylaxis) during the first week after TBI decreases the incidence of early posttraumatic seizures [86], although this does not appear to reduce mortality, long-term neurological disability, or the risk of late posttraumatic seizures [86]. More important in the acute rehabilitation setting is the now well-established finding that prophylactic administration of anticonvulsants after the first week post-TBI does not prevent the development of late posttraumatic seizures, reduce short- or long-term neurological disability, or influence post-TBI mortality [86]. Additionally, many of these agents – particularly phenytoin [87, 88] and carbamazepine [88] – worsen cognitive and motor function in this population. Despite its increasingly common use as an alternate "seizure prophylactic" in this setting [89, 90], levetiracetam has not been shown to be effective for the prophylaxis of either early or late posttraumatic seizures and is known to produce agitation and other neurobehavioral disturbances ("psychiatric adverse events") [91, 92]. Valproate is less problematic with respect to its effects on cognition after TBI [93]; accordingly, when prophylaxis against early posttraumatic seizures is undertaken or if an anticonvulsant is used for behavior- or mood-stabilizing purposes, valproate is preferable to phenytoin, carbamazepine, and levetiracetam for this purpose. However, continued use of any of these or other anticonvulsants as prophylaxis against new-onset seizures after the first week post injury (i.e., late posttraumatic seizures) is discouraged [94].

A variety of similarly problematic medications are administered commonly to persons with TBI during the acute hospital and inpatient neurorehabilitation phases of care. Antagonists of type-2 dopamine (D2) receptors and/or benzodiazepines are used in many settings as treatments for posttraumatic delirium (particularly agitation and aggression) [95] and as agents with which to improve compliance with mechanical ventilation [96]. Agents that attenuate noradrenergic function, including clonidine, propranolol, and other antihypertensives, are commonly used for medical and/or behavioral purposes as well. However, dopaminergic and noradrenergic antagonists delay neuronal recovery and impair neuronal plasticity [97–103]. Among persons with TBI, typical antipsychotics exacerbate cognitive impairments [104] and prolong the period of PTA [105]. Benzodiazepines are well known to impair memory and other aspects of cognition [106] in healthy adults and among persons with TBI [107]. In light of these findings, use of agents with potent antidopaminergic, antinoradrenergic, and/or GABA-ergic properties is best avoided during the neurorehabilitative care of persons with TBI. When evaluating neuropsychiatrically patients receiving these agents, considering their potential effects on neurological and cognitive function before making definitive diagnostic or prognostic statements is prudent.

With respect to the effects of other agents on posttraumatic neuropsychiatric function, medications possessing potent in vivo anticholinergic properties are of concern as well. These medications are commonly prescribed for posttraumatic dizziness and urinary incontinence. Antidepressants with potent anticholinergic properties (e.g., tricyclic and tetracyclic antidepressants and also paroxetine [108]) are often prescribed by rehabilitation physicians for pain, headaches, and emotional disturbances. However, TBI produces acute and chronic disturbances of cerebral cholinergic function [56], and cholinergic deficits become prominent and functionally significant in many patients over the first several weeks after TBI. As a result of these deficits, patients with TBI are vulnerable to the adverse cognitive and behavioral effects of agents with anticholinergic properties. In general, prescription of agents with potent anticholinergic properties for persons with TBI should be avoided whenever possible.

Finally, pain and spasticity are common problems among persons with TBI, most often as a result of injury to the head or other orthopedic or soft tissue injuries that are sustained concurrently with TBI. Among the agents used for these problems, opiate analgesics are particularly likely to adversely affect cognitive and neuropsychiatric function. At typical analgesic doses, these agents produce impairments in memory among persons without TBI of severities comparable to those encountered among persons in PTA [109]. These agents may exacerbate, prolong, or mimic posttraumatic coma, posttraumatic delirium, PTA, and the posttraumatic dysexecutive syndrome. Using the minimum necessary dose of any of these agents for as brief a time as is feasible clinically, or, better, avoiding or eliminating these whenever possible, is recommended.

Conclusion

TBI is a significant public health problem that produces substantial neurological and neuropsychiatric morbidity. The biomechanical and cytotoxic processes incited by TBI produce a predictable injury profile that involves anterior, and predominantly ventral, frontal, and temporal cortex, frontal subcortical white matter, and midbrain areas. Damage to these structures explains, in large part, the anatomic contributions to the neurobehavioral sequelae of TBI, including alterations of arousal, attention, processing speed, memory, functional communication, executive function, emotional regulation, and behavior.

As discussed in this chapter, the period of neuropsychiatric disturbance that immediately follows TBI is understood usefully as posttraumatic encephalopathy (PTE), a condition with several stages through which patients proceed during recovery from TBI. These stages include, in typical sequence, posttraumatic coma, posttraumatic delirium, posttraumatic amnesia (PTA), posttraumatic dysexecutive syndrome, and full recovery. Among these, duration of PTA is particularly useful to measure accurately: duration of PTA is strongly predictive of short- and long-term neurorehabilitation outcomes. Additionally, data developed on our neuropsychiatric consultation service suggest that several elements of the neuropsychiatric assessment, including the number of SNS (paratonia, primitive reflexes) and also a brief bedside neurobehavioral status examination (normatively interpreted MMSE and FAB), yield data that allow neuropsychiatrists to assess functional status, functional prognosis, and rehabilitation lengths of stay among persons with TBI receiving inpatient neurorehabilitative care.

Treatment approaches based on data yielded by the neuropsychiatric assessment vary widely among institutions, both nationally and internationally. These treatment issues are beyond the scope of this chapter but are well described elsewhere [57, 110–117]. Independent of specific treatment recommendations, the principles of neuropsychiatric assessment of TBI in the neurorehabilitation setting described in this chapter apply broadly. Well informed and equipped with this information, neuropsychiatrists will contribute importantly and effectively to multidisciplinary teams working to improve the neuropsychiatric and functional outcomes of persons with TBI.

References

1. Thurman D, Guerrero J (1999) Trends in hospitalization associated with traumatic brain injury. JAMA 282:954–957
2. Thurman DJ, Alverson C, Dunn KA et al (1999) Traumatic brain injury in the United States: a public health perspective. J Head Trauma Rehabil 14:602–615
3. Selassie AW, Zaloshnja E, Langlois JA et al (2008) Incidence of long-term disability following traumatic brain injury hospitalization, United States, 2003. J Head Trauma Rehabil 23:123–131
4. Levin HS (1995) Neurobehavioral outcome of closed head injury: implications for clinical trials. J Neurotrauma 12:601–610
5. severe head injury. Experience of the Traumatic Coma Data Bank. J Neurosurg 73:699–709
6. Rapoport M, McCauley S, Levin H et al (2002) The role of injury severity in neurobehavioral outcome 3 months after traumatic brain injury. Neuropsychiatry Neuropsychol Behav Neurol 15:123–132
7. Hart T, Whyte J, Polansky M et al (2003) Concordance of patient and family report of neurobehavioral symptoms at 1 year after traumatic brain injury. Arch Phys Med Rehabil 84:204–213
8. Kaufman HH, Levin HS, High WM Jr et al (1985) Neurobehavioral outcome after gunshot wounds to the head in adult civilians and children. Neurosurgery (Baltim) 16:754–758
9. Dikmen S, Machamer J, Miller B et al (2001) Functional status examination: a new instrument for assessing outcome in traumatic brain injury. J Neurotrauma 18:127–140

10. Dikmen SS, Machamer JE, Powell JM et al (2003) Outcome 3 to 5 years after moderate to severe traumatic brain injury. Arch Phys Med Rehabil 84:1449–1457
11. Hall KM, Bushnik T, Lakisic-Kazazic B et al (2001) Assessing traumatic brain injury outcome measures for long-term follow-up of community-based individuals. Arch Phys Med Rehabil 82:367–374
12. Doctor JN, Castro J, Temkin NR et al (2005) Workers' risk of unemployment after traumatic brain injury: a normed comparison. J Int Neuropsychol Soc 11:747–752
13. Guilmette TJ, Paglia MF (2004) The public's misconception about traumatic brain injury: a follow up survey. Arch Clin Neuropsychol 19:183–189
14. Swift TL, Wilson SL (2001) Misconceptions about brain injury among the general public and non-expert health professionals: an exploratory study. Brain Inj 15:149–165
15. Marr AL, Coronado VG (2002) Central Nervous System Injury Surveillance Data Submission Standards – 2002
16. Kraus JF, Rice TM, Peek-Asa C et al (2003) Facial trauma and the risk of intracranial injury in motorcycle riders. Ann Emerg Med 41:18–26
17. Johnston JJ (2007) The Galasko report implemented: the role of emergency medicine in the management of head injuries. Eur J Emerg Med 14:130–133
18. Palchak MJ, Holmes JF, Vance CW et al (2003) A decision rule for identifying children at low risk for brain injuries after blunt head trauma. Ann Emerg Med 42:492–506
19. Borg J, Holm L, Cassidy JD et al (2004) Diagnostic procedures in mild traumatic brain injury: results of the WHO Collaborating Centre Task Force on Mild Traumatic Brain Injury. J Rehabil Med (Suppl 43):61–75
20. Teasdale G, Jennett B (1974) Assessment of coma and impaired consciousness. a practical scale. Lancet 2:81–84
21. Clifton GL, Hayes RL, Levin HS et al (1992) Outcome measures for clinical trials involving traumatically brain-injured patients: report of a conference. Neurosurgery (Baltim) 31:975–978
22. Cowen TD, Meythaler JM, Devivo MJ et al (1995) Influence of early variables in traumatic brain injury on functional independence measure scores and rehabilitation length of stay and charges. Arch Phys Med Rehabil 76:797–803
23. Gabbe BJ, Cameron PA, Finch CF (2003) The status of the Glasgow Coma Scale. Emerg Med (Fremantle) 15:353–360
24. Russell WR, Smith A (1961) Post-traumatic amnesia in closed head injury. Arch Neurol 5:4–17
25. Arciniegas DB, McAllister TW (2008) Neurobehavioral management of traumatic brain injury in the critical care setting. Crit Care Clin 24:viii, 737–viii, 765
26. Levin HS, O'Donnell VM, Grossman RG (1979) The Galveston Orientation and Amnesia Test. A practical scale to assess cognition after head injury. J Nerv Ment Dis 167:675–684
27. Jackson WT, Novack TA, Dowler RN (1998) Effective serial measurement of cognitive orientation in rehabilitation: the Orientation Log. Arch Phys Med Rehabil 79:718–720
28. Novack TA, Dowler RN, Bush BA et al (2000) Validity of the Orientation Log, relative to the Galveston Orientation and Amnesia Test. J Head Trauma Rehabil 15:957–961
29. Frey KL, Rojas DC, Anderson CA et al (2007) Comparison of the O-Log and GOAT as measures of posttraumatic amnesia. Brain Inj 21:513–520
30. Kay T, Harrington DE, Adams RE et al (1993) Definition of mild traumatic brain injury: Report from the Mild Traumatic Brain Injury Committee of the Head Injury Interdisciplinary Special Interest Group of the American Congress of Rehabilitation Medicine. J Head Trauma Rehabil 8:86–87
31. McMillan TM, Jongen EL, Greenwood RJ (1996) Assessment of post-traumatic amnesia after severe closed head injury: retrospective or prospective? J Neurol Neurosurg Psychiatry 60:422–427
32. Williams DH, Levin HS, Eisenberg HM (1990) Mild head injury classification. Neurosurgery (Baltim) 27:422–428

33. van der Naalt J, Hew JM, van Zomeren AH et al (1999) Computed tomography and magnetic resonance imaging in mild to moderate head injury: early and late imaging related to outcome. Ann Neurol 46:70–78
34. Zafonte RD, Mann NR, Millis SR et al (1997) Posttraumatic amnesia: its relation to functional outcome. Arch Phys Med Rehabil 78:1103–1106
35. Jennett B, Bond M (1975) Assessment of outcome after severe brain damage. Lancet 1:480–484
36. Katz DI, Alexander MP (1994) Traumatic brain injury. Predicting course of recovery and outcome for patients admitted to rehabilitation. Arch Neurol 51:661–670
37. Ellenberg JH, Levin HS, Saydjari C (1996) Posttraumatic amnesia as a predictor of outcome after severe closed head injury. Prospective assessment. Arch Neurol 53:782–791
38. Brooks DN, Aughton ME, Bond MR et al (1980) Cognitive sequelae in relationship to early indices of severity of brain damage after severe blunt head injury. J Neurol Neurosurg Psychiatry 43:529–534
39. Geffen GM, Encel JS, Forrester GM (1991) Stages of recovery during post-traumatic amnesia and subsequent everyday memory deficits. NeuroReport 2:105–108
40. Haslam C, Batchelor J, Fearnside MR et al (1994) Post-coma disturbance and post-traumatic amnesia as nonlinear predictors of cognitive outcome following severe closed head injury: findings from the Westmead Head Injury Project. Brain Inj 8:519–528
41. Sherer M, Sander AM, Nick TG et al (2002) Early cognitive status and productivity outcome after traumatic brain injury: findings from the TBI model systems. Arch Phys Med Rehabil 83:183–192
42. Avesani R, Salvi L, Rigoli G et al (2005) Reintegration after severe brain injury: a retrospective study. Brain Inj 19:933–939
43. Doig E, Fleming J, Tooth L (2001) Patterns of community integration 2-5 years post-discharge from brain injury rehabilitation. Brain Inj 15:747–762
44. Bigler ED (2007) Anterior and middle cranial fossa in traumatic brain injury: relevant neuroanatomy and neuropathology in the study of neuropsychological outcome. Neuropsychology 21:515–531
45. Sabet AA, Christoforou E, Zatlin B et al (2008) Deformation of the human brain induced by mild angular head acceleration. J Biomech 41:307–315
46. Besenski N (2002) Traumatic injuries: imaging of head injuries. Eur Radiol 12:1237–1252
47. Ryan GA, McLean AJ, Vilenius AT et al (1994) Brain injury patterns in fatally injured pedestrians. J Trauma 36:469–476
48. Misra JC, Chakravarty S (1984) A study of rotational brain injury. J Biomech 17:459–466
49. Fijalkowski RJ, Stemper BD, Pintar FA et al (2007) New rat model for diffuse brain injury using coronal plane angular acceleration. J Neurotrauma 24:1387–1398
50. Margulies SS, Thibault LE, Gennarelli TA (1990) Physical model simulations of brain injury in the primate. J Biomech 23:823–836
51. Meythaler JM, Peduzzi JD, Eleftheriou E et al (2001) Current concepts: diffuse axonal injury-associated traumatic brain injury. Arch Phys Med Rehabil 82:1461–1471
52. Black KL, Hanks RA, Wood DL et al (2002) Blunt versus penetrating violent traumatic brain injury: frequency and factors associated with secondary conditions and complications. J Head Trauma Rehabil 17:489–496
53. Povlishock JT, Katz DI (2005) Update of neuropathology and neurological recovery after traumatic brain injury. J Head Trauma Rehabil 20:76–94
54. Bigler ED (2003) Neurobiology and neuropathology underlie the neuropsychological deficits associated with traumatic brain injury. Arch Clin Neuropsychol 18:595–621
55. Phillips LL, Reeves TM (2001) Interactive pathology following traumatic brain injury modifies hippocampal plasticity. Restor Neurol Neurosci 19:213–235
56. Arciniegas DB (2003) The cholinergic hypothesis of cognitive impairment caused by traumatic brain injury. Curr Psychiatry Rep 5:391–399
57. Arciniegas DB, Silver JM (2006) Pharmacotherapy of posttraumatic cognitive impairments. Behav Neurol 17:25–42

58. Markianos M, Seretis A, Kotsou S et al (1992) CSF neurotransmitter metabolites and short-term outcome of patients in coma after head injury. Acta Neurol Scand 86:190–193
59. Markianos M, Seretis A, Kotsou A et al (1996) CSF neurotransmitter metabolites in comatose head injury patients during changes in their clinical state. Acta Neurochir (Wien) 138:57–59
60. McAllister TW, Flashman LA, Sparling MB et al (2004) Working memory deficits after traumatic brain injury: catecholaminergic mechanisms and prospects for treatment – a review. Brain Inj 18:331–350
61. Povlishock JT (1992) Traumatically induced axonal injury: pathogenesis and pathobiological implications. Brain Pathol 2:1–12
62. Salmond CH, Chatfield DA, Menon DK et al (2005) Cognitive sequelae of head injury: involvement of basal forebrain and associated structures. Brain 128:189–200
63. American Psychiatric Association (2000) Diagnostic and Statistical Manual of Mental Disorders, Text Revision, 4th edn. American Psychiatric Association, Washington, DC
64. Rappaport M (2005) The Disability Rating and Coma/Near-Coma scales in evaluating severe head injury. Neuropsychol Rehabil 15:442–453
65. Trzepacz PT, Mittal D, Torres R et al (2001) Validation of the Delirium Rating Scale-Revised-98: comparison with the delirium rating scale and the cognitive test for delirium. J Neuropsychiatry Clin Neurosci 13:229–242
66. Sherer M, Nakase-Thompson R, Yablon SA et al (2005) Multidimensional assessment of acute confusion after traumatic brain injury. Arch Phys Med Rehabil 86:896–904
67. Hagen C, Malkmus D, Durham P (1972) Rancho Los Amigos Scale. http://www.rancho.org/patient_education/bi_cognition.pdf
68. Wortzel HS, Frey KL, Anderson CA, Arciniegas DB (2009). Subtle neurological signs predict the severity of subacute cognitive and functional impairments after traumatic brain injury. J Neuropsychiatry Clin Neurosci 21:463–466
69. Folstein MF, Folstein SE, McHugh PR (1975) Mini-mental state: a practical method for grading the cognitive state of patients for the clinician. J Psychiatry Res 12:189–198
70. Dubois B, Slachevsky A, Litvan I et al (2000) The FAB: a frontal assessment battery at bedside. Neurology 55:1621–1626
71. Crum RM, Anthony JC, Bassett SS et al (1993) Population-based norms for the mini-mental state examination by age and education level. JAMA 269:2386–2391
72. Appollonio I, Leone M, Isella V et al (2005) The frontal assessment battery (FAB): normative values in an Italian population sample. Neurol Sci 26:108–116
73. Arciniegas DB, Frey K, Alderfer B et al (2006) Impairments of frontally-mediated cognition characterize posttraumatic encephalopathy following resolution of posttraumatic amnesia. J Neuropsychiatry Clin Neurosci 18:281
74. Vanier M, Mazaux JM, Lambert J et al (2000) Assessment of neuropsychologic impairments after head injury: interrater reliability and factorial and criterion validity of the Neurobehavioral Rating Scale – Revised. Arch Phys Med Rehabil 81:796–806
75. McCauley SR, Levin HS, Vanier M et al (2001) The neurobehavioural rating scale-revised: sensitivity and validity in closed head injury assessment. J Neurol Neurosurg Psychiatry 71:643–651
76. Royall DR, Mahurin RK, Gray KF (1992) Bedside assessment of executive cognitive impairment: the executive interview. J Am Geriatr Soc 40:1221–1226
77. Grigsby J, Kaye K, Robbins LJ (1992) Reliabilities, norms and factor structure of the Behavioral Dyscontrol Scale. Percept Mot Skills 74:883–892
78. Kaye K, Grigsby J, Robbins LJ et al (1990) Prediction of independent functioning and behavior problems in geriatric patients. J Am Geriatr Soc 38:1304–1310
79. Cummings JL, Mega M, Gray K et al (1994) The Neuropsychiatric Inventory: comprehensive assessment of psychopathology in dementia. Neurology 44:2308–2314
80. Kalmar K, Novack TA, Nakase-Richardson R et al (2008) Feasibility of a brief neuropsychologic test battery during acute inpatient rehabilitation after traumatic brain injury. Arch Phys Med Rehabil 89:942–949
81. Hanks RA, Millis SR, Ricker JH et al (2008) The predictive validity of a brief inpatient neuropsychologic battery for persons with traumatic brain injury. Arch Phys Med Rehabil 89:950–957

82. Akiyama Y, Miyata K, Harada K et al (2009) Susceptibility-weighted magnetic resonance imaging for the detection of cerebral microhemorrhage in patients with traumatic brain injury. Neurol Med Chir (Tokyo) 49:97–99
83. Arciniegas DB, Anderson CA, Rojas DC (2005) Electrophysiological techniques. In: Silver JM, McAllister TW, Yudofsky SC (eds) Textbook of traumatic brain injury. American Psychiatric Publishing, Washington, DC
84. Rothman MS, Arciniegas DB, Filley CM et al (2007) The neuroendocrine effects of traumatic brain injury. J Neuropsychiatry Clin Neurosci 19:363–372
85. Frey LC (2003) Epidemiology of posttraumatic epilepsy: a critical review. Epilepsia 44(suppl 10):11–17
86. Schierhout G, Roberts I (2000) Anti-epileptic drugs for preventing seizures following acute traumatic brain injury. Cochrane Database Syst Rev 4:CD000173
87. Dikmen SS, Temkin NR, Miller B et al (1991) Neurobehavioral effects of phenytoin prophylaxis of posttraumatic seizures. JAMA 265:1271–1277
88. Smith KR Jr, Goulding PM, Wilderman D et al (1994) Neurobehavioral effects of phenytoin and carbamazepine in patients recovering from brain trauma: a comparative study. Arch Neurol 51:653–660
89. Szaflarski JP, Meckler JM, Szaflarski M et al (2007) Levetiracetam use in critically ill patients. Neurocrit Care 7:140–147
90. Ruegg S, Naegelin Y, Hardmeier M et al (2008) Intravenous levetiracetam: treatment experience with the first 50 critically ill patients. Epilepsy Behav 12:477–480
91. Mula M, Trimble MR, Yuen A et al (2003) Psychiatric adverse events during levetiracetam therapy. Neurology 61:704–706
92. Mula M, Trimble MR, Sander JW (2004) Psychiatric adverse events in patients with epilepsy and learning disabilities taking levetiracetam. Seizure 13:55–57
93. Dikmen SS, Machamer JE, Winn HR et al (2000) Neuropsychological effects of valproate in traumatic brain injury: a randomized trial. Neurology 54:895–902
94. Marion DW (2006) Evidenced-based guidelines for traumatic brain injuries. Prog Neurol Surg 19:171–196
95. Fugate LP, Spacek LA, Kresty LA et al (1997) Measurement and treatment of agitation following traumatic brain injury: II. A survey of the Brain Injury Special Interest Group of the American Academy of Physical Medicine and Rehabilitation. Arch Phys Med Rehabil 78:924–928
96. Milbrandt EB, Kersten A, Kong L et al (2005) Haloperidol use is associated with lower hospital mortality in mechanically ventilated patients. Crit Care Med 33:226–229
97. Goldstein LB (1993) Basic and clinical studies of pharmacologic effects on recovery from brain injury. J Neural Transplant Plast 4:175–192
98. Goldstein LB (1999) Pharmacological approach to functional reorganization: the role of norepinephrine. Rev Neurol (Paris) 155:731–736
99. Goldstein LB (2003) Neuropharmacology of TBI-induced plasticity. Brain Inj 17:685–694
100. Goldstein LB (2006) Neurotransmitters and motor activity: effects on functional recovery after brain injury. NeuroRx 3:451–457
101. Hoffman AN, Cheng JP, Zafonte RD et al (2008) Administration of haloperidol and risperidone after neurobehavioral testing hinders the recovery of traumatic brain injury-induced deficits. Life Sci 83:602–607
102. Kline AE, Hoffman AN, Cheng JP et al (2008) Chronic administration of antipsychotics impede behavioral recovery after experimental traumatic brain injury. Neurosci Lett 448:263–267
103. Kline AE, Massucci JL, Zafonte RD et al (2007) Differential effects of single versus multiple administrations of haloperidol and risperidone on functional outcome after experimental brain trauma. Crit Care Med 35:919–924
104. Stanislav SW (1997) Cognitive effects of antipsychotic agents in persons with traumatic brain injury. Brain Inj 11:335–341

105. Rao N, Jellinek HM, Woolston DC (1985) Agitation in closed head injury: haloperidol effects on rehabilitation outcome. Arch Phys Med Rehabil 66:30–34
106. Buffett-Jerrott SE, Stewart SH (2002) Cognitive and sedative effects of benzodiazepine use. Curr Pharm Des 8:45–58
107. Bleiberg J, Garmoe W, Cederquist J et al (1993) Effects of dexedrine on performance consistency following brain injury: a double-blind placebo crossover case study. Neuropsychiatry Neuropsychol Behav Neurol 6:245–248
108. Schmitt JA, Kruizinga MJ, Riedel WJ (2001) Non-serotonergic pharmacological profiles and associated cognitive effects of serotonin reuptake inhibitors. J Psychopharmacol 15:173–179
109. McCarter RJ, Walton NH, Moore C et al (2007) PTA testing, the Westmead post traumatic amnesia scale and opiate analgesia: a cautionary note. Brain Inj 21:1393–1397
110. Warden DL, Gordon B, McAllister TW et al (2006) Guidelines for the pharmacologic treatment of neurobehavioral sequelae of traumatic brain injury. J Neurotrauma 23:1468–1501
111. Cicerone KD, Dahlberg C, Kalmar K et al (2000) Evidence-based cognitive rehabilitation: recommendations for clinical practice. Arch Phys Med Rehabil 81:1596–1615
112. Cicerone KD, Dahlberg C, Malec JF et al (2005) Evidence-based cognitive rehabilitation: updated review of the literature from 1998 through 2002. Arch Phys Med Rehabil 86:1681–1692
113. Cappa SF, Benke T, Clarke S et al (2005) EFNS guidelines on cognitive rehabilitation: report of an EFNS task force. Eur J Neurol 12:665–680
114. Cappa SF, Benke T, Clarke S et al (2003) EFNS guidelines on cognitive rehabilitation: report of an EFNS task force. Eur J Neurol 10:11–23
115. Tate RL, Moseley A, Perdices M et al (2006) Update on Cicerone's systematic review of cognitive rehabilitation: the PsycBITE perspective. Arch Phys Med Rehabil 87:446
116. Cicerone KD, Mott T, Azulay J et al (2008) A randomized controlled trial of holistic neuropsychologic rehabilitation after traumatic brain injury. Arch Phys Med Rehabil 89:2239–2249
117. Cicerone KD, Mott T, Azulay J et al (2004) Community integration and satisfaction with functioning after intensive cognitive rehabilitation for traumatic brain injury. Arch Phys Med Rehabil 85:943–950

Part V
Vascular and Inflammatory Disorders

Neuropsychiatric Aspects of Vascular Cognitive Impairment

Ingmar Skoog

Abstract Neuropsychiatric disorders such as dementia and depression are common in the elderly. After the age of 85, the prevalence of dementia is 30%, that of depression 10%, and that of psychotic symptoms 10%. The lifetime prevalence of depression approaches 50% in women and 25% in men. Cognitive dysfunction is common both in depression and in individuals with psychotic symptoms, and it is the core manifestation in dementia disorders, such as Alzheimer's disease. Cognitive symptoms are also included in the criteria for major depression in the DSM-IV. There is controversy about whether depression is a risk factor for dementia, but depression is common in individuals with dementia. Cognitive dysfunction in elderly individuals may also be caused by prodromal symptoms of dementia. Cerebrovascular diseases are also common in the elderly and are related to both cognitive impairment and depression. Vascular cognitive impairment is a term encompassing vascular causes of cognitive impairment, including dementia. The two most common cerebrovascular diseases are stroke and ischemic white matter lesions (WMLs). Stroke and ischemic WMLs increase the risk for dementia and depression. The latter is a reason for the introduction of the concept of vascular depression in the elderly. However, most depressions in the elderly are not related to vascular disease. Adding to the complexity, associations between cerebrovascular and neuropsychiatric disorders may also go in the opposite direction, as several studies report that depression may increase the risk for stroke. There is thus a complex interaction between depression, dementia, and vascular diseases. It is important to detect neuropsychiatric syndromes in patients with cardiovascular diseases as this has implications for their management and prognosis. Vascular disorders and risk factors are also important to detect as they are targets for prevention of dementia and depression.

Keywords Alzheimer's disease • Cerebrovascular disease • Dementia • Depression • White matter lesions

---

I. Skoog (✉)
Neuropsychiatric Epidemiology Unit, Department of Psychiatry, Institute of Neuroscience and Physiology, Sahlgrenska Academy at Göteborg University, Göteborg, Sweden
e-mail: ingmar.skoog@neuro.gu.se

K. Miyoshi et al. (eds.), *Neuropsychiatric Disorders*,
DOI 10.1007/978-4-431-53871-4_11, © Springer 2010

Background

Cognitive function declines with increasing age. This decline differs between individuals, probably as a consequence of genetic predisposition and educational and professional background. The decline may be accelerated by different insults to the brain, for example, cardiovascular and cerebrovascular diseases, other brain disorders, preclinical dementia, and terminal decline. The cognitive dysfunction in individuals with cardiovascular and cerebrovascular disease is often subsumed under the term vascular cognitive impairment (VCI) [1]. Neuropsychiatric conditions, such as Alzheimer's disease (AD), depression, and psychotic disorders, are also related to cognitive dysfunction, and in addition they have all been associated with cardiovascular and cerebrovascular diseases. AD and cerebrovascular disease often coexist in the same patient, being then labeled mixed dementia [2]. Vascular depression is the term for coexistent depression and cerebrovascular disease [3].

Neuropsychiatric Disorders Associated with Cognitive Impairment

Alzheimer's Disease

The typical clinical picture of AD is dementia with insidious onset and a slowly progressive loss of memory and other cognitive functions, such as language, visuospatial abilities, executive function, orientation, praxis, and behavior. NINCDS-ADRDA criteria [4] state that the diagnosis of probable AD requires the absence of systemic disorders or other brain diseases that alone could account for dementia. Clinical AD has a long preclinical phase [5, 6]. Thus, some cognitive dysfunctions in elderly nondemented persons are caused by preclinical AD.

AD in the brain is characterized by marked neuronal and synaptic degeneration and the presence of extensive amounts of senile plaques, neurofibrillary tangles, and deposition of the beta-amyloid peptide in specific regions of the brain [7]. However, a large proportion of individuals who were cognitively normal before death have numerous histopathological hallmarks of AD in the brain at autopsy [8–11]. Several population-based neuropathological studies suggest that only approximately 50% of individuals who fulfill neuropathological criteria for AD had dementia or significant cognitive decline during life [8, 9, 12]. These neuropathological findings have recently been confirmed by positron emission tomography studies using the Pittsburgh compound B to detect amyloid deposition in living individuals [13]. In this study, 21% of normal elderly showed beta-amyloid deposition compatible with AD. Based on known figures on age-related prevalence of dementia, this finding indicates that less than 50% of individuals with AD in the brain show cognitive impairment during life. This finding implies that AD often does not present with the clinical picture of dementia.

Depression

A depressive syndrome includes symptoms of depressed mood, tearfulness, diminished pleasure or interest, excessive guilt feelings, low self-esteem, feelings of worthlessness, hopelessness, pessimism, and emotional flatness, poor appetite, weight loss, low energy or increased fatigue, sleep problems, poor concentration, difficulty making decisions, intellectual problems, psychomotor retardation or agitation, reduced talkativeness, and suicidal ideations [14].

Most cross-sectional studies report that the prevalence of depression is around 10% [15–24], with higher prevalence in women than in men. The lifetime prevalence of depression in persons reaching the age of 85 is 45% in women and 23% in men [25]. Cognitive symptoms are one of the core symptoms of major depression according to DSM-IV [14]. In line with this, population studies show that nondemented individuals with depression perform worse on cognitive testing [26]. Whether depression also increases the risk for later development of dementia is not clear. Three prospective population studies did not find an increased rate of depression before the onset of dementia [27–30]. In contrast, a meta-analysis including 22 studies suggested that depression increased the risk for later development of dementia [31]. However, this meta-analysis included a mixture of population-based studies and studies from memory clinics, which made it difficult to evaluate whether depression increases risk for dementia in cognitively intact individuals from the general population.

Psychotic Symptoms

Psychotic symptoms, such as hallucinations and delusions, are common in demented elderly [32–34] but are reported to be uncommon in the nondemented elderly. However, these symptoms may be underrated in traditional epidemiological studies, which generally rely on self-reports. We examined psychotic symptoms in 85-year-olds using several sources of information, including self-report, key-informant interviews, and medical record reviews [35], and found that 10% of nondemented 85-year-olds had psychotic symptoms and 7% had paranoid ideation during the preceding year. Hallucinations were found in 7% and delusions in 6%. These figures were considerable higher than findings that had been reported previously in the nondemented elderly. With the same method, we also found high rates in nondemented 95-year-olds [36], whereas the prevalence was considerably lower in 70-year-olds [37]. Nondemented 85-year-olds with psychotic symptoms or paranoid ideation performed worse on psychometric tests measuring verbal ability, inductive logical reasoning/problem solving, and tests of spatial ability [38]. Hallucinations, delusions, and paranoid ideation at age 85 were each related to an increased incidence of dementia from age 85 to 88 years, but only one-third of those with these symptoms developed dementia [35]. Paranoid ideation was associated with myocardial infarction in this study.

Cerebrovascular Diseases Associated with Cognitive Impairment and Neuropsychiatric Conditions

Many different cerebrovascular diseases have been related to cognitive decline, dementia, and other neuropsychiatric conditions. These cerebrovascular disorders include stroke, silent infarcts, ischemic white matter lesions (WMLs), hereditary cerebral hemorrhage with amyloidosis, granular cortical atrophy, hypertensive encephalopathy, cerebral amyloid angiopathy, and cerebral vasculitis [39]. Most often there is a mixture of different cerebrovascular changes, which could be expected as different cerebrovascular diseases share similar risk factors. The two most common cerebrovascular diseases are stroke and ischemic WMLs.

Cerebrovascular disorders are generally believed to be the second most common cause of dementia, after AD. Dementia caused by cerebrovascular disease is often labeled vascular dementia (VaD). AD and cerebrovascular disease often coexist in the same patient. This condition is termed mixed dementia [2]. Cerebrovascular disorders are also associated with cognitive decline that does not reach the diagnostic threshold for dementia [40–44]. The term VCI was introduced by Bowler and Hachinski [1] to capture the whole range of cognitive dysfunction associated with vascular disease. This term thus includes VaD, mixed dementia, and other forms of cognitive decline caused by cerebrovascular and cardiovascular diseases. Cerebrovascular diseases have also been associated with other neuropsychiatric manifestations, mainly depression

It is important to recognize that cognitive impairment and neuropsychiatric conditions associated with cerebrovascular or cardiovascular disorders are potentially preventable or treatable.

Stroke

Stroke patients typically have history of stroke or transit ischemic attacks (TIA), including acute focal neurological symptoms and signs, such as hemiparesis or acute aphasia [39]. The symptoms must be present for 24 h or more for a diagnosis of stroke. If they are present for a shorter duration, a diagnosis of TIA is given. The cerebral infarcts are most often caused by thromboembolism from extracranial arteries and the heart and are often related to large vessel disease. Other cardiovascular manifestations, including myocardial infarction and hypertension, are common in the patients. The most important risk factors for stroke are hypertension, diabetes mellitus, atherosclerosis, atrial fibrillation, smoking, overweight, and hypercholesterolemia, especially high levels of low-density lipoprotein cholesterol [45]. All these risk factors are potentially preventable or treatable.

Most epidemiological studies report an increased frequency of dementia in individuals with stroke. In the studies by Tatemichi et al. [46–48], relatively young individuals with ischemic stroke had at least nine times greater risk for dementia than stroke-free controls. Those persons with dementia after stroke had a higher mortality rate and worse prognosis than those without dementia, which was independent of stroke severity. Also, Pohjasvaara et al. [49] reported an increased prevalence of dementia in stroke victims, as well as a decrease in independent living for those with dementia. Lindén et al. [44] reported that stroke victims aged above 70 had an odds ratio of 4.7 for dementia. The odds for dementia was higher in those aged 70 to 80 [odds ratio (OR), 6.7] than in those aged over 80 years, but the frequency of dementia after stroke was higher after age 80 (34% vs. 18%). In addition, 60% of nondemented stroke victims had some cognitive dysfunction, showing that very few elderly stroke victims are free from cognitive disturbances. In a population study on 85-year-olds, Liebetrau et al. [50] reported that the odds ratio for dementia in stroke was 4.3 and the prevalence of dementia after stroke was 57%. It may be that the increased risk for dementia with stroke decreases with age at the same time as the prevalence increases, both among those with and those without a history of stroke.

The pathogenesis of stroke-related dementia is not settled. The main hypothesis is that dementia is related to the location or the volume of the infarcts, but there are also other possibilities. The risk factors for dementia in individuals with stroke can be divided into stroke-related and non-stroke-related factors [51]. The stroke-related factors are similar to those in stroke, such as male sex, hypertension, diabetes mellitus, smoking, and cardiac diseases. Non-stroke-related risk factors are similar to those found in sporadic AD and include higher age, lower level of formal education, family history of dementia, and the presence of cerebral atrophy. This combination of risk factors supports the view that stroke-related dementia often is a consequence of both stroke and preexisting AD pathology. According to neuropathological studies, pure VAD, without any AD brain changes, is rare [52].

Stroke is an essential part of most criteria for VaD or VCI. The typical clinical course of stroke-related dementia is sudden onset, stepwise deterioration, and a fluctuating course. In the early stages, the cognitive symptoms may vary between individuals depending on the site of the lesions. A large proportion of patients with cerebrovascular disease have a gradual onset of dementia with a slowly progressive course [53], with or without focal signs or infarcts on brain imaging, which makes it difficult to differentiate from AD or other types of dementia. Changing risk factor patterns (e.g., decrease in the frequency of smoking, better treatment of hypertension) have decreased the incidence of stroke and may thus decrease the frequency of VaD. On the other hand, more individuals survive after stroke, which may act in the opposite direction. It is not yet known if the prevalence or incidence of VaD increases or decreases.

The associations may also go in the opposite direction, as individuals with cognitive impairment may be at increased risk for stroke and cerebral infarction. Three studies [54–56] reported that elderly individuals with decreased cognitive ability and without previous stroke at baseline were at increased risk for later incidents of stroke. In addition, one of these studies reported that also mild dementia at baseline was associated with an increased incidence of new strokes [56]. One reason may be that these individuals already had silent cerebrovascular disease, such as silent infarcts or WMLs.

Depression is common after stroke [57], both in the acute [58], subacute [59–61], and long-term perspective [62–64]. The frequency estimates varies from 25% to

48% in the acute stage, from 14% to 50% at 1–12 months after stroke, and from 12% to 42% after a year or more following stroke [62]. In the study by Linden et al. [62], stroke was related to an odds ratio (OR) for depression of 3.2 in women and 4.0 in men 1.5 years after the index stroke. A systematic review from 51 observational studies [65, 66] found a pooled estimate of 33% for depression after stroke. Depression is important to detect in stroke patients, as it has been associated with worse outcome in numerous studies [67–69]. Depressed stroke patients have more cognitive impairments [61], spend more days in hospital [70], utilize more care, and are more often institutionalized than the nondepressed [71]. The etiology of depression after stroke is debated. Some authors suggest biological factors, such as disruption of frontostriatal [72] or left-sided prefrontosubcortical pathways [73], or infarcts in strategic locations, such as right hemisphere strokes [74]. However, a meta-analysis found no consistent location of infarcts to be associated with depression after stroke [75]. Others suggest that depression could be a reaction to disability and loss of autonomy after stroke [76]. However, frequency of depression is increased after stroke, also when controlling for stroke severity and disability [62].

Also, this association may go in the opposite direction, as several studies have shown that depression increases the risk for first incidence stroke [77–79]. Reasons include that depression has been associated with risk factors for stroke, such as myocardial arrhythmia [80], increased platelet activation [81] and increased insulin resistance [82]. However, in the study by Liebetrau et al. [78], depression was related to lower diastolic blood pressure, and not to any other vascular factors. Another explanation may be that late-life depression has been suggested to be related to silent cerebrovascular diseases, such as ischemic WMLs, which may increase the incidence of stroke.

Silent Infarcts

Cerebral infarcts often occur without focal symptoms. The frequency of these silent infarcts increases with age [83]. These lesions were until recently believed to be benign incidental findings on brain imaging. It has now been shown that individuals with silent infarcts are at increased risk for clinical stroke [83] and dementia [84]. Among 85-year-olds, 10% had silent infarcts on CT, and these lesions doubled the prevalence of dementia [85]. These lesions are thus important to detect, as treatment of vascular risk factors, such as hypertension, may decrease the risk of new strokes and thus potentially delay the onset of dementia in these high-risk patients.

White Matter Lesions

White matter lesions (WMLs) are common in the elderly [86]. Subcortical areas of both hemispheres are affected by marked or diffuse ischemic demyelination and moderate loss of axons with astrogliosis and incomplete infarction. In addition, arteriosclerotic changes with thickening of the vessel walls and narrowing of the lumina of the small penetrating arteries and arterioles caused by hyalinization or fibrosis are also present [87, 88].

The cause of WMLs is probably that long-standing hypertension causes lipohyalinosis and thickening of the vessel walls with narrowing of the lumen of the small perforating arteries and arterioles that nourish the deep white matter [87]. It has been suggested that the arterial changes are caused by the exposure of vessel walls to increased pressure over time. The greater the pressure and/or lifespan, the more likely are these changes to be present; this may be one reason for the observed increase with age reported in most studies. Episodes of hypotension may lead to further hypoperfusion and hypoxia-ischemia, leading to more loss of myelin in subcortical areas. The deep white matter has few collaterals, which makes it more vulnerable to ischemia than the cortex. Furthermore, myelin is probably more vulnerable than axons to ischemia [89]. The cortex, the subcortical U-fibers, and corpus callosum are thus generally well preserved [89].

The main risk factors for WMLs are high age, hypertension, and hypertension clustering factors [90]. It was recently shown that increased diastolic blood pressure and mean arterial pressure in midlife were related to the presence of WMLs in late life, supporting both the theory that long-standing high blood pressure is significant and that resistance of the smaller arteries and microvascular network is important [91].

In living individuals, WMLs can be detected on brain imaging. On computerized tomography (CT) scans they appear as low-density areas and on magnetic resonance imaging (MRI) as hyperdense areas. MRI and CT may not always capture the same WMLs. WMLs on MRI often show no correlation with cognitive decline and dementia and correspond to several different histological findings, for example, état crible. WMLs on CT are most often related to cognitive impairment and dementia and generally correspond to the histopathological picture described above [92]. Furthermore, it has been shown that CT is better than MRI in predicting symptomatic cerebrovascular disease in individuals with AD [93]. MRI is thus more sensitive than CT to detect changes in the white matter but has a lower specificity in relation to neuropathological and clinical manifestations.

On CT, WMLs were found in 35% of nondemented 85-year-olds in a study conducted in 1986–1987 [92], but a study conducted in 2000 found that 55% of individuals aged 70–84 years had WMLs [94], illustrating that CT is becoming more sensitive. MRI studies generally report much higher rates of WMLs than CT studies. The Rotterdam population study [41] reported that 11% in the age strata 65–69 years, 21% in those aged 70–74 years, 27% in those aged 70–79 years, and 54% in those aged 80–84 years had WMLs on MRI. A recent population-based neuropathological study reported that 94% of demented subjects had WMLs [86], and another neuropathological study found that 60% of individuals with AD had WMLs [88].

WMLs have been related to dementia both according to neuropathology [86, 88] and in population-based CT studies [92], and among the nondemented it has been related to visuo-spatial difficulties and psychomotor slowness [41, 43]. It has also been found to be more common in individuals with AD than in individuals without dementia [88, 92]. Investigations using CT of the brain in a population study of

85-year-olds revealed that one-third of the nondemented and about two-thirds of the AD patients had WMLs [92]. A similar proportion of AD patients had neuropathological evidence of ischemic WMLs when examined post mortem [88]. Based on an autopsy study of nondemented individuals who had extensive AD neuropathology, it was suggested that white matter degeneration precedes cortical atrophy in AD [95]. A longitudinal population study also reported that WMLs predicted later development of dementia [96]. Thus, WMLs seems to be strongly related to cognitive decline and dementia in the elderly. It has even been suggested that individuals with subcortical cerebrovascular disease show more decline in cognitive function than those with cortical strokes [97].

The dementia related to WMLs often has an insidious onset and a slowly progressive course [88, 97], which makes it difficult to distinguish from AD. WMLs seldom occur as the sole cause of dementia, and the clinical picture may vary depending on what other causes contribute to the dementia. Punctate WMLs on MRI do not progress, whereas confluent white matter abnormalities are progressive, and are thus more malignant in the long term [98].

Ischemic WMLs are also related to late-life depression [99]. Two prospective population-based studies using MRI report that white matter changes increase the risk of subsequent occurrence of depression [100, 101]. In the latter study, it was suggested that part of the relationship between white matter changes and depression was mediated by loss of functional ability [101]. Also, cross-sectional studies report that changes in the white matter detected with MRI are related to depression [102]. The association between WMLs on CT and depression is less clear. Cross-sectional studies from our group showed that WMLs on CT were associated with dementia but not with depression [92]. WMLs in the frontal region have been associated with depression in elderly patients [102], suggesting that WMLs disrupt the frontostriatal circuitry and thereby lead to the development of depression. All these findings are in line with the vascular depression hypothesis [3].

WMLs in depressed individuals may also influence outcome of depression. It has been reported that severe WMLs on MRI predicted a shorter time to relapse in elderly depressed individuals [103]. Furthermore, depressed individuals with WMLs may also have a poorer response to antidepressant monotherapy than those without WMLs [104].

Depression may also influence the development of WMLs. One recent study reported that depression at baseline was associated with faster progression of WMLs during follow-up [105].

Mixed Pathology

As already mentioned, only about half of individuals who fulfill neuropathological and positron emission tomography (PET) criteria for AD are demented during life [10, 13]. Furthermore, a considerable proportion of individuals who meet the clinical criteria for a diagnosis of probable AD have mixed pathologies [106–108].

Concomitant cerebrovascular diseases may increase the possibility that individuals with AD lesions in their brains will express a dementia syndrome [8, 12].

Furthermore, vascular pathology in AD may contribute to the clinical variability in symptomatology and clinical course in individuals diagnosed with AD during life [109]. To what extent cerebrovascular disease contributes to the clinical picture of dementia in each individual case is impossible to determine both at clinical and at neuropathological examination. A cerebrovascular disease may be the primary cause of dementia in an individual, but it may also be the event that finally overcomes the compensatory capacity of a brain that is already affected by AD pathology. In many instances, a combination of minor pathologies related to both disorders may cause dementia, when these minor pathologies would not have done so individually [110]. Thus, AD and cerebrovascular disease, which for long were regarded to be distinct and separate entities, often coexist and aggravate each other [111]. The complexity of the diagnosis in cases with mixed pathology may be one reason why the use of different diagnostic criteria for VaD result in substantial differences in the proportion of demented individuals diagnosed with VAD or AD [112–114]. The mixed cases are probably underestimated and may be the most common cause of dementia. Their relation to depression is not known.

Conclusion

The reported association between cerebrovascular diseases and neuropsychiatric disorders such as dementia and depression may teach us more about the pathogenesis of these disorders, but may also have implications for the clinical management. It is important to search for treatable cardiovascular and cerebrovascular diseases in the evaluation of patients with neuropsychiatric disorders, as these may influence the expression and clinical manifestations of the disease. It is also important to detect neuropsychiatric syndromes in patients with cardiovascular diseases as this recognition has implications for management and prognosis and may decrease patients' compliance with treatment.

Vascular disorders and risk factors, which are common in the elderly, are therefore important targets for prevention of dementia and depression. Thus, even if they only result in a moderately increased risk of neuropsychiatric disorders, such as dementia and depression, they may have an immense effect on the total number of affected individuals [115].

References

1. Bowler JV, Hachinski V (1995) Vascular cognitive impairment: a new approach to vascular dementia. Baillieres Clin Neurol 4:357–376
2. Langa KM, Foster NL, Larson EB (2004) Mixed dementia. Emerging concepts and therapeutic implications. JAMA 292:2901–2908

3. Alexopoulos GS, Meyers BS, Young RC et al (1997) 'Vascular depression' hypothesis. Arch Gen Psychiatry 54:915–922
4. McKhann G, Drachman D, Folstein M et al (1984) Clinical diagnosis of Alzheimer's disease: Report of the NINCDS-ADRDA work group under the auspices of department of health and human services task force on Alzheimer's disease. Neurology 34:939–944
5. Sacuiu S, Sjögren M, Gustafson D et al (2005) Prodromal cognitive signs of dementia in 85-year-olds using four sources of information. Neurology 65:1894–1900
6. Sacuiu S, Gustafson D, Johansson B et al (2009) The pattern of cognitive symptoms predicts time to dementia onset. Alzheimers Dement 5:199–206
7. Tomlinson B, Henderson G (1976) Some quantitative cerebral findings in normal and demented old people. In: Terry RD (ed) Neurobiology of aging. Raven, New York
8. White L, Petrovich H, Hardman J et al (2002) Cerebrovascular pathology and dementia in autopsied Honolulu-Asia Aging Study participants. Ann NY Acad Sci 977:9–23
9. Group N (2001) Medical Research Council Cognitive Function and Aging Study. Pathological correlates of late-onset dementia in a multicentre, community-based population in England and Wales. Lancet 357:169–175
10. Davies L, Wolska B, Hilbich C et al (1988) A4 amyloid protein deposition and the diagnosis of Alzheimer's disease: prevalence in aged brains determined by immunocytochemistry compared with conventional neuropathologic techniques. Neurology 38:1688–1693
11. Delaère P, He Y, Fayet G et al (1993) bA4 deposits are constant in the brain of the oldest old: an immunocytochemical study of 20 French centenarians. Neurobiol Aging 14:191–194
12. Snowdon D, Greiner L, Mortimer J et al (1997) Brain infarction and the clinical expression of Alzheimer disease. The Nun Study. JAMA 277:813–817
13. Aizenstein HJ, Nebes RD, Saxton JA et al (2008) Frequent amyloid deposition without significant cognitive impairment among the elderly. Arch Neurol 65:1509–1517
14. American Psychiatric Association (1994) Diagnostic and statistical manual of mental disorders, 4th edn. American Psychiatric Association, Washington, DC
15. Skoog I (2008) Mental disorders associated with aging. In: Heggenhougen K, Quah S (eds) International encyclopedia of public health, vol 6. Academic, San Diego, pp 174–182
16. Ernst C, Angst J (1995) Depression in old age. Is there a real decrease in prevalence? A review. Eur Arch Psychiatry Clin Neurosci 245:272–287
17. Riedel-Heller SG, Busse A, Angermeyer MC (2006) The state of mental health in old-age across the 'old' European Union – a systematic review. Acta Psychiatr Scand 113:388–401
18. Skoog I, Nilsson L, Landahl S et al (1993) Mental disorders and the use of psychotropic drugs in an 85-year-old urban population. Int Psychogeriatr 5:33–48
19. Beekman ATF, Deeg DJH, van Tilburg T et al (1995) Major and minor depression in later life: a study of prevalence and risk factors. J Affect Disord 36:65–75
20. Ritchie K, Artero S, Beluche I et al (2004) Prevalence of DSM-IV psychiatric disorder in the French elderly population. Br J Psychiatry 184:147–152
21. McDougall FA, Kvaal K, Matthews FE et al (2007) Medical Research Council Cognitive Function and Ageing Study. Prevalence of depression in older people in England and Wales: the MRC CFA Study. Psychol Med 37:1787–1795
22. Steffens DC, Skoog I, Norton MC et al (2000) Prevalence of depression and its treatment in an elderly population: the Cache County study. Arch Gen Psychiatry 57:601–607
23. Jorm AF (2000) Does old age reduce the risk of anxiety and depression? A review of epidemiological studies across the adult life span. Psychol Med 30:11–22
24. Palsson S, Skoog I (1997) The epidemiology of affective disorders in the elderly: a review. Int Clin Psychopharm 12(suppl 2):S3–S13
25. Palsson SP, Östling S, Skoog I (2001) The incidence of first-onset depression in a population followed from the age of 70 to 85. Psychol Med 31:1159–1168
26. Palsson S, Johansson B, Berg S et al (2000) A population study on the influence of depression on neuropsychological functioning in 85-year-olds. Acta Psychiatr Scand 101:185–193

27. Persson G, Skoog I (1992) Subclinical dementia: relevance of cognitive and affective symptoms and signs. A nine year prospective study. J Geriatr Psychiatry Neurol 5:172–178
28. Copeland JRM, Davidson IA, Dewey ME et al (1992) Alzheimer's disease, other dementias, depression and pseudodementia: prevalence, incidence and three-year outcome in Liverpool. Br J Psychiatry 161:230–239
29. Henderson AS, Korten AE, Jacomb PA et al (1997) The course of depression in the elderly: a longitudinal community-based study in Australia. Psychol Med 27:119–129
30. Palsson S (2000) Population studies on depression in the elderly. Prevalence, incidence and relation to cognitive function and dementia. Dissertation, University of Gothenburg
31. Ownby RL, Crocco E, Acevedo A et al (2006) Depression and risk for Alzheimer disease: systematic review, meta-analysis, and metaregression analysis. Arch Gen Psychiatry 63:530–538
32. Skoog I (1993) The prevalence of psychotic, depressive and anxiety syndromes in demented and non-demented 85-year-olds. Int J Geriatr Psychiatry 8:247–253
33. Savva GM, Zaccai J, Matthews FE et al (2009) Medical Research Council Cognitive Function and Ageing Study. Prevalence, correlates and course of behavioural and psychological symptoms of dementia in the population. Br J Psychiatry 194:212–219
34. Petrovic M, Hurt C, Collins D et al (2007) Clustering of behavioural and psychological symptoms in dementia (BPSD): a European Alzheimer's disease consortium (EADC) study. Acta Clin Belg 62:426–432
35. Östling S, Skoog I (2002) Psychotic symptoms and paranoid ideation in a nondemented population-based sample of the very old. Arch Gen Psychiatry 59:53–59
36. Östling S, Börjesson-Hansson A, Skoog I (2007) Psychotic symptoms and paranoid ideation in a population-based sample of 95-year-olds. Am J Geriatr Psychiatry 15:999–1004
37. Sigström R, Skoog I, Sacuiu S et al (in press) The prevalence of psychotic symptoms and paranoid ideation in a non-demented population sample of 70-82 year olds. Int J Geriatr Psychiatry
38. Östling S, Johansson B, Skoog I (2004) Cognitive test performance in relation to psychotic symptoms and paranoid ideation in non-demented 85-year-olds. Psychol Med 34:443–450
39. Skoog I (2006) Vascular dementia. In: Pathy MSJ, Sinclair AJ, Morley JE (eds) Principles and practice of geriatric medicine, 4th edn. Wiley, Chichester, pp 1103–1110
40. Breteler MMB, Claus JJ, Grobbee DE et al (1994) Cardiovascular disease and distribution of cognitive function in elderly people: the Rotterdam Study. BMJ 308:1604–1608
41. Breteler MMB, van Swieten JC, Bots ML et al (1994) Cerebral white matter lesions, vascular risk factors, and cognitive function in a population-based study: the Rotterdam Study. Neurology 44:1246–1252
42. Breteler MMB, van Amerongen NM, van Swieten JC et al (1994) Cognitive correlates of ventricular enlargement and cerebral white matter lesions on magnetic resonance imaging. The Rotterdam Study. Stroke 25:1109–1115
43. Skoog I, Berg S, Johansson B et al (1996) The influence of white matter lesions on neuropsychological functioning in demented and non-demented 85-year-olds. Acta Neurol Scand 93:142–148
44. Linden T, Skoog I, Fagerberg B et al (2004) Cognitive impairment and dementia 20 months after stroke. Neuroepidemiology 23:45–52
45. Qiu C, Skoog I, Fratiglioni L (2002) Occurrence and determinants of Vascular Cognitive Impairment. In: Erkinjuntti T, Gauthier S (eds) Vascular cognitive impairment. Martin Dunitz, London, pp 61–83
46. Tatemichi TK, Desmond DW, Mayeux R et al (1992) Dementia after stroke: baseline frequency, risks, and clinical features in a hospitalized cohort. Neurology 42:1185–1193
47. Tatemichi TK, Desmond DW, Paik M et al (1993) Clinical determinants of dementia related to stroke. Ann Neurol 33:568–575
48. Tatemichi TK, Paik M, Bagiella E et al (1994) Dementia after stroke is a predictor of long-time survival. Stroke 25:1915–1919

49. Pohjasvaara T, Erkinjuntti T, Vataja R et al (1997) Dementia three months after stroke. Baseline frequency and effect of different definitions of dementia in the Helsinki Stroke Aging Memory (SAM) cohort. Stroke 28:785–792
50. Liebetrau M, Steen B, Skoog I (2003) Stroke in 85-year-olds. Prevalence, incidence, risk factors and relation to mortality and dementia. Stroke 34:2617–2622
51. Skoog I (1998) Guest editorial. Status of risk factors for vascular dementia. Neuroepidemiology 17:2–9
52. Barker WW, Luis CA, Kashuba A et al (2002) Relative frequencies of Alzheimer disease, Lewy body, vascular and frontotemporal dementia, and hippocampal sclerosis in the State of Florida Brain Bank. Alzheimer Dis Assoc Disord 16:203–212
53. Fischer P, Gatterer G, Marterer A et al (1990) Course characteristics in the differentiation of dementia of the Alzheimer type and multi-infarct dementia. Acta Psychiatr Scand 81:551–553
54. Ferrucci L, Guralnik J, Salive M et al (1996) Cognitive impairment and risk of stroke in the older population. J Am Geriatr Soc 44:237–241
55. Gale C, Martyn C, Cooper C (1996) Cognitive impairment and mortality in a cohort of elderly people. Br Med J 312:608–611
56. Zhu L, Fratiglioni L, Guo Z et al (2000) Incidence of stroke in relation to cognitive function and dementia in the Kungsholmen Project. Neurology 54:2103–2107
57. Folstein MF, Maiberger R, McHugh PR (1977) Mood disorder as a specific complication of stroke. J Neurol Neurosurg Psychiatry 40:1018–1020
58. Rao R, Jackson S, Howard R (2001) Depression in older people with mild stroke, carotid stenosis and peripheral vascular disease: a comparison with healthy controls. Int J Geriatr Psychiatry 16:175–183
59. Burvill PW, Johnson GA, Jamrozik KD et al (1995) Prevalence of depression after stroke: the Perth Community Stroke Study. Br J Psychiatry 166:320–327
60. Ng KC, Chan KL, Straughan PT (1995) A study of post-stroke depression in a rehabilitative center. Acta Psychiatr Scand 92:75–79
61. Pohjasvaara T, Leppavuori A, Siira I et al (1998) Frequency and clinical determinants of poststroke depression. Stroke 29:2311–2317
62. Linden L, Blomstrand C, Skoog I (2007) Depressive disorders after 20 months in elderly stroke patients. A case-control study. Stroke 38:1860–1863
63. Astrom M, Adolfsson R, Asplund K (1993) Major depression in stroke patients. A 3-year longitudinal study. Stroke 24:976–982
64. Kauhanen ML, Korpelainen JT, Hiltunen P et al (2000) Aphasia, depression, and non-verbal cognitive impairment in ischaemic stroke. Cerebrovasc Dis 10:455–461
65. Hackett ML, Yapa C, Parag V et al (2005) Frequency of depression after stroke: a systematic review of observational studies. Stroke 36:1330–1340
66. Hackett ML, Anderson CS (2005) Predictors of depression after stroke: a systematic review of observational studies. Stroke 36:2296–2301
67. Ramasubbu R, Robinson RG, Flint AJ et al (1998) Functional impairment associated with acute poststroke depression: the Stroke Data Bank Study. J Neuropsychiatry Clin Neurosci 10:26–33
68. Schulz R, Beach SR, Ives DG et al (2000) Association between depression and mortality in older adults: the Cardiovascular Health Study. Arch Intern Med 160:1761–1768
69. Pohjasvaara T, Vataja R, Leppavuori A et al (2001) Depression is an independent predictor of poor long-term functional outcome post-stroke. Eur J Neurol 8:315–319
70. Schubert DS, Taylor C, Lee S et al (1992) Detection of depression in the stroke patient. Psychosomatics 33:290–294
71. Kotila M, Numminen H, Waltimo O et al (1999) Post-stroke depression and functional recovery in a population-based stroke register. The Finnstroke study. Eur J Neurol 6:309–312
72. Beblo T, Wallesch CW, Herrmann M (1999) The crucial role of frontostriatal circuits for depressive disorders in the postacute stage after stroke. Neuropsychiatry Neuropsychol Behav Neurol 12:236–246
73. Vataja R, Pohjasvaara T, Leppavuori A et al (2001) Magnetic resonance imaging correlates of depression after ischemic stroke. Arch Gen Psychiatry 58:925–931

74. Starkstein SE, Robinson RG, Honig MA et al (1989) Mood changes after right-hemisphere lesions. Br J Psychiatry 155:79–85
75. Carson AJ, MacHale S, Allen K et al (2000) Depression after stroke and lesion location: a systematic review. Lancet 356:122–126
76. Kneebone II, Dunmore E (2000) Psychological management of post-stroke depression. Br J Clin Psychol 39:53–65
77. Bos MJ, Lindén T, Koudstaal PJ et al (2008) Depressive symptoms and risk of stroke: the Rotterdam Study. J Neurol Neurosurg Psychiatry 79:997–1001
78. Liebetrau M, Steen B, Skoog I (2008) Depression as a risk factor for the incidence of first-ever stroke in 85-year-olds. Stroke 39:1960–1965
79. Salaycik KJ, Kelly-Hayes M, Beiser A et al (2007) Depressive symptoms and risk of stroke: the Framingham Study. Stroke 38:16–21
80. Frasure-Smith N, Lesperance F, Talajic M (1995) Depression and 18-month prognosis after myocardial infarction. Circulation 91:999–1005
81. Musselman DL, Tomer A, Manatunga AK et al (1996) Exaggerated platelet reactivity in major depression. Am J Psychiatry 153:1313–1317
82. Okamura F, Tashiro A, Utumi A et al (2000) Insulin resistance in patients with depression and its changes during the clinical course of depression: minimal model analysis. Metabolism 49:1255–1260
83. Vermeer SE, Koudstaal PJ, Oudkerk M et al (2002) Prevalence and risk factors of silent brain infarcts in the population-based Rotterdam Scan Study. Stroke 33:21–25
84. Vermeer SE, Prins ND, Den Heijer T et al (2003) Silent brain infarcts and the risk of dementia and cognitive decline. N Engl J Med 348:1215–1222
85. Liebetrau M, Steen B, Hamann GF et al (2004) Silent and symptomatic infarcts on cranial computerized tomography in relation to dementia and mortality. A population-based study in 85-year-olds. Stroke 35:1816–1820
86. Fernando MS, Ince PG, on behalf of the MRC Cognitive function and Ageing Neuropathology Study Group (2004) Vascular pathologies and cognition in a population-based cohort of elderly people. J Neurol Sci 226:13–17
87. Román GC (1987) Senile dementia of the Binswanger type. A vascular form of dementia in the elderly. JAMA 258:1782–1788
88. Brun A, Englund E (1986) A white matter disorder in dementia of the Alzheimer type: A pathoanatomical study. Ann Neurol 19:253–262
89. Englund E, Brun A (1990) White matter changes in dementia of Alzheimer's type. The difference in vulnerability between cell compartments. Histopathology (Oxf) 16:433–439
90. Skoog I, Gustafson D (2003) Hypertension, hypertension-clustering factors and Alzheimer's disease. Neurol Res 25:675–680
91. Guo X, Pantoni L, Simoni M et al (2009) Midlife blood pressure and late-life white matter lesions: the Prospective Population Study of Women in Gothenburg, Sweden. Hypertension 54:57–62
92. Skoog I, Palmertz B, Andreasson L-A (1994) The prevalence of white matter lesions on computed tomography of the brain in demented and non-demented 85-year-olds. J Geriatr Psychiatry Neurol 7:169–175
93. Lopez OL, Becker JT, Jungreis CA et al (1995) Computed tomography–but not magnetic resonance imaging–identified periventricular white-matter lesions predict symptomatic cerebrovascular disease in probable Alzheimer's disease. Arch Neurol 52:659–664
94. Simoni M, Pantoni L, Pracucci G et al (2008) Prevalence of CT-detected cerebral abnormalities in an elderly Swedish population sample. Acta Neurol Scand 118:260–267
95. De la Monte S (1989) Quantitation of cerebral atrophy in preclinical and end-stage Alzheimer's disease. Ann Neurol 25:450–459
96. Prins ND, van Dijk EJ, den Heijer T et al (2004) Cerebral white matter lesions and the risk of dementia. Arch Neurol 61:1531–1534
97. Gunstad J, Brickman AM, Paul RH et al (2005) Progressive morphometric and cognitive changes in vascular dementia. Arch Clin Neuropsychol 20:229–241
98. Schmidt R, Enzinger C, Ropele S et al (2003) Austrian Stroke Prevention Study. Progression of cerebral white matter lesions: 6-year results of the Austrian Stroke Prevention Study. Lancet 361:2046–2048

99. Herrmann LL, Le Masurier M, Ebmeier KP (2008) White matter hyperintensities in late life depression: a systematic review. J Neurol Neurosurg Psychiatry 79:619–624
100. Steffens DC, Krishnan KR, Crump C et al (2002) Cerebrovascular disease and evolution of depressive symptoms in the cardiovascular health study. Stroke 33:1636–1644
101. Teodorczuk A, Firbank MJ, Pantoni L et al (2009) Relationship between baseline white-matter changes and development of late-life depressive symptoms: 3-year results from the LADIS study. Psychol Med 12:1–8
102. Greenwald BS, Kramer-Ginsberg E, Krishnan KR et al (1998) Neuroanatomic localization of magnetic resonance imaging signal hyperintensities in geriatric depression. Stroke 29:613–617
103. O'Brien J, Ames D, Chiu E et al (1998) Severe deep white matter lesions and outcome in elderly patients with major depressive disorder: follow up study. BMJ 317:982–984
104. Simpson S, Baldwin RC, Jackson A et al (1998) Is subcortical disease associated with a poor response to antidepressants? Neurological, neuropsychological and neuroradiological findings in late-life depression. Psychol Med 28:1015–1026
105. Chen PS, McQuoid DR, Payne ME et al (2006) White matter and subcortical gray matter lesion volume changes and late-life depression outcome: a 4-year magnetic resonance imaging study. Int Psychogeriatr 18:445–456
106. Lim A, Tsuang D, Kukull W et al (1999) Clinico-neuropathological correlation of Alzheimer's disease in a community-based case series. J Am Geriatr Soc 47:564–569
107. Nagy Z, Esiri M, Jobst K et al (1997) The effects of additional pathology on the cognitive deficit in Alzheimer disease. J Neuropathol Exp Neurol 56:165–170
108. Heyman A, Fillenbaum G, Welsh-Bohmer K et al (1998) Cerebral infarcts in patients with autopsy-proven Alzheimer's disease: CERAD, part XVIII. Consortium to Establish a Registry for Alzheimer's Disease. Neurology 51:159–162
109. Etiene D, Kraft J, Ganju N et al (1998) Cerebrovascular pathology contributes to the heterogeneity of Alzheimer's disease. J Alzheimers Dis 1:119–134
110. Erkinjuntti T, Hachinski V (1993) Dementia post stroke. In: Teasell R (ed) Physical medicine and rehabilitation: state of the art reviews, vol 7. Hanley & Belfus, Philadelphia, pp 195–212
111. Pasquier F, Leys D (1997) Why are stroke patients prone to develop dementia? J Neurol 244:135–142
112. Skoog I, Nilsson L, Palmertz B et al (1993) A population-based study of dementia in 85-year-olds [see comments]. N Engl J Med 328:153–158
113. Wetterling T, Kanitz R-D, Borgis K-J (1996) Comparison of different diagnostic criteria for vascular dementia (ADDTC, DSM-IV, ICD-10, NINDS-AIREN). Stroke 27:30–36
114. Amar K, Wilcock G, Scott M (1996) The diagnosis of vascular dementia in the light of the new criteria. Age Ageing 25:51–55
115. Skoog I, Gustafson D (2006) Lessons learned from primary prevention trials in dementia. In: Rockwood K, Gauthier S (eds) Trial designs and outcomes in dementia therapeutic research. Taylor & Francis, Abingdon, pp 189–211

Neuropsychiatric Complications of Cerebrovascular Disease

Moises Gaviria and Rhonda DePaul Verzal

Abstract This rendition delves into several of the neuropsychiatric manifestations of cerebrovascular events, including mania, anxiety, apathy, disturbance of the sleep–wake cycle, fatigue, sexual dysfunction, cognitive impairment, empathic impairment, theory of mind, social-emotional dysfunction, involuntary emotional expression disorder, irritability, psychosis, agitation, and depression. The focus is on the manifestations of these presentations for proper diagnosis, as well as the lesion localization particular to the respective symptomatology. Furthermore, the hope is that this contribution allows for a greater awareness regarding the complications of stroke and brings attention to the sequelae from which its victims suffer.

Keywords Cerebrovascular disease • Involuntary emotional expression disorder • Neuropsychiatric complications • Stroke • Theory of mind

Introduction

Stroke is the third leading cause of death in the United States, the second leading cause of death worldwide, and a major cause of long-term physical and mental disability in stroke survivors. With estimates by the American Stroke Association of 750,000 strokes occurring annually in the United States, there are likely about 4.5 million stroke survivors in America today [1]. Additionally, economic costs of

M. Gaviria (✉) and R.D. Verzal
University of Illinois at Chicago, 1853 West Polk Street, Room 130 CMW, Mail Code 784, Chicago, IL, 60612, USA
e-mail: moi.gaviria@usa.net

M. Gaviria
Advocate Christ Medical Center, 4440 West 95th Street, Oak Lawn, IL, 60453, USA
and
14636 Golf Road, Orland Park, IL, 60462-7427, USA

R.D. Verzal
133 Edgewater Drive, Crystal Lake, IL, 60014, USA
e-mail: rhonda.depaul@gmail.com

K. Miyoshi et al. (eds.), *Neuropsychiatric Disorders*,
DOI 10.1007/978-4-431-53871-4_12, © Springer 2010

stroke in the United States have been estimated to be at least $43 billion each year [2]. A major portion of these costs are allocated toward the treatment of secondary complications, especially disability caused by depression, cognitive impairment, and other neuropsychiatric complications.

The symptomatology of stroke survivors is an array of comorbid symptoms, many of which were previously assumed to be of the same etiology or interrelated. However, given recent research among this patient population, more understanding has been gathered regarding the individual pathogenesis for many of these complications. Some of the neuropsychiatric sequelae secondary to cerebrovascular disease and their hypothesized mechanisms will be discussed here as the individual entities that they are. It is in this way that the clinician can more closely examine each symptom the individual patient suffers from and appropriately treat the exact cause of that symptom rather than approaching collective complaints and applying a generalized treatment plan. This approach may prove to be useful in the rehabilitation and treatment of neuropsychiatric complications in stroke patients leading to historical recovery in the quality of life of these patients and their loved ones.

Mania

Mania secondary to stroke, given its rarity and likely underdiagnosis, has limited appearance throughout the neuropsychiatric literature. In prior studies looking at neuropsychiatric complications following stroke, enrolled patients uncommonly suffered from poststroke mania in comparison to other psychiatric complaints [1]. Of two major studies investigating poststroke complications, one following 700 consecutive stroke patients [3] and another looking at 661 stroke survivors [4], only 6 patients in total between the two studies presented with mania secondary to stroke. Additionally, in two other considerably large community studies, the Oxfordshire Community Stroke Project and the Perth Community Stroke Project, both of which were investigating the prevalence of neuropsychiatric disorders following stroke, zero patients were found to suffer from poststroke mania [1]. When witnessed, however, mania secondary to stroke demonstrates very similar symptomatology in comparison to patients suffering from primary mania. These frequently include elation, pressured speech, insomnia, grandiosity, and flight of ideas with racing thoughts. Although the prognostic characteristics of poststroke mania are limited, it does appear that a family history of mood disorder is correlated with a higher risk of mania after stroke [1].

Despite the infrequency of poststroke mania, the lesion localization in patients suffering from secondary mania is more definitively understood. Most hypotheses related to mania and stroke location concur that right hemispheric strokes are likely responsible for the manifestation of this symptom. Prior studies have discussed that lesions in the right hemisphere lead to anterior limbic circuit dysfunction involving the orbitofrontal and basotemporal cortex in addition to the head of the caudate and dorsomedial thalamic nucleus. It has been hypothesized that a more generalized cerebral distribution may be responsible for the rarity of this symptom, given that both subcortical and limbic involvement is necessary for manic symptoms [1].

The neuropathology of poststroke manic symptoms appears to be due to a contralateral release phenomenon. It is likely that after a right hemispheric lesion there is subsequent activation of the contralateral left hemisphere. Both Starkstein and Robinson, as well as Mimura et al., have discussed the concept of left hemisphere release in postlesion mania [5]. This hypothesized pathogenesis originated during a case involving a patient who suffered from acute onset of poststroke mania after a right hemispheric infarction in the middle cerebral artery distribution. This patient's prestroke medical records included a single-photon emission computed tomography (SPECT) study, which provided a postinfarction comparison. In evaluation of these SPECT studies, it became evident that there was a definite pattern of left-sided orbitofrontal hyperperfusion associated with severe right frontal hypoperfusion only observed during the patient's poststroke manic episodes [5].

Given the rarity of this complication, information regarding its treatment is limited. Lithium has been the most commonly used therapy for patients suffering from mania secondary to stroke. However, pharmaceutical studies focused on poststroke mania are scarce to none, leaving only published case reports as the single source of reference relating to its therapy. Treatment modalities discussed throughout the literature include the use of olanzapine, carbamazepine, and valproic acid, the last of which has demonstrated the greatest documented therapeutic results. Filardi da Rocha et al. reported the use of 750 mg/day of valproic acid with good improvement of symptomatology in their 57-year-old male patient with mania secondary to a severe right temporal-parietal lobe stroke [6]. Because of the infrequency of reports investigating poststroke mania, clinicians must continue to thoroughly evaluate their stroke patients in order to ensure that this diagnosis is not missed. Once the diagnosis of mania is made, much benefit could be gained for future stroke survivors if effective treatment options are compared and documented by the neuropsychiatrists treating these patients.

Anxiety

The DSM-IV-TR criteria for primary generalized anxiety disorder includes the presence of a sustained worrying state, in addition to a minimum of three other anxiety symptoms, such as concentration difficulties, irritability, muscle tension, sleep disturbances, restlessness, and decreased energy, for a period of at least 6 months.

Although not as prevalent as poststroke depression (PSD), anxiety has also come to be regarded as a major neuropsychiatric complication severely impacting the daily functioning and quality of life of stroke survivors. In 1997, Robinson reported a mean prevalence of poststroke anxiety to be 14.4%, with some studies reporting up to 28%; however, with improved screening and diagnosis, this value is surely more common today [7]. Recent studies have demonstrated that patients who present with anxiety disorder after suffering a stroke are more likely to have impairment in psychosocial functioning and activities of daily living (AODL) than patients with generalized anxiety disorder not suffering from cerebrovascular disease [7]. Additionally, these patients were at a greater risk of comorbid insomnia and depression than their nonstroke counterparts. These findings are not only significant for the increased burden of disease on the patient but have ramifications regarding the prescribing of sleep-promoting and anxiolytic drugs, which also contribute to further difficulty in daily functioning.

In contrast to studies investigating PSD, a previous history of migraines and/or epilepsy before the insighting cerebrovascular event seem to increase the risk of poststroke anxiety [7]. In addition, anxiety secondary to stroke was related to the following demographic and clinical factors: smoking, migraine, epilepsy, previous mental disorders, comorbid depression and insomnia, stroke severity, and impairment in psychosocial functioning and in AODL. Women also seem to be more likely to suffer anxiety secondary to stroke than men, although reasons for this finding are still under investigation.

Patients diagnosed with generalized anxiety disorder secondary to stroke demonstrated lesion localization predominantly in the territory supplied by anterior circulation. Stroke survivors who suffered a lesion in the anterior circulation demonstrated worse scores on the anxiety scale than those survivors with lesions in the posterior circulation [8]. This finding may support recent hypotheses that suggest a distinction between the mechanism of poststroke anxiety and generalized anxiety. Several recent studies report that although left hemispheric strokes were found to cause comorbid depression and anxiety disorders, isolated anxiety secondary to stroke was localized to right hemispheric lesions [5], although a more specific lesion localization has yet to be identified.

Treatment modalities used for patients suffering from poststroke anxiety have primarily been based on those implicated for patients with primary generalized anxiety disorder. Studies on therapy for anxiety secondary to stroke are limited. Thus far, the recommended treatment is benzodiazepines, excluding the elderly population given reports of significant side effects. The preferable therapeutic modality in elderly patients who are unable to tolerate benzodiazepines are buspirone and selective serotonin uptake inhibitors (SSRIs).

Apathy

Apathy can be defined as lack of emotion, feeling, or concern, not attributable to an alteration in consciousness or cognition. It is prevalent in both the general psychiatric patient population, as well as in stroke survivors, with implications in the functional recovery and rehabilitation of these patients. In patients who have suffered from first-ever and/or recurrent strokes, there exists a frequency of apathy of approximately 23% [9]. This effect can be evaluated through the interpretation of the Apathy Scale proposed by Starkstein et al., which is a modified version of the apathy evaluation scale originally designed by Marin et al. Interestingly, the occurrence of depression is not significantly different when comparing patients with and without apathy, as one might expect. Poststroke apathy has been demonstrated more commonly in older patients when compared to nonapathetic stroke survivors, as well as in those who suffered from an ischemic, rather than a hemorrhagic, stroke [10].

Symptomatic lesions have been found in even distribution bilaterally throughout the brain among apathetic and nonapathetic stroke patients. Continued research is warranted by the recurrent inconsistencies regarding lesion localization in patients suffering from poststroke apathy. Chemerinski et al. reported a collective literature review demonstrating the occurrence of 93 left-sided lesions, 77 right-sided lesions, and 94 bilateral strokes resulting in secondary apathy [1]. Several factors that have been previously correlated with apathy following stroke include cognitive dysfunction, advanced age, deficits in AODL, decreased attention and information processing, and poor fluency [1]. When examining the functional level of stroke survivors, apathetic patients demonstrate a significantly lower recovery level in aspects of self-care. This aspect is of great importance when evaluating caregiver burden and the long-term ramifications that these patients and their families face during stroke rehabilitation.

Treatment recommendations for poststroke apathy include the use of various stimulating antidepressants, such as fluoxetine, for first-line therapy. Additionally, other stimulating agents, such as amphetamine, methylphenidate, selegiline, and bupropion have been used successfully to treat apathy; however, only in case reports. Recent studies have examined the role of cholinesterase inhibitors in the treatment of apathy given the activating properties of these agents and the correlation with poststroke apathy and cholinergic deficits [11].

Disturbance of the Sleep–Wake Cycle

Sleep disorders have recently become an area of medical interest given their significant impact on a patient's daily living. Pathology of sleep is a spectrum of abnormalities that affect sleep time, the sleep cycle, and breathing and activity during sleep. One example includes dyssomnias, such as insomnia and hypersomnia, in which a patient has an alteration in the amount of time asleep within a given 24-h period. On average, 7–9 h of sleep per night is considered adequate by the National Sleep Foundation in the United States, although there are some normal variants that slightly deviate from this amount. Chen et al. defined short-sleep duration as a night's sleep of 6 h or less and a long-sleep duration as more than 9 h of sleep [12]. Other sleep disorders involve disruption in the normal pattern of the sleep cycle between non-REM and REM (rapid eye movement sleep). Abnormalities within either the amount or cycling of the sleep cycle can consequentially lead to deficits in attention, memory, daily functioning, an increase in accidents, and a diminishment of overall health.

In patients who have suffered stroke, the reduction in quality of life has evoked great focus. Although the etiology of this change is multifactorial, disturbance of the sleep–wake cycle in these patients appears to be a significant contributor. Long-term follow-up of stroke survivors who have suffered from both ischemic stroke and/or subarachnoid hemorrhage reveals difficulty in initiation of sleep, irritability, loss of interests, poor concentration, fatigue, and falling asleep at inappropriate times throughout the day. Assessment of functional outcome, and therefore quality of life, has been evaluated in stroke patients using the Rankin Scale, a 6-point handicap scale focusing on restrictions of lifestyle in coordination with polysomnographic studies.

It appears that up to one-third of stroke survivors suffer from either insomnia, excessive daytime sleepiness, or both, resulting in lower values when scoring quality of life. It is important to note that sleep disturbances caused by stroke must be differentiated from sleep disturbances that are secondary to other neuropsychiatric complications of stroke, such as depression. For example, Schuiling et al. reported that sleep disturbances resulting from depression are characteristically demonstrated by short-REM sleep latency and an increased amount of REM sleep overall, whereas sleep disturbances that do not show this pattern, but occur after stroke, are more likely a result of the stroke alone and may secondarily lead to the initiation of sleep disturbance depression [13]. Landau et al. demonstrated lesion localization in patients with sleep disturbances secondary to stroke concentrated in the right pons, followed by bilateral pontine strokes, and then left pontine lesions [14]. In patients diagnosed with restless leg syndrome following stroke, Kim et al. demonstrated lesion topography predominantly in subcortical regions, such as the pyramidal tract and basal ganglia–brainstem axis [15]. This result reinforces that compromise of cerebral perfusion in areas of the brain controlling motor function and the sleep–wake cycles may result in restlessness symptoms. Treatment modalities available for these symptoms include dopamine agonists, which have delivered relatively significant relief in symptoms [15].

Fatigue

Fatigue has been known to be a common sequelae in stroke survivors, with a prevalence ranging from 38% to 68% [16]. Treating this phenomenon has proven to be quite challenging given the lack of established standards in its measurement and difficulty in determining its exact etiology. Additionally, the diagnostician must take into consideration other possible contributing factors associated with fatigue from which numerous stroke patients suffer from months to years after the inciting event; these include mental factors, such as depression and anxiety, but also might be related to physical deconditioning and gross motor deficits. Because the etiology of fatigue has proven to be so complex, it is not until recently that research has began to control for some of these confounding factors and evaluate a more central origin of fatigue in stroke survivors.

In a study investigating fatigue in stroke survivors, patients who suffered from minor strokes were compared to those who experienced a transient ischemic attack (TIA). While previous studies suggested that fatigue after stroke was attributable to compensatory behaviors related to gross neurological deficits, the comparison used in this study demonstrated that poststroke fatigue may be of central origin rather than physical sequelae secondary to increased effort required after suffering a stroke [16]. By investigating patients who suffered from minor rather than major strokes, there were minimal to no residual neurological deficits to which secondary poststroke fatigue might be attributable. These results were the first set of published data investigating fatigue in relationship to stroke using this approach.

The study evaluated 149 patients: 73 status post minor stroke and 67 status post TIA. Demographic characteristics, recent life events, vascular risk factors, medications, and mental and physical disabilities were all variables that were controlled among the two patient groups. Fatigue was evaluated at 6 months after minor stroke or TIA using the Chalder Fatigue Scale [17]. The results of the study demonstrated that patients who suffered from a minor stroke had a 56% fatigue prevalence in comparison to the TIA patients with a prevalence of 29%. This finding is one that should serve to motivate neuropsychiatrists and other clinicians to move toward the consideration of a central mechanism underlying fatigue in patients who have suffered a stroke. Additionally, collaborative efforts between researchers, physicians, and pharmaceutical experts should investigate central-acting treatment modalities for these patients. Treatment is mainly symptomatic, with the use of stimulating agents, in addition to treating concurrent neuropsychiatric complaints.

Sexual Dysfunction

In adult patients, cerebrovascular disease causes greater secondary impairment than any other major illness in the United States. Perhaps one of the most limited areas of investigation among poststroke complications is that of sexual dysfunction. Historically, the pathogenesis of sexual dysfunction was viewed as predominantly a psychogenic disorder; however, after more closely investigating patients suffering from various sexual impairments, additional hypotheses have begun to reveal themselves. Prior studies have demonstrated that sexual dysfunction after stroke is multifactorial, with both organic and psychological etiologies at its origin. Organic influences on sexual function include certain comorbid medical conditions, such as diabetes, hypertension, and cardiac disease. Psychosocial factors include loss of self-esteem, fear of another stroke, and changes within the spousal relationship [18]. More recently, physicians have recognized that in stroke patients there likely exists both a psychogenic and neurogenic pathophysiology to erectile dysfunction.

Although most research on sexual dysfunction has involved male patients, there is no doubt that this is a complication experienced by both male and female patients. One Scandinavian study reported a decline in sexual desire in three-quarters of male stroke patients and two-thirds of female stroke patients [19]. From previous studies, it is evident that major complications of concern include decreased sexual desire in both male and female patients, diminished vaginal lubrication and orgasm in female patients, and impairment in erection and ejaculation in men [18]. Additionally, these poststroke consequences extend beyond the individual to also affect their intimate relationships with their partners.

A recent study investigating sexual dysfunction in male stroke patients was aimed at correlating this impairment with brain localization of the stroke lesions [20]; this appears to be the first study to correlate specific aspects of sexual dysfunction with localization of strokes. The comparison was made between 109 male stroke patients and 109 aged-matched controls. A five-item version of the International Index of Erectile Function was use to evaluate changes in sexual desire, ejaculatory function, and sexual satisfaction after stroke. These results were then analyzed with the location of the respective patients' brain lesions.

Overall, the study demonstrated a significant decrease in erectile function in the stroke patient group. Frequency of sexual intercourse and sexual desire were both significantly reduced in this patient group. The diminished frequency in intercourse was found to be most commonly (almost 60%) secondary to the lack of sexual desire after stroke. More specifically, stroke patients suffering from ejaculation disorders demonstrated lesions in the right cerebellum. Additionally, patients experiencing decreases in sexual desire showed imaging correlations such that their brain lesions were concentrated to the left basal ganglia. Overall, these findings were able to localize patterns with certain aspects of sexual dysfunction. A larger and more inclusive study would likely be helpful in confirming these associations between sexual dysfunction and the respective neuroanatomy.

The common implication among studies evaluating poststroke sexual dysfunction is such that these impairments should be more frequently addressed and aggressively treated during the rehabilitation process in stroke survivors so that they can enjoy a healthier quality of life and continue to share and participate in intimate relationships with their partners. Although poststroke rehabilitation has shown to help in the recovery of sexual functioning, additional therapies used for sexual dysfunction unrelated to stroke may also be used.

Cognitive Performance

Neuroscience has demonstrated the association between increased cognitive impairment following infarction; however, the pathophysiology by which infarcts result in this cognitive dysfunction is incompletely understood. A popular hypothesis involves the disruption of the cerebral circuitry with resultant deficits in cognition, usually with the frontal-subcortical circuits being affected. Injury to these circuits results in deficits in memory, information processing, and executive dysfunction. Additionally, disruption of cerebro-cerebellar circuits often causes problems in higher cognitive functions.

In particular, many studies have examined the impact of location and number of infarcts on cognitive impairment. In a recent study by Saczynski and colleagues, three separate cognitive domains were investigated following the diagnosis of cerebral infarct: processing speed, memory, and executive dysfunction. In the 4,030 nondemented participants enrolled in the Age Gene/Environment Susceptibility – Reykjavik Study, it was found that those patients who suffered infarcts in multiple locations had slower processing speed, poorer performance in memory, and executive dysfunction in comparison to patients with infarcts concentrated to a single location. Interestingly, those participants who did suffer multiple infarcts within one region did not demonstrate any cognitive discrepancies from the noninfarct control group after model adjustment [21]. These findings are all independent of white matter lesions, brain atrophy, cardiovascular comorbidities, and depressive symptoms. Treatment modalities for post-stroke cognitive impairment include the use of acetylcholinesterase inhibitors, in addition to recent developments, such as the use of repetitive transcranial magnetic stimulation (TMS). A focal lesion such as a stroke may produce a state of hemispheric imbalance. TMS can be used to repair this disequilibrium between the ipsi-lesional and contra-lesional cerebrum.

Involuntary Emotional Expression Disorder

The expression of human emotion allows individuals the potential to communicate feelings to those around them; however, the pathology of emotional expression can be consequentially devastating to an individual's relationship with loved ones, the overall functional quality of life, and the ability to relate, cope, and form new bonds. Although this emotional disinhibition syndrome is observed in association with numerous neurological conditions, its application to poststroke patients has become a growing area of interest and research. Given the importance of identifying and properly treating this neuropsychiatric condition, Cummings and colleagues proposed terminology and diagnostic criteria to be applied to this involuntary emotional expression disorder (IEED) [22]. IEED is defined as uncontrollable bouts of emotional expression that are incongruent with or disproportionate to how the patient actually feels at the time of the episode.

The current definition of IEED likely results from a single pathological mechanism but is inclusive of the following clinical observations: pathological crying and laughing, emotional affective lability, emotionalism, emotional incontinence, emotion or affective pathology, and emotional dyscontrol. This syndrome has previously been referred to as pseudobulbar affect, given its origin and possible relationship to lesions damaging the neural networks or white matter tracts connecting the frontal lobes, limbic system, brainstem, and cerebellum [22]. However, because additional studies have shown that the majority of these cases of bilateral corticobulbar or corticopontine infarcts are not associated with upper motor neuron lesions, this term has more frequently been replaced by pathological affect [1]. It is crucial that the diagnostician differentiate between the aforementioned neurological disorder and others that may have a similar presentation, such as gelastic or dacrystic epilepsy (ictal laughing and crying, respectively); this emotional lability is associated with a seizure or as part of an aura [23].

The diagnostic criteria for IEED include episodes of involuntary emotional displays, such as laughing or crying, that are attributable to brain disease or injury and deviate from the patient's affective behavior before the onset of brain disease or injury [22]. The episodes are either incongruent with the patient's mood or are congruent but occur with significant exaggeration. Additionally, they may occur without any preceding stimulus. The emotional symptoms cannot be attributable to another neuropsychiatric disorder nor can they be secondary to substance use [22]. Additional clinical observations may also aid in the diagnosis of IEED, such as symptomatology stemming from geographically close cerebral pathology. This definition includes the presence of autonomic changes, as well as pseudobulbar palsy signs, such as increased jaw jerk and gag reflex, dysarthria, dysphagia, and tongue weakness [22]; however, the absence of these associated symptoms must not exclude this diagnosis as most patients with corticobulbar infarcts will present without them [1]. With the use of the Pathological Laughter and Crying Scale, previous studies have demonstrated the effectiveness of using nortriptyline for 4–6 weeks to treat patients with IEED [24]. Additionally, a double-blind drug trial using citalopram in patients with poststroke IEED also demonstrated a reduction in the number of crying spells by more than 50% [25].

Irritability

Irritability remains one of the predominant neuropsychiatric complications of stroke, with recent studies reporting close to 33% of poststroke patients suffering from irritability [26]. Irritability is one of the most common chief complaints of patients and patient's families when presenting to the neuropsychiatrist. Poststroke irritability is characterized by impatience with situations requiring delays and waiting, flashes of anger, frequent and rapid mood fluctuations, and quarreling.

Cerebrovascular disease is a pathology that not only has serious consequences for the patient himself, but also for members of the family, loved ones, or caretakers of the patient. Certain neuropsychiatric complications of stroke have a greater impact on the patient than the family; however, poststroke irritability oftentimes has a greater impact on those people who interact with the patient than the patient himself. With this consideration, identifying and properly treating poststroke irritability can significantly diminish caregiver burden. One study evaluated the caregiving experience using both the Brain Impairment Behavior Inventory (BIBI) and the companion Brain Impairment Behavior Bother Scale (BIBBS) revealing the three greatest stressors to them as caregivers. The results of this study demonstrated that patient irritability was the greatest stressor for caregivers of stroke survivors [27].

The localization of lesions in patients presenting with poststroke irritability are most commonly within the orbitofrontal lobe, the left cerebral cortex (greater than right), anterior temporal lobes (amygdale), and the limbic system [28]. Risk factors associated with increased rates of poststroke irritability include being aphasic and younger at the occurrence of the stroke. Aphasia increased the irritability rate fourfold, and patients younger than 65 years old had 2.5 times the incidence of poststroke irritability as their older counterparts [26]. Additionally, it has been observed that irritable symptoms of stroke patients usually increase at 1 year poststroke [26]; therefore, if the clinician suspects poststroke irritability, screening should take place at this time. Treatment regimens include mood stabilizers.

Psychosis

In comparison to many of the other neuropsychiatric complications of stroke, psychotic symptoms, such as hallucinations and delusions, are rare. Only five patients followed in a 9-year longitudinal study demonstrated symptoms consistent with poststroke psychosis [29]. Another study following stroke patients up to 11 years later found a total of eight patients who exhibited psychotic symptoms after right-sided temporoparieto-occipital infarcts [30]. Many of these stroke patients also experienced seizures close to the time at which psychosis was observed. Improvement of their psychotic symptoms was noted after treatment with antiepileptic medications [30].

A frontal lobe syndrome and psychosis have been observed after infarction in the brainstem dopaminergic nuclei, specifically at the ponto-mesencephalic junction. Stereotactic lesion localization on MRI in addition to concordant analysis of regional cerebral blood flow demonstrated that infarction within these nuclei likely has resultant disruption of the ascending dopaminergic projections to the frontal-subcortical circuit components [31]. In addition, a longitudinal study of stroke patients demonstrated that right frontoparietal lesions and subcortical atrophy were significant risk factors for psychosis following stroke given that nonpsychotic stroke survivors did not have these findings [29].

Agitation

Agitation following stroke is observed in approximately 28% of patients who have suffered from a cerebrovascular event. Poststroke agitation manifests primarily by stubbornness (81%), noncompliance, such as with rehabilitation, refusal to cooperate with the patient's caregiver (75%), crying and cursing (75%), and less commonly violence toward objects, such as slamming doors (2%), and never violence toward people [26]. Lesions resulting in poststroke agitation are neuroanatomically confined to the bitemporal lobes and/or the amygdale [28]. The current treatment recommendation includes mood stabilizing agents.

Depression

Given that depression is the most prevalent neuropsychiatric complication of cerebrovascular disease with the greatest quantity of studies and publications, this discussion will devote less to it.

Depression is a frequent complication of stroke, affecting 185,000 stroke survivors in the United States annually. Patients with PSD demonstrate less evidence of recovery from the functional impairments of stroke in comparison to their nondepressed counterparts, and these patients are 3.4 times more likely to die during the first 10 years following stroke [32]. Everson and colleagues [32] found that, in patients with stroke, five or more depressive symptoms at baseline were associated with significantly increased risk of mortality after adjusting for age, sex, ethnicity, education, alcohol consumption, smoking, body mass index, hypertension, and diabetes mellitus. Many patients with PSD also suffer from significant disability and an inability to carry out AODL.

PSD, with documented frequencies of up to 79% [33] of patients who have suffered a cerebrovascular accident, manifests primarily as feelings of uselessness and being a burden on caregivers and family (97%). It also frequently includes feelings of sadness (85%), crying (85%), and less commonly, pessimism and suicidal ideations, both of which are more common in primary depressive disorders [26].

Current evidence suggests that lesions in the basal ganglia or left frontal lobe have a greater association with PSD. Narushima et al. [34] performed a meta-analysis of patients with PSD and noted that there was a significant inverse correlation between severity of depression and distance of the lesion from the frontal pole among 163 patients with left hemispheric stroke, but not among other 106 patients with right hemispheric stroke. PSD is a reflection of failed functioning of critical neural networks, and neurotrophic factors such as brain-derived neurotrophic factor (BDNF) may induce antidepressant effects through neuronal plasticity and recovery of neuronal networks [34]. The most successful treatment regimens for PSD include the use of fluoxetine, followed by nortriptyline, and in some cases, citalopram, trazadone and methylphenidate [11] (Table 1).

Conclusion

This current rendition highlights some of the significant complications resulting from cerebrovascular disease. It brings to attention the importance of correct identification of these conditions to improve the quality of life, as well as the economical and social effects on stroke patients and their families. With greater awareness regarding these diagnoses, hospitalizations and caregiver burden can be decreased, and the proper diagnosis will aid in the appropriate treatment of these conditions.

References

1. Chemerinski E, Levine SR (2006) Neuropsychiatric disorders following vascular brain injury. Mt Sinai J Med 73(7):1006–1014
2. Hadidi N, Treat-Jacobson DJ, Lindquist R (2009) Poststroke depression and functional outcome: a critical review of literature. Heart Lung 38(2):151–162
3. Starkstein SE, Boston J, Robinson RG (1988) Mechanisms of mania after brain injury: 12 case reports and review of the literature. J Nerv Ment Dis 176:87–100
4. Dunne JW, Leedman PJ, Edis RH (1986) Inobvious stroke: a cause of delirium and dementia. Aust N Z J Med 16(6):771–778
5. Braun CMJ, Daigneault R, Gaudelet S (2008) DSMIV symptoms of mania: which ones result more often from right than left hemisphere lesions? Compr Psychiatry 49:441–459
6. Filardi da Rocha F, Horizonte B, Carneiro JG (2008) Poststroke manic symptoms: an unusual neuropsychiatric condition. Rev Bras Psiquiatr 30(2):168–176
7. Leppavuori A, Pohjasvaara T, Vataja R et al (2003) Generalized anxiety disorders three to four months alter ischemic stroke. Cerebrovasc Dis 16:257–264

Table 1 Neuropsychiatric symptoms and lesion localization (modified from [3])

Neuropsychiatric symptoms	Lesion localization	Treatment
Depression	L cerebral cortex, frontal lobe, frontosubcortical circuits, basal ganglia and limbic system	Fluoxetine, followed by nortriptyline, and in some cases, citalopram, trazadone, and methylphenidate
Mania	Anterior region of bilateral hemispheres, R temporal lobe, R caudate nucleus, R subcortical region, R ventral pons, L basal ganglia	Olanzapine, carbamazepine, and valproic acid
Apathy	Frontal lobe, cingulate gyrus, supplemental motor area, amygdala, capsule, insula, caudate nucleus/nuclei, bilateral anterior thalamic nuclei	Stimulating a ntidepressants, i.e., fluoxetine. Stimulating agents, i.e., amphetamine, methylphenidate, selegiline, bupropion. AChE-I
IEED	Bilateral corticobulbar tracts, L frontal cortex	Nortriptyline, citalopram
Psychosis	R hemisphere, especially temporo-parieto-occipital or frontoparietal, and thalamus	Antiepileptics
Agitation	Bitemporal, amygdala	Mood stabilizing agents
Disturbance of sleep–wake cycle	Pons (R > bilateral > L), subcortical regions such as the pyramidal tract and basal ganglia–brainstem axis	Dopamine agonists
Irritability	Orbitofrontal lobe, anterior temporal lobe (amygdala), limbic system, L cerebral cortex	Mood stabilizers
Anxiety	L cerebral hemisphere	Benzidiazepines; in elderly, SSRIs, buspirone
Sexual dysfunction	L basal ganglia, R cerebellum	Poststroke rehabilitation, nonstroke sexual dysfunction meds
Cognitive impairment	Frontal-subcortical circuits, cerebro-cerebellar circuits	Acetylcholinesterase inhibitors, TMS
Fatigue	No specific localization	Stimulating agents

IEED involuntary emotional expression disorder; *AChE-I* acetylcholinesterase inhibitors; *SSRI* selective serotonin uptake inhibitors; *TMS* transcranial magnetic stimulation

8. Dennis M, O'Rrourke S, Lewis S, Sharpe M, Warlow C (2000) Emotional outcomes after stroke: factors associated with poor outcome. J Neurol Neurosurg Psychiatry 68:47–52
9. Starkstein SE, Fedoroff JP, Price TR et al (1993) Apathy following cerebrovascular lesions. Stroke 24:1625–1631
10. Santa N, Sugimori H, Kusuda K et al (2008) Apathy and functional recovery following first-ever stroke. Int J Rehabil Res 31(4):321–326
11. Paranthaman G, Balwin R (2006) Treatment of psychiatric syndromes due to cerebrovascular disease. Int Rev Psychiatry 18(5):453–470
12. Chen JC, Brunner RL, Ren H et al (2008) Sleep duration and ischemic stroke in older women. Stroke 39:315–3192
13. Schuiling WJ, Rinkel GJE, Walchenbach R et al (2005) Disorders of sleep and wake in patients after SAH. Stroke 36:578–582
14. Landau ME, Maldonado JY, Jabbari B (2005) The effects of isolated brainstem lesions on human REM sleep. Sleep Med 6:37–40
15. Lee SJ, Kim JS, Song IU (2009) Poststroke restless legs syndrome and lesion location: anatomical considerations. Mov Disord 24(1):77–84
16. Winward C et al (2009) Fatigue after TIA and minor stroke. Stroke 40(3):757–766
17. Chalder T, Berelowitz G, Pawlikowska T et al (1993) Development of a fatigue scale. J Psychosom Res 37(2):147–153
18. Tamtam Y, Tamtam L, Akil E et al (2008) Post-stroke sexual functioning in first stroke patients. Eur J Neurol 15:660–666
19. Sjogren K, Damber JE, Liliequist B (1983) Sexuality after stroke with hemiplegia: aspects of sexual function. Scand J Rehabil Med 15:55–61
20. Jung J-H, Kam S-C, Choi S-M (2008) Sexual dysfunction in male stroke patients: correlation between brain lesions and sexual function. Urology 71:99–103
21. Saczynski JS, Sigurdsson S, Jonsdottir MK et al (2009) Cerebral infarcts and cognitive performance. Stroke 40:677–682
22. Cummings JL, Arciniegas DB, Brooks BR (2006) Defining and diagnosing involuntary emotional expression disorder. CNS Spectr 11(6 suppl 6):1–7
23. Cummings JL (2007) Involuntary emotional expression disorder: definition, diagnosis and measurement scales. CNS Spectr 12(4 suppl 5):11–16
24. Robinson RG, Parikh RM, Lipsey JR et al (1993) Pathological laughing and crying following stroke: validation of a measurement scale and double-blind treatment study. Am J Psychiatry 150:286–293
25. Andersen G, Verstergaard K, Riis JO et al (1993) Citalopram for post-stroke pathological crying. Lancet 342:837–839
26. Angelelli P, Paolucci S, Bivona U et al (2004) Development of neuropsychiatric symptoms in poststroke patients: a cross-sectional study. Acta Psychiatr Scand 110:55–63
27. Williams A (1994) What bothers caregivers of stroke victims? J Neurosci Nurs 26(3):155–161
28. Luna-Matos M, McGrath H, Gaviria M (2007) Neuropsychiatric manifestations in cerebrovascular diseases. Rev Chil Neuro-Psiquiatr 45(2):129–140
29. Rabins PV, Starkstein SE, Robinson RG (1991) Risk factors for developing atypical (schizophreniform) psychosis following stroke. J Neuropsychiatry Clin Neurosci 3:6–9
30. Levin DN, Finklestein S (1982) Delayed psychosis after right temporoparietal stroke or trauma: relation to epilepsy. Neurology 32:267–273
31. Nishio Y, Ishii K, Kazui H (2007) Frontal-lobe syndrome and psychosis after damage to the brainstem dopaminergic nuclei. J Neurol Sci 260:271–274
32. Everson SA, Robertson RE, Goldberg DE (1998) Depressive symptoms and increased risk of stroke mortality over a 29-year period. Arch Intern Med 158:1133–1138
33. Hadidi N, Treat-Jacobson DJ, Lindquist R (2009) Poststroke depression and functional outcome: a critical review of litreature. Issues Neurol 38(2):151–162
34. Narushima K, Kosier JT, Robinson RG (2003) A reappraisal of PSD, intra- and inter-hemispheric lesion location using meta-analysis. J Neuropsychiatry Clin Neurosci 15:422–430

Systemic Inflammation and Cognition in the Elderly

Julian Trollor and Emmeline Agars

Abstract A complex inflammatory cascade is an established part of the pathophysiology of Alzheimer's disease (AD), and preliminary studies have suggested a link between systemic inflammation and AD. Recent research has extended this theme by examining the influence of systemic inflammation on cognitive function in community-dwelling elderly. Preliminary findings suggest that elevated levels of some inflammatory markers such as interleukin-6 (IL-6) and C-reactive protein (CRP) are associated with poorer cognition at cross-sectional assessment. Longitudinal studies suggest an impact of raised IL-6 and CRP, in terms of both cognitive decline and outcome of dementia. Although findings vary considerably between studies, systemic inflammation may have relevance for cognitive function and cognitive decline in late life. Further comprehensive studies are required to further explore the relationship between systemic inflammation and cognition in the elderly.

Keywords Cognition • Cytokines • Dementia • Inflammation • Mild cognitive impairment

---

E. Agars and J. Trollor
Brain and Ageing Program, School of Psychiatry, University of New South Wales, Sydney, NSW 2052, Australia

J. Trollor (✉)
Department of Developmental Disability Neuropsychiatry, School of Psychiatry, University of New South Wales, Sydney, NSW 2052, Australia
and
University of New South Wales, 34 Botany Street, UNSW, Sydney, NSW 2052, Australia
e-mail: j.trollor@unsw.edu.au

K. Miyoshi et al. (eds.), *Neuropsychiatric Disorders*,
DOI 10.1007/978-4-431-53871-4_13, © Springer 2010

Introduction

Systemic inflammation has been associated with increased risk of age-related disorders such as AD. The cross-sectional relationship between systemic inflammation and cognition in nondemented elders is less clear. Furthermore, whether systemic inflammation has relevance for change in cognition over time remains uncertain. The way in which systemic inflammation influences cognition in ageing and age-related cognitive disorders is complex and is likely modified by interplay among many factors such as physical health, lifestyle, nutrition, and genes. Given the findings in AD, it is important to clarify the relationship between systemic inflammation and risk of cognitive decline in late life. If a significant relationship is identified, moderation of systemic inflammation may be an important therapeutic target that may ultimately reduce the burden of age-related neuropsychiatric disorders. This chapter reviews the literature that examines the impact of systemic inflammation and cognition in community-dwelling elders.

Background

Inflammation and Alzheimer's disease

A link between inflammation and cognition was hypothesized after discovery of upregulated inflammatory processes in post-mortem Alzheimer's disease (AD) brain specimens [1, 2]. Subsequent research has suggested a pivotal role of inflammation in Alzheimer pathology involving activation of microglia, astrocytes, and the complement system as well as increased cytokine expression and acute-phase protein response [3, 4]. Support for a role of inflammation in AD also comes from epidemiological studies that demonstrate a protective effect of anti-inflammatory agents for AD [5]. A meta-analysis of seven small case-control studies [6] determined a substantially reduced odds ratio (0.556, $P<0.0001$) for development of AD in arthritis patients, but nonsteroidal anti-inflammatory drug trials in dementia have thus far been unsuccessful [7].

The relationship between systemic inflammation and dementia has been investigated in several cross-sectional studies. Among the most consistent findings are an association between cytokines such as interleukin-1α (IL-1α), IL-6, and tumor necrosis factor-α (TNF-α) with dementia in clinical populations [8–12]. The relationship between inflammatory factors and dementia subtype has varied among studies [11–13]. Recent work has also suggested a cross-sectional link between TNF-α and mild cognitive impairment (MCI) [9].

Additional evidence for the role of inflammatory modulators in the pathogenesis of AD comes from studies that show the risk of AD is affected by genetic variation in inflammatory modulators such as IL-1α, interleukin-1β (IL-1β), IL-6, TNF-α, α2-macroglobulin, and α1-antichymotrypsin [14]. Polymorphic variation in the

IL-6 gene is associated with lower risk of developing AD [15], and IL-6 mRNA levels may also predict the clinical progression of the disease [16]. Of interest is the demonstration of interactive effects with other alleles known to confer risk for AD. For example, McCusker et al. [17] demonstrated that, in those carrying the apolipoprotein E4 (ApoEε4) allele, TNF-α substantially increased the risk of AD. Nicoll et al. [18] demonstrated that simultaneous inheritance of the high-risk alleles for IL-1α (IL-1α-889) and IL-β (IL-β+3953) increased the odds of developing AD by 10.8 [18]. Taken together, available data suggest that AD risk may be influenced by inflammatory factors in relationship to both serum measures and "genetic susceptibility profile." The data not only underscore the importance of inflammation in AD but raise the possibility that inflammatory processes may be relevant to cognitive ageing in nonclinical populations. The relevance of inflammation in this context is best examined in community-dwelling ageing populations, which are the main focus in this chapter.

"Inflammaging"

The term "inflammaging" has been used to describe the progressive increase in systemic inflammation with advancing age and is characterized by a decline in adaptive immune mechanisms, upregulation of the innate immune system, and a resultant low-grade, chronic inflammatory response. Central to this process is the overactivation of mononuclear phagocytes, which results in elevation of cytokine levels [19, 20]; this comes at a time when the brain may be more susceptible to adverse effects of inflammation. For example, animal studies demonstrate an increased susceptibility of the aged brain to oxidative stress and inflammation [21], affording a greater potential impact of inflammation on cognitive function. The brain has been traditionally viewed as an immune-privileged site. However, recent research indicates the peripheral immune system and the central nervous system (CNS) communicate extensively [22]. Such communication raises a number of possibilities regarding the relationship between cognitive function and inflammation. For example, peripherally generated inflammation may be a response or contributor to CNS inflammation and pathology [7].

Whether "inflammaging" or increased susceptibility to its effects translates into meaningful change in cognitive function or confers greater risk of cognitive decline is uncertain and is the subject of this review. To explore this issue, a MEDLINE search was conducted using the MESH term "inflammation" or keyword "inflammatory markers" and MESH terms "cognition" or "cognition disorders." The search strategy identified those articles published in the English language until July 2009. Articles were examined in detail only if the participants were drawn from nonclinical populations, and only if the study included participants ≥65 years of age. Reference lists were cross-checked for additional articles not initially identified by the search strategy. The cross-sectional and longitudinal data from studies fulfilling the selection criteria are summarized in Tables 1 and 2, respectively.

Table 1 Cross-sectional studies of circulating inflammatory markers and cognitive function in community-dwelling elderly populations

	Inflammatory marker/s	Study population	Cognitive tests	Outcomes	Covariates	Results
Alley et al.[23]	IL-6 CRP	851 Community-dwelling elders, 70–79 years, USA	Similarities subset of Wechsler Adult Intelligence Scale-Revised, copying geometric figures, delayed recognition Span test, modified Boston Naming test, incidental recall on naming items, abbreviated short portable mental status questionnaire	Individual cognitive tests/domains and global cognitive function	Age, sex, race, education, income, DM, MI, stroke, hip #, BP, HbA1c, HDL, waist circumference, NSAIDs, alcohol, smoking, physical activity	Before covariate inclusion, raised IL-6 and CRP were inversely associated with abstraction and language ability ($P<0.05$) and global cognition ($P<0.001$); IL-6 alone associated with poor spatial ability ($P<0.01$) and CRP with short portable mental status questionnaire ($P<0.01$); all results nonsignificant after inclusion of covariates
Baune et al.[24]	IL-1β sIL-4R IL-6 IL-8 IL-10 IL-12 TNF-α	369 Community-dwelling participants, >65 years, mean age 72.6 years, Germany	Three word recall test (Tulving and Colotla lag measures), word fluency, Stroop color-word test, Wechsler Adult Intelligence scales digit symbol test, Purdue Pegboard test, MMSE	Individual cognitive tests/domains	Age, gender, education, smoking, depressive symptoms, TIA, stroke, DM	Increased IL-8 inversely associated with memory ($P<0.01$), cognitive speed ($P<0.001$) and motor function ($P<0.01$)

Sweat et al. [25]	CRP	125 Community-dwelling 42–82-year-olds, categorized by BMI, USA	California Verbal Learning test, Wechsler Memory Scale-Revised, Digit Span Backwards, Visual Memory Span Backwards, Colorado Assessment tests: Tower of London, Shipley Institute of Living Scale	Individual cognitive tests/domains	Age, education, DM, statins	Significant inverse association between CRP and cognition only in overweight and obese women: executive function and figural memory ($P<0.01$), estimated IQ and general cognitive functioning ($P<0.05$)
Schram et al.[26]						
1. Rotterdam Study	IL-6 CRP α1-Antichymo-trypsin	3,874 Community-dwelling elderly, mean age, 72 years, Netherlands	MMSE, abbreviated Stroop test part 3, Letter Digit Substitution Task, word fluency, Geriatric Mental Status schedule	Individual cognitive tests/domains	Age, sex, education	CRP and IL-6 inversely associated with global cognition and executive functioning ($P<0.01$), IL-6 was also inversely associated with MMSE score ($P<0.05$)
2. Leiden 85-plus Study	IL-6 CRP	491 Community-dwelling 85-year-olds, Netherlands	MMSE, abbreviated Stroop test part 3, Letter Digit Substitution Task, Geriatric Mental Status schedule, 12-Picture Learning test	Individual cognitive tests/domains	Age, sex, education	No significant association
Fischer et al.[27]	CRP Homocysteine Fibrinogen	606 Community-dwelling 75-year-olds, Austria	MMSE	Global cognitive function	Sex, BP, total cholesterol, LDL, HDL, TG, antihypertensive medications, statins, smoking	No significant association

(continued)

Table 1 (continued)

	Inflammatory marker/s	Study population	Cognitive tests	Outcomes	Covariates	Results
Dik et al. [28]	IL-6 CRP α1-Antichymotrypsin Albumin	1,284 Community dwelling 62–85-year-olds, Netherlands	MMSE, Auditory Verbal Learning task, Raven's colored progressive matrices, Alphabet coding task-15	Individual cognitive tests/domains	Age, sex, education	Serum α1-antichymotrypsin inversely associated with delayed recall ($P<0.05$) and albumin inversely associated with MMSE score ($P=0.05$)
Ravaglia et al. [29]	CRP	540 Cognitively intact elders, mean age, 73 years, Italy	MMSE	Global cognitive function	Age, sex, education, fibrinogen, leukocyte count, albumin, BMI, DM, IHD, PVD, cerebrovascular disease, chronic pulmonary disease, peptic ulcer, edentulism	Raised CRP inversely associated with MMSE score
Elwan et al. [30]	IL-6 ICAM-1 ApoE genotyping	94 Neurologically intact healthy Egyptians, age range, 40–82 years, mean, 58.5 years	Paced Auditory Serial Addition test, Intentional and Incidental memory test, Digit Symbol Substitution test, Trail Making test A and B, Eysenck Personality questionnaire	Individual cognitive tests/domains	Age, sex, education	Raised IL-6 inversely associated with attention and intentional (sensory) memory ($P<0.05$); ApoEε4 genotype associated with significantly poorer intentional memory ($P<0.05$)

Teunissen et al. [31]	IL-6 IL-6 receptor CC16 CRP Haptoglobin	65 Community-dwelling subjects, mean age, 54 years baseline, Netherlands	MAAS protocol: Auditory Verbal Learning task, Letter Digit coding test, Stroop color-word test	Individual cognitive tests/domains	Age, sex, education	Serum haptoglobin and CRP inversely correlated with Stroop test and delayed recall ($P<0.05$)
Weaver et al. [32]	IL-6	779 Community-dwelling 70–79-year-olds, USA	Boston naming test, delayed verbal memory test, delayed recognition Span test, similarities subset of the Weschler Adult intelligence Scale-revised, copying of geometric figures	Individual cognitive tests/domains	Age, sex, income, education, ethnicity, alcohol, physical activity, BMI, HbA1c, DM, cancer	No significant associations
Bruunsgaard et al. [33]	IL-6 TNF-α CRP sTNFR-II	126 Centenarians, 45 81-year-olds, 23 55–65-year-olds, 38 18–30-year-olds, Denmark	MMSE, Lawton's instrumental ADL scale, caregiver's information, categorized by CDR scale	Dementia severity	Age, cancer, acute and chronic inflammatory illness, anti-inflammatory drugs, antibiotics, stroke, TIA, atherosclerosis, leukocyte subsets	TNF-α levels correlated with dementia severity ($P<0.05$)

IL interleukin; *CRP* C-reactive protein; *USA* United States of America; *DM* diabetes mellitus; *MI* myocardial infarction; *Hip #* hip fracture; *BP* blood pressure; *HbA1c* glycated hemoglobin; *HDL* high-density lipoprotein; *NSAIDs* nonsteroidal anti-inflammatory drugs; *sIL-4R* serum interleukin-4 receptor; *TNF-α* tumor necrosis factor-alpha; *MMSE* mini-mental state examination; *BMI* body mass index; *TIA* transient ischemic attack; *HT* hypertension; *CVD* cardiovascular disease; *ApoEε4* apolipoprotein E4; *CERAD* Consortium to Establish a Registry for Alzheimer's disease; *LDL* low-density lipoprotein; *TG* triglycerides; *IHD* schemic heart disease; *PVD* peripheral vascular disease; *ICAM-1* intracellular adhesion molecule-1; *sTNFR-II* serum tumor necrosis factor receptor-II; *WHO ICD-10* World Health Organization International Classification of Diseases, tenth revision; *ADL* activities of daily living; *CDR* clinical dementia rating

Note: Where unspecified, results are after adjustment for covariates listed

Table 2 (continued)

	Duration	Inflammatory marker/s	Study population	Cognitive tests/ diagnostic tools	Outcomes	Covariates	Results
Ravaglia et al. [38]	4 years	IL-6 CRP α1-Antichymotrypsin	804 Participants 65 years and older, mean 74 years baseline, Italy	DSM-IV (Dementia), NINCDS-ADRDA (AD), NINDS-AIREN (VaD)	All cause dementia, AD, VaD	Age, sex, education, ApoEε4, physical activity, stroke, CVD, BMI, total homocysteine, creatinine, folate, vitamin B12	Combination of raised CRP and IL-6 predicted all cause dementia [HR = 1.57 (1.03–2.41)] and VaD [HR = 2.56 (1.21–5.50)]; combination CRP, IL-6 and α1-antichymotrypsin also predicted all cause dementia [HR = 1.70 (1.05–2.75)], whilst elevated CRP predicted VaD [HR = 2.93 (1.39–6.18)]. No inflammatory marker predicted AD risk
Schram et al. [26]							
1. Rotterdam Study	Mean 4.6 years	IL-6 CRP α1-Antichymotrypsin	3,874 Community dwelling elderly, mean age 72 years, Netherlands	MMSE, abbreviated Stroop test part 3, Letter Digit Substitution Task, word fluency, Geriatric Mental Status schedule	Individual cognitive tests/ domains	Age, sex, education	No significant associations
2. Leiden 85-plus Study	Mean 3.4 years	IL-6 CRP	491 Community dwelling 85 year olds, Netherlands	MMSE, abbreviated Stroop test part 3, Letter Digit Substitution Task, Geriatric Mental Status	Individual cognitive tests/ domains	Age, sex, education	Elevated IL-6 associated with decline in memory function ($P < 0.05$), in ApoEε4

				schedule, 12-Picture Learning test			carriers IL-6 and CRP more strongly associated with annual decline in global cognition and memory function than non-carriers ($P<0.05$)
Tan et al. [39]	Mean 7 years	IL-6CRP	691 Cognitively intact, community dwelling participants, mean age 79 years, USA	MMSE, CDR, DSM-I, dementia symptoms >6 months	AD	Age, sex, APOEε4, stroke, education, smoking, homocysteine, BMI, statins	Neither serum CRP nor IL-6 were related to AD risk
van den Biggelaar et al. [40]	5 years	CRP	267 Cognitively intact, community dwelling 85 year old participants, Netherlands	MMSE, Geriatric depression scale (GDS-15)	Global cognitive decline, depression	Sex, education, MMSE	No relationship between CRP and cognitive decline. Higher baseline CRP predicted increase in depressive symptoms ($P<0.001$)
Weuve et al. [41]	4.4–7.8 years	CRP	4,231 Female health professionals aged 60–90 years, USA	Telephone interview for cognitive status: East Boston Memory test, Wechsler Memory Scale – Revised Logical Memory subsets, delayed recall	Individual cognitive tests/ domains	Age, education, income, alcohol, HT, BMI, strenuous physical activity, smoking, hormone replacement therapy, total cholesterol:HDL, TG, DM, MI	CRP not associated with decline in cognitive function

(continued)

Table 2 (continued)

	Duration	Inflammatory marker/s	Study population	Cognitive tests/ diagnostic tools	Outcomes	Covariates	Results
Dik et al. [28]	3 years	IL-6 CRP α1-Antichymotrypsin Albumin	1,284 Community dwelling 62–85 year olds, Amsterdam	MMSE, Auditory Verbal Learning task, Raven's coloured progressive matrices, alphabet coding task-15	Individual cognitive tests/ domains	Age, sex, education	Serum α1-antichymotrypsin associated with decline in MMSE, OR = 1.60, 95% CI (1.05–2.43); CRP, IL-6 and albumin not related to cognitive decline
Tilvis et al. [42]	10 years	CRP	650 Community dwelling 75, 80 and 85 year olds, Finland	MMSE, CDR	Dementia severity	Age, sex, baseline MMSE score	Elevated CRP associated with drop in CDR class at 5 years (RR = 2.32, 95% CI (1.01–5.46) but not at 10 years
Yaffe et al. [43]	4 years	IL-6 CRP TNF-a	2,632 Community dwelling black and white elders, mean age 74 years, USA	Modified mini-mental state examination (3MSE)	Global cognitive function	Age, race, sex, education, alcohol, stroke, depressive symptoms, statins, baseline cognitive score	Only in participants with metabolic syndrome were raised inflammatory markers significantly associated with cognitive decline (RR = 1.66, 95% CI (1.19–2.32) those with metabolic syndrome and low inflammation (RR = 1.08, 95% CI (0.89–1.30)

							and those without metabolic syndrome and high inflammation (RR = 0.81, 95% CI (0.60–1.08) were not at elevated risk of decline
Engelhart et al. [44]	4–9 years	IL-6 CRP α1-Antichymotrypsin ICAM-1 VCAM-1	727 (Random subcohort of 6,713) and 188 cases classified dementia at follow-up Community dwelling population, Netherlands, mean age 71.7 years, dementia free at baseline	MMSE, Geriatric Mental State Schedule, Cambridge examination for mental disorders in elderly persons, DSM-III-R, NINCDS-ADRDA (AD), NINDS-AIREN (VaD)	All cause dementia, AD, VaD	Age, sex, education level, smoking, anti-inflammatory medications, statins, BMI, SBP, DM, Ankle-brachial index, intima media thickness of carotid artery, carotid plaques (measured 6 locations)	Elevated α1-antichymotrypsin and IL-6 associated with increased risk dementia, AD, VaD; less strong association present CRP, no association ICAM or VCAM
Schmidt et al. [45]	25 years	CRP	1,050 Japanese American men, 49–70 years at baseline, USA	Cognitive Abilities Screening instrument, Informant questionnaire on Cognitive Decline in the Elderly, CERAD battery, DSM-III-R (dementia), NINS-ADRDA (AD)	All cause dementia, AD, VaD	Age, education, ApoEε4, BMI, smoking, BP, total cholesterol, stroke, coronary heart disease, LV hypertrophy, AF, DM, ABI	Elevated CRP inversely related with incidence of all cause dementias, AD and VaD ($P<0.01$)

(continued)

Table 2 (continued)

	Duration	Inflammatory marker/s	Study population	Cognitive tests/ diagnostic tools	Outcomes	Covariates	Results
Weaver et al. [32]	2.5 and 7 years	IL-6	779 Community dwelling 70–79 year olds, USA	Boston naming test, delayed verbal memory test, delayed recognition Span test, similarities subset of the Weschler Adult intelligence Scale-revised, copying of geometric figures	Individual cognitive tests/ domains	Age, sex, income, education, ethnicity, alcohol, physical activity, BMI, HbA1c, DM, cancer	Highest tertile IL-6 associated with cognitive decline at 2.5 (OR = 2.03, 95% CI (1.30–3.19) and 7 year (OR = 1.90, 95% CI (1.14–3.18) follow-up

IL interleukin; *CRP* C-reactive protein; *USA* United States of America; *DM* diabetes mellitus; *MI* myocardial infarction; *Hip #* hip fracture; *BP* blood pressure; *HbA1c* glycated hemoglobin; *HDL* high-density lipoprotein; *NSAIDs* nonsteroidal anti-inflammatory medications; *OR* odds ratio; *CI* confidence interval; ApoEε4 apolipoprotein; *CIND* cognitive impairment no dementia; *DSM-IVR* Diagnostic and Statistical Manual of Mental Disorders, fourth revision; *NINCDS–ADRDA* National Institute for Neurological and Communicative Disorders and Stroke–Alzheimer's Disease and Related Disorder Association; *AD* Alzheimer's disease; *LDL* low-density lipoprotein; *MMSE* mini-mental states examination; *CERAD* Consortium to Establish a Registry for Alzheimer's Disease; *HT* hypertension; *BMI* body mass index; *ICAM-1* intracellular adhesion molecule-1; *VCAM-1* vascular cell adhesion molecule-1; *VaD* vascular dementia; *CVD* cardiovascular disease; *HR* hazard ratio; *CDR* clinical dementia rating; *TG* triglycerides; *RR* risk ratio; *LV* left ventricle; *AF* atrial fibrillation; *ABI* ankle–brachial index

Cross-Sectional Studies

Eleven studies report the relationship between various inflammatory markers and cognitive function (see Table 1) from cross-sectional analyses. The studies vary in size, ranging from a small Egyptian study ($n=94$) [30] to a large study of community-dwelling elders ($n=3,874$) [26]. Studies involve a diverse range of ethnic groups [24, 29, 30, 35]. Some studies include participants from mid to late life [25, 30].

The most consistently reported finding is a cross-sectional association between elevated levels of IL-6 and C-reactive protein (CRP) and poorer cognitive performance [23, 26, 32, 36]. The MacArthur Study of Successful Aging ($n=851$) assessed IL-6 and CRP in 70–79-year-olds [23]. Participants were selected on the basis of minimal cognitive disability and intact functional status. Global cognitive function was derived from a composite of five neuropsychological tests. Cross-sectional analysis revealed that both CRP and IL-6 levels were inversely related to global cognitive function ($P<0.001$) as well as individual tests of abstraction and language ($P<0.05$). IL-6 levels were inversely related to spatial ability, and CRP was inversely related to the score on the short portable mental status questionnaire. However, after inclusion of covariates in the analysis, the results of the analyses were no longer significant for IL-6 or CRP.

Schram et al. [26] investigated inflammatory markers and cognitive function in two large community-derived cohorts with conflicting results. Both were conducted in the Netherlands: the Rotterdam Study investigated 3,874 individuals aged 55 years and over (age range, 55–99 years; mean, 72) and the Leiden 85-plus Study investigated 491 individuals aged 85 years at baseline. Circulating levels of IL-6 and CRP were measured in both studies, with the addition of α1-antichymotrypsin in the Rotterdam Study. Neuropsychological testing measured mini-mental state examination score (MMSE), individual measures of executive function and memory, and a global score derived from summation of individual neuropsychological test scores. In cross-sectional analysis, the Rotterdam Study revealed that IL-6 and CRP were inversely related to global cognition and executive function ($P<0.01$) and IL-6 was inversely associated with MMSE ($P<0.05$). The Leiden 85-plus Study demonstrated no significant cross-sectional associations between inflammatory markers and cognition. This variability in results highlights the impact of methodological issues in the wider literature and may arise from differences in cohort size and age, cytokine assays (e.g., high-sensitivity CRP measured in Rotterdam Study, whole blood rather than plasma in Leiden 85-plus analysis), and inclusion of different cognitive tests.

The Longitudinal Aging Study Amsterdam reported by Dik et al. [28] was a similarly large prospective population-based cohort study. This study measured α1-antichymotrypsin, albumin, CRP, and IL-6 in participants aged 65–88 years ($n=1,284$; mean age, 75.4 years). Cognitive testing included global cognition and individual neuropsychological domains such as information processing speed, fluid intelligence, and memory (see Table 1). After adjustment, only α1-antichymotrypsin and albumin were significantly associated with delayed recall and MMSE, respectively ($P<0.05$). Similarly to observations by Schram et al. [26], Dik et al. [28] found no effect of ApoEε4 on cross-sectional analysis. Dik et al. [28] categorized markers into tertiles and dichotomized IL-6 around the detection limit to compensate for reduced assay sensitivity. However, disparities in cytokine measurement and analysis may in part explain the lack of significant results in this study. A number of other studies of community-dwelling elders have failed to establish a relationship between cognitive function and CRP [27, 28, 33]. The negative findings by Fischer et al. [27] may relate to a number of methodological problems including a very high dropout rate (60%), and the study by Bruunsgaard et al. [33] used a limited range of cognitive tests and, as it contained a large sample of centenarians, was biased toward a very old population.

Interaction between inflammatory factors, gender, and other risk variables has been demonstrated in some studies. For example, in a study of 125 community-dwelling subjects 42–82 years old, Sweat et al. [25] demonstrated an association between raised CRP and cognitive impairment in women only. As the relationship was stronger in overweight and obese subjects [body mass index (BMI) > 25] and was particularly notable for frontal-executive function, the authors suggested vascular mediation of the relationship.

Few studies have evaluated the relationship between cognitive function and a comprehensive array of inflammatory markers while controlling for possible covariates. A notable exception is the study by Baune et al. [24], which found an isolated association between IL-8 levels and poorer memory, processing speed, and motor function in a cohort of 369 older Germans [24]. This same study failed to find an association between cognitive function and IL-6 or TNF-α.

Of additional note is that our literature search also identified a small number of studies that explored the relationship between proinflammatory cytokines and cognition in midlife (not tabulated). A small initial study [31] suggested an association between higher CRP levels and poorer performance on a test of episodic verbal memory in middle-aged participants. Another study in 460 middle-aged participants demonstrated an association between higher IL-6 levels and poorer performance on tests of attention, working memory, and executive function. More recently, in a large study (n = 4,200) of predominantly male office staff aged between 35 and 55 years, Gimeno et al. [46] demonstrated an association between higher levels of CRP and poorer memory function and between higher IL-6 levels and performance on a semantic fluency task.

Longitudinal Studies

Sixteen studies reported on the relationship between inflammatory markers and longitudinal cognitive outcome (see Table 2). Higher IL-6 levels at baseline have been associated with cognitive decline in some longitudinal studies of elderly subjects [23, 26, 32, 35, 37, 43, 44] but not in others [26, 28, 38, 39]. The variability in findings in regard to IL-6 and long-term cognitive outcome is hard to explain. Although obvious methodological differences exist between studies, there are few consistent patterns that unite those studies with and without significant results. For example, those studies that failed to find a relationship were of similar overall duration, included participants of similar ages, and included similar covariates in analyses as those which found a significant relationship between IL-6 at baseline and long-term cognitive outcome. Of note is that several studies failing to find an association between cognition and IL-6 levels tended to use a less detailed cognitive battery or employed less sensitive cognitive measures such as MMSE [26, 39].

Two studies evaluated IL-6 levels at baseline in nondemented community-dwelling elders and specifically related this to dementia diagnosis at follow-up [38, 39]. The Conselice Study of Brain Aging [38] investigated the role of inflammatory markers on development of dementia in a community cohort of 804 elderly Italians cognitively intact at baseline (mean age, 74 years). After 4 years, combination IL-6 and CRP predicted all-cause dementia and vascular dementia (VaD) but not AD [hazard ratio, 2.56; 95% confidence interval (CI), 1.21–5.20]. IL-6 alone did not predict AD diagnosis. Tan et al. [39] followed 691 elders in the United States for a mean of 7 years but found no relationship between IL-6 and AD diagnosis. The small number of studies in this area makes firm conclusions impossible. However, taken together these results suggest that IL-6 levels at baseline are not strongly predictive of AD on follow-up. There is some preliminary support for a longitudinal association between IL-6 and VaD, which would be in keeping with a cross-sectional study by Zuliani et al. [11] in a clinical cohort of 222 patients derived from outpatient clinics in which higher IL-6 was associated with VaD but not AD ($P<0.05$).

Fifteen studies have examined the relationship between raised CRP at baseline and cognitive outcome at longitudinal follow-up in community-dwelling elders who were nondemented at initial assessment. Studies are divided regarding the presence of an association, with eight studies finding an association [23, 34, 36, 41–45] and seven studies failing to find an association [26, 28, 35, 37–40]. There is no specific pattern of methodological differences between those studies that did or did not find an association between CRP and cognitive outcome. Those studies that have found an association between baseline CRP and change in cognition have highlighted an association with decline in global measures of cognition [26, 43], memory function [36], dementia diagnosis [34, 38, 45], or dementia severity [42]. A specific association with dementia subtype has not been observed, but available data suggest that raised CRP at baseline is more strongly associated with VaD rather than AD [38]. This issue is complicated by the association between CRP and other known vascular risk factors, and can only be resolved by studies that comprehensively control for common vascular risks.

An interaction between CRP and some other risk variables for cognitive decline has been observed. For example, Yaffe et al. [43] observed that inflammatory markers only impacted on cognition in those with metabolic syndrome. An interaction between CRP and ApoEε4 genotype in which CRP has greater impact on cognitive decline in the presence of ApoEε4 genotype [26] has also been observed, but a contrary finding has also been published [34].

A limited number of other inflammatory markers have been examined in community samples to determine any longitudinal impact on cognitive function. Serum amyloid A (SAA) was measured in one study [35] but had no bearing on long-term cognition. The acute-phase protein α1-antichymotrypsin has been linked to cognitive decline in one study [28], but two other studies did not find an association [26, 38]. Two studies have evaluated the effect of vascular cell adhesion molecule-1 (VCAM-1) and intercellular adhesion molecule-1 (ICAM) [37, 44]. No association between VCAM and cognitive decline has been demonstrated, but one study [37] did show an association between ICAM and decline in global cognitive measures and nonverbal reasoning after 4 years of follow-up.

It is noteworthy that a small number of longitudinal studies have examined the relationship between inflammatory markers and cognition in midlife (not tabulated). A very large cohort of 4,200 office staff aged 35–55 years was examined by Gimeno et al. [46], but no association was found between IL-6 or CRP and cognitive outcome after 11 years follow-up. In contrast, a small study [31] ($n=65$) found that CRP level was inversely related to memory function after 6 years follow-up. This study did not control for lifestyle, cardiovascular, and metabolic variables commonly associated with both raised CRP and cognitive function. The effect of CRP on cognitive function may only be apparent after a lengthy period of elevation and may increase with age and vascular burden.

Discussion

The review highlights a degree of inconsistency in results of studies that examine the relationship between systemic inflammation and cognition. The most common cross-sectional finding has been the relationship between cognition and both IL-6 and CRP. Longitudinal studies suggest an impact of raised IL-6 and CRP in terms of both cognitive decline and outcome of dementia. The overall impression is that systemic inflammation may have relevance for both cross-sectional cognitive function and decline in cognition in late life. Furthermore, it is apparent that important interactions with other risk factors for cognitive disorders (e.g., ApoEε4 genotype) are only just beginning to be explored.

As can be appreciated from Tables 1 and 2, considerable methodological variation exists between studies, and this in part may account for variability in reported findings. Key issues that this review has highlighted and which could contribute to this variability include the discrepancies in study populations (ethnicity, sample size, and age); the varying sensitivity of assays for inflammatory markers; the highly variable sophistication of the neuropsychological test battery; and, for longitudinal studies, variable duration of follow-up.

One of the main issues in understanding the conflicting studies is appreciating the complexity of systemic inflammation. Peripheral measures of systemic inflammation represent the sum total influence of multiple interacting factors, ranging from inflammatory disorders to metabolic factors such as obesity through to lifestyle factors such as diet and exercise and medications being consumed. Of key importance for researchers is how to deal with multiple interacting factors as covariates in analysis. Close examination of the data to determine the relationship between the inflammatory marker of interest and other key demographic, medical, or lifestyle variables should form part of an initial approach to analysis so that the researcher can determine the range of covariates to be entered into the analysis. A consistent approach is lacking in the literature in this regard.

Another issue in progressing research in this area is enhancement of the range of inflammatory markers being studied. A more comprehensive approach could assist in identifying an array of inflammatory variables that may have an impact on cognition. Comprehensive investigations have rarely been undertaken, particularly in regard to longitudinal studies of cognition. It may be possible to build a picture of an "at-risk" inflammatory profile if a clearer understanding of the range of factors influencing cognition was appreciated. Furthermore, cohorts should ideally be characterized in a comprehensive way so that data on physical health status, lifestyle, nutritional status, and genetics can be examined and linked to inflammatory status.

Conclusion

Elevated levels of some systemic markers of inflammation, particularly CRP and IL-6, may be associated with poorer cognitive function at baseline and decline in cognition with time in the community-dwelling, nondemented elderly. Studies so far are inconsistent in findings. Preliminary literature extending to midlife populations also suggests a cross-sectional association between poorer cognitive function and elevated levels of IL-6 and CRP. Further longitudinal studies are required that include more comprehensive measures of inflammation and cognition. In particular, studies in which detailed clinical, lifestyle, and genetic data are available would help to elucidate the relationship between systemic inflammation and risk of cognitive decline.

References

1. Ishii T, Haga S, Shimizu F (1975) Identification of components of immunoglobulins in senile plaques by means of fluorescent antibody technique. Acta Neuropathol 32:157–162
2. Rogers J, Luber-Narod J, Styren SD et al (1988) Expression of immune system-associated antigens by cells of the human central nervous system: relationship to the pathology of Alzheimer's disease. Neurobiol Aging 9:339–349
3. McGeer PL, Rogers J, McGeer E (2006) Inflammation, anti-inflammatory agents and Alzheimer disease: the last 12 years. J Alzheimers Dis 9:271–276
4. Akiyama H, Bargers S, Barnum S et al (2000) Inflammation and Alzheimer's disease. Neurobiol Aging 21:383–421
5. Breitner JC (1996) Inflammatory processes and antiinflammatory drugs in Alzheimer's disease: a current appraisal. Neurobiol Aging 17:789–794
6. McGeer PL, Schulzer M, McGeer EG (1996) Arthritis and anti-inflammatory agents as possible protective factors for Alzheimer's disease: a review of 17 epidemiologic studies. Neurology 47:425–432

7. Wyss-Coray T (2006) Inflammation in Alzheimer's disease: driving force, bystander or beneficial response? Nat Med 12(9):1005–1015
8. Bermejo P, Martin-Aragon S, Benedi J et al (2008) Differences of peripheral inflammatory markers between mild cognitive impairment and Alzheimer's disease. Immunol Lett 117(2):198–202
9. Alvarez A, Cacabelos R, Sanpedro C et al (2007) Serum TNF-alpha levels are increased and correlate negatively with free IGF-I in Alzheimer's disease. Neurobiol Aging 28:533–536
10. Dimopoulos N, Piperi C, Salonicioti A et al (2006) Indices of low-grade chronic inflammation correlate with early cognitive deterioration in an elderly Greek population. Neurosci Lett 398(1–2):118–123
11. Zuliani G, Ranzini M, Guerra G et al (2007) Plasma cytokines profile in older subjects with late-onset Alzheimer's disease or vascular dementia. J Psychiatr Res 41:686–693
12. Licastro F, Pedrini S, Caputo L et al (2000) Increased plasma levels of interleukin-1, interleukin-6 and α1-antichymotrypsin in patients with Alzheimer's disease: peripheral inflammation or signals from the brain? J Neuroimmunol 103:97–102
13. Singh VK, Guthikonda P (1997) Circulating cytokines in Alzheimer's disease. J Psychiatr Res 31(6):657–660
14. McGeer PL, McGeer EG (2001) Polymorphisms in inflammatory genes and the risk of Alzheimer disease. Arch Neurol 58:1790–1792
15. Papassotiropolous A (1999) A genetic variation of the inflammatory cytokine interleukin-6 delays the initial onset and reduces the risk for sporadic Alzheimer's disease. Ann Neurol 45:666–668
16. Luterman JD, Haroutunian V, Yemul S et al (2000) Cytokine gene expression as a function of the clinical progression of Alzheimer disease dementia. Arch Neurol 57:1153–1160
17. McCusker SM, Curran MD, Dynan KB (2001) Association between polymorphism in regulatory region of gene encoding tumour necrosis factor alpha and risk of Alzheimer's disease and vascular dementia: a case-control study. Lancet 357(9254):436–439
18. Nicoll JA, Mrak RE, Graham DI et al (2000) Association of interleukin-1 gene polymorphisms with Alzheimer's disease. Ann Neurol 47(3):365–368
19. Franceschi C, Capri M, Monti D et al (2007) Inflammaging and anti-inflammaging: a systemic perspective on aging and longevity emerged from studies in humans. Mech Ageing Dev 128:92–105
20. Giunta B, Fernandez F, Nikolic WV et al (2008) Inflammaging as a prodrome to Alzheimer's disease. J Neuroinflammation 5:51–66
21. Sparkman NL, Johnson RW (2008) Neuroinflammation associated with aging sensitizes the brain to the effects of infection and stress. Neuroimmunomodulation 15:323–330
22. Wilson CJ, Finch CE, Cohen HJ (2002) Cytokines and cognition: the case for a head-to-toe paradigm. J Am Geriatr Soc 50:2041–2056
23. Alley DE, Crimmins EM, Karlamangla A et al (2008) Inflammation and rate of cognitive change in high-functioning older adults. J Gerontol A Biol Sci Med Sci 63A(1):50–55
24. Baune BT, Ponath G, Golledge J et al (2008) Association between IL-8 cytokine and cognitive performance in an elderly general population: the MEMO-study. Neurobiol Aging 29:937–944
25. Sweat V, Starr V, Bruehl H (2008) C-reactive protein is linked to lower cognitive performance in overweight and obese women. Inflammation 31(3):198–207
26. Schram MT, Euser SM, de Craen AJM et al (2007) Systemic markers of inflammation and cognitive decline in old age. J Am Geriatr Soc 55:708–716
27. Fischer P, Zehetmayer S, Bauer K et al (2006) Relation between vascular risk factors and cognition at age 75. Acta Neurol Scand 114:84–90
28. Dik MG, Jonker C, Hack CE et al (2005) Serum inflammatory proteins and cognitive decline in older persons. Neurology 64:1371–1377
29. Ravaglia G, Forti P, Maioli F et al (2005) Serum C-reactive protein and cognitive function in healthy elderly Italian community dwellers. J Gerontol A Biol Sci Med Sci 60A(8):1017–1021

30. Elwan O, Madkour O, Elwan F et al (2003) Brain aging in normal Egyptians: cognition, education, personality, genetic and immunological study. J Neurol Sci 211:15–22
31. Teunissen CE, van Boxtel MPJ, Bosma H et al (2003) Inflammation markers in relation to cognition in a healthy aging population. J Neuroimmunol 134:142–150
32. Weaver JD, Huang MH, Albert M et al (2002) Interleukin-6 and risk of cognitive decline: MacArthur studies of successful aging. Neurology 59:371–378
33. Bruunsgaard H, Andersen-Ranberg K, Jeune B et al (1999) A high plasma concentration of TNF-α is associated with dementia in centenarians. J Gerontol A Biol Sci Med Sci 54A(7):357–364
34. Haan MN, Aiello AE, West NA et al (2008) C-reactive protein and rate of dementia in carriers and non carriers of apolipoprotein APOE4 genotype. Neurobiol Aging 29:1774–1782
35. Jordanova V, Stewart R, Davies E et al (2007) Markers of inflammation and cognitive decline in an African-Caribbean population. Int J Geriatr Psychiatry 22:966–973
36. Komulainen P, Lakka TA, Kivipelto M et al (2007) Serum high sensitivity C-reactive protein and cognitive function in elderly women. Age Ageing 36:443–448
37. Rafnsson SB, Deary IJ, Smith FB et al (2007) Cognitive decline and markers of inflammation and hemostasis: the Edinburgh artery study. J Am Geriatr Soc 55:700–707
38. Ravaglia G, Forti P, Maioli F et al (2007) Blood inflammatory markers and risk of dementia: the Conselice study of brain aging. Neurobiol Aging 28:1810–1820
39. Tan ZS, Beiser AS, Vasan RS et al (2007) Inflammatory markers and the risk of Alzheimer's disease: the Framingham study. Neurology 68:1902–1908
40. Van den Biggelaar AHJ, Gussekloo J, de Craen AJM et al (2007) Inflammation and interleukin-1 signaling network contribute to depressive symptoms but not cognitive decline in old age. Exp Gerontol 42:693–701
41. Weuve J, Ridker PM, Cook NR et al (2006) High-sensitivity C-reactive protein and cognitive function in older women. Epidemiology 17:183–189
42. Tilvis RS, Kahonen-Vare MH, Jolkkonen J et al (2004) Predictors of cognitive decline and mortality of aged people over a 10-year period. J Gerontol A Biol Sci Med Sci 59A(3):268–274
43. Yaffe K, Kanaya A, Lindquist K et al (2004) The metabolic syndrome, inflammation, and risk of cognitive decline. JAMA 292(18):2237–2242
44. Engelhart M, Geerlings MI, Meijer J et al (2004) Inflammatory proteins in plasma and the risk of dementia. Arch Neurol 61:668–672
45. Schmidt R, Schmidt H, Curb D et al (2002) Early inflammation and dementia: a 25-year follow-up of the Honolulu-Asia aging study. Ann Neurol 52:168–174
46. Gimeno D, Marmot MG, Singh et al (2008) Inflammatory markers and cognitive function in middle-aged adults: the Whitehall II study. Psychoneuroendocrinology 33:1322–1334

Part VI
Neurodegenerative Disorders

Diagnosis and Clinical Relevance of Depression and Apathy in Alzheimer's Disease

Sergio E. Starkstein and Simone Brockman

Abstract Depression is one of the most common psychiatric disorders in Alzheimer's disease (AD), and depression is associated with poorer quality of life, greater disability in activities of daily living, faster cognitive decline, and higher frequency of depression and burden in caregivers. Depression in AD in usually underdiagnosed, which may be related to the lack of validated diagnostic criteria and specific instruments to assess depression in dementia. Left untreated, major depression in AD may last for about 12 months. Apathy is increasingly recognized as a major behavioral disorder in neuropsychiatric diseases, but confusion still exists as to its proper definition and assessment and whether apathy should be considered a symptom or a syndrome. Nevertheless, a variety of instruments have been developed to rate the severity of apathy in dementia, and a structured clinical interview has been recently validated. Moreover, there is now international consensus for a set of standardized diagnostic criteria to diagnose apathy in AD. Finally, apathy is a significant predictor of faster functional, mood, and motor decline.

Depression and apathy are among the most common behavioral and psychological disorders in AD. Both disorders have a strong negative impact on patients' quality of life and are related to increased burden and stress among caregivers. One of the limitations in dealing with apathy and depression in dementia is that their respective diagnoses are not straightforward. Several scales to rate the severity of depression and apathy have been validated for use in AD, but standardized diagnostic criteria have only recently been proposed. This chapter addresses different strategies currently used to diagnose depression and apathy in AD and discusses the diagnostic criteria recently proposed. Another aim of this chapter is to discuss the frequency and clinical correlates of depression and apathy in AD.

S.E. Starkstein (✉) and S. Brockman
School of Psychiatry and Clinical Neurosciences,
University of Western Australia, WA, Australia
e-mail: ses@cyllene.uwa.edu.au
and
Fremantle Hospital, Education Building T-7,
Fremantle 6959, WA, Australia

K. Miyoshi et al. (eds.), *Neuropsychiatric Disorders*,
DOI 10.1007/978-4-431-53871-4_14, © Springer 2010

Keywords Anxiety • Apathy • Dementia • Depression • Motivation

Depression in Alzheimer's Disease

Diagnosis of Depression in AD

One of the major challenges in neuropsychiatry is how to obtain a valid and reliable diagnosis of a psychiatric disorder when its symptoms overlap with the symptoms of the neurological condition. Another limitation is that common disorders such as depression in Alzheimer's disease (AD) are rarely isolated phenomena and usually coexist with other psychiatric conditions such as anxiety, apathy, pathological affective display, psychotic symptoms, and poor insight. These confounding factors may account for the lack of general consensus on the most valid and reliable method to diagnose depression in AD.

Four different strategies have been used to diagnose depression in chronic degenerative disorders. The "inclusive approach" [1] diagnoses depression based on symptoms that may or may not be related to the physical illness. This approach is the most commonly used diagnostic strategy in neuropsychiatry. The "exclusive approach," on the other hand, does not include for diagnosis those symptoms considered to be related to the physical illness [2]. The "substitutive approach" replaces overlapping symptoms of depression with psychological symptoms [3]. Finally, the "specific symptom approach" only considers for diagnosis those symptoms that were identified as belonging to a "depressive cluster" using specific statistical techniques, such as latent class analysis. In a recent study Verkaik and coworkers [4] examined potential confounders for the diagnosis of depression in AD. One main confounder is that some studies diagnosed depression on the basis of a cutoff score on a depression scale (the "continuous method") whereas other studies diagnosed depression using standardized diagnostic criteria (the "categorical method"). Other confounders identified by the authors are (1) the grouping of different types of dementia, (2) different criteria to diagnose AD, (3) different instruments to assess the severity of AD and depression, and (4) heterogeneous samples in terms of size and sociodemographic characteristics.

Diagnostic Criteria for Depression in AD

Lyketsos and coworkers were the first to propose standardized criteria to diagnose depression in AD [5]. They assessed a large sample of individuals living in the community using the Neuropsychiatric Inventory (NPI). A latent class analysis produced three clusters, one of which was characterized by depression, anxiety, irritability, and apathy. Based on this cluster, Lyketsos and coworkers proposed the diagnostic criteria summarized in Table 1. One limitation of the study lies with the use of the NPI,

Table 1 Diagnostic criteria for Alzheimer's disease (AD)-associated neuropsychiatric disturbance (adapted from [5])

A. Meeting National Institutes of Neurology and Communicative Disorders/Alzheimer's Disease and Related Disorders Association (NINCDS/ADRDA) criteria for probable AD.
B. A prominent disturbance of affect, disruptive to the patient or the care environment, and representing a change from the patient's baseline, as evidenced by the presence of one or more of the following symptoms:
   (1) Depression
   (2) Irritability
   (3) Anxiety
   (4) Euphoria
C. One or more of the following associated symptoms must be present:
   (1) Aggression
   (2) Psychomotor agitation
   (3) Delusions
   (4) Hallucinations
   (5) Sleep disturbance
   (6) Appetite disturbance
D. Symptoms from B and C co-occur most days, and the disturbance has a duration of at least 2 weeks.
E. The disturbance has its first onset within 2 years or after the onset of dementia.
F. The disturbance cannot be explained in its entirety by another cause (e.g., a general medical condition, medications, life stressors).

a useful screening instrument but without the phenomenological detail necessary to diagnose depression using diagnostic criteria such as in the DSM-IV.

A workgroup conveyed by the National Institutes of Mental Health (NIMH) proposed standardized diagnostic criteria for depression in AD (NIMH-dAD) based on expert advice [6] (Table 2). These criteria are similar to the DSM-IV criteria for major depression; but with the inclusion of irritability and social withdrawal to replace loss of libido, and loss of pleasure in response to social contact to replace loss of interest. Finally, the NIMH-dAD diagnostic criteria require only three symptoms for the diagnosis of depression, and these symptoms do not have to be present every day.

An early study from our group assessed a consecutive series of AD patients attending a memory clinic using the structured clinical interview for the DSM-III-R (SCID) [7]. The main finding was that the presence of sad mood was significantly associated with most symptoms of depression assessed by the Hamilton depression scale, such as guilt, suicidal ideation, insomnia, loss of interest, psychomotor retardation, worrying, anxiety, loss of libido, and loss of energy. The question arises as to the specificity of symptoms of depression in AD, that is, whether AD patients have symptoms of depression in the absence of sad mood or loss of interest/anhedonia (masked depression). We found that only 2% of 233 AD patients had enough symptoms to meet the DSM-IV criteria for major depression in the absence of sad mood or loss of interest/anhedonia. Moreover, we also found that AD patients who reported no sad mood had no more symptoms of depression than a group of age-comparable healthy controls.

Table 2 Provisional diagnostic criteria for depression of AD (adapted from [6])

A. Three or more of the following symptoms have been present during the same 2-week period and represent a change from previous functioning: at least one of the symptoms is either (1) depressed mood or (2) decreased positive affect or pleasure:
   (1) Clinically significant depressed mood
   (2) Decreased positive affect or pleasure in response to social contacts and usual activities
   (3) Social isolation or withdrawal
   (4) Disruption in appetite
   (5) Disruption in sleep
   (6) Psychomotor changes
   (7) Irritability
   (8) Fatigue or loss of energy
   (9) Feelings of worthlessness, hopelessness, or excessive or inappropriate guilt
   (10) Recurrent thoughts of death, suicidal ideation, plan, or attempt

B. All criteria met for dementia of the Alzheimer type.

C. The symptoms cause clinically significant distress or disruption in functioning.

D. The symptoms do not occur exclusively during the course of a delirium.

E. The symptoms are not caused by the direct physiological effects of a substance.

F. The symptoms are not better accounted for by other psychiatric conditions.

Specify if:

Co-occurring onset: if onset antedates or co-occurs with the AD symptoms
Post-AD onset: if onset occurs after AD symptoms

Specify:

With psychosis of AD
With other significant behavioral signs or symptoms
With past history of mood disorders

Taken together, these findings suggest that symptoms of depression are not rife among euthymic AD patients. It is important to note that AD patients may have poor insight into their own depressive symptoms and tend to minimize or deny their presence. Therefore, it is important to obtain collateral information when assessing patients' mood.

In a more recent study we assessed the construct of major and minor depression in a series of 670 patients with AD [8]. In this cross-sectional study, we found that 26% had major depression and an identical percentage had minor depression. The percentage of patients with three or more symptoms of depression (as required by the NIMH-dAD diagnostic criteria) but without sad mood was 22% among patients with mild AD, 23% among patients with moderate AD, and 41% among patients with severe AD, suggesting that the NIMH-dAD may have high sensitivity but poor specificity.

Another strategy to clarify the phenomenology of depression in AD is to assess the pattern of symptom improvement on the remission of depression. To this end, we examined a series of 65 patients with AD and depression who received a follow-up assessment 1–3 years later [9]. At follow-up, 33 patients had a full remission of depression whereas 32 patients continued to be depressed (with major or minor depression). The main finding was that patients with a full remission of depression had a significantly lower score on the Hamilton depression scale for the symptoms of sad mood, guilt, suicide ideation, insomnia, loss of interest, psychomotor changes, loss of energy, social withdrawal, and loss of appetite/weight as compared to patients with no remission of depression. Moreover, patients on remission also showed a significant decrease in the severity of anxiety. On the other hand, there were no significant between-group differences in the severity of apathy, supporting previous findings that showed that apathy and depression are overlapping but independent syndromes in AD [10].

Frequency of Depression in AD

Before discussing the frequency of depression in AD, it is important to note that estimates of depression in AD depend on sampling issues, diagnostic methods, and clinical manifestations. The prevalence of major and minor depression has been estimated to range between 30% and 50% [3]. Population studies reported a prevalence of dysphoria of 20% and an 18-month incidence of 18% [11, 12]. A population case-report study from the United Kingdom diagnosed major depression in 24% of their sample [13], and similar frequencies were reported in a recent study from Maastricht [14].

Clinical Correlates of Depression in AD

Depression in AD has been associated with worse quality of life, greater impairments in activities of daily living, decrease in caregiver's well-being [15], faster cognitive decline, greater health care utilization [16], higher mortality rates [17], and higher rates of nursing home placement [18]. Our group [8] found that patients meeting DSM-IV criteria for either minor or major depression had more severe social dysfunction and greater impairment in activities of daily living than AD patients without depression. Furthermore, AD patients with major depression had more severe anxiety, apathy, delusions, and parkinsonism than patients with minor depression, suggesting that the severity of psychopathological and neurological impairments in AD increases with increasing severity of depression. On the other hand, patients with either major or minor depression had similar deficits on activities of daily living and social functioning, suggesting that even mild levels of depression are significantly associated with increased functional impairment in AD. Depression among nursing home patients with AD has been associated with relatively more severe malnutrition, behavioral problems, noncompliance with treatment, increased nursing staff time, and excessive mortality rate [19].

Conclusion

Depression is among the most frequent psychiatric disorders in AD. One important limitation to the diagnosis of depression in AD is the lack of valid and reliable criteria.

Recent studies proposed standardized diagnostic criteria for depression in AD for empirical validation. Our group demonstrated the validity of the DSM-IV criteria for major depression in several studies [7, 8]. Depression is associated with a poor quality of life for both patients and caregivers [15]. Depressed AD patients have a faster functional decline, earlier admission to nursing homes, and higher mortality. Future studies should examine whether the successful treatment of depression in AD may have a beneficial impact upon the comorbid conditions of depression.

Apathy in AD

Apathy is defined as a psychiatric syndrome characterized by deficits in goal-directed behaviors as manifested by the simultaneous diminution of cognitive and emotional concomitants of goal-directed behavior [20]. A similar division of apathy into emotional, cognitive and behavioral domains was proposed by van Reekum and coworkers [21]. More recently, Levy and Dubois suggested that apathy should be defined as an observable behavioral syndrome consisting of a quantitative reduction in self-generated voluntary and purposeful behaviors [22].

One of the limitations for the diagnosis of apathy in AD is that this syndrome is subsumed under different terms such as athymormia, psychic akinesia, abulia, and the negative syndrome. There is also a paucity of structured interviews to diagnose apathy in dementia, and specific diagnostic criteria have only recently been validated. We discuss here the different instruments and strategies to diagnose apathy in AD, and we also discuss the major comorbid disorders of apathy in dementia.

Diagnosis of Apathy in AD

Although the ICD-10 makes no reference to apathy, the DSM-IV mentions apathy as a subtype of personality disorder caused by a General Medical Condition. Our group has validated a set of standardized criteria for the diagnosis of apathy in AD [23]. To this aim, we assessed a series of 319 patients with AD using the apathy scale (a severity rating scale) and found that 13% of the sample met our ad hoc criteria for apathy. These criteria have been recently updated by Starkstein and Leentjens [24] (Table 3). On the other hand, none of a series of 46 age-comparable healthy controls demonstrated apathy. It is important to note the overlap between depression and apathy in AD: 13% of the AD sample had apathy and no depression, but 24% had both depression and apathy. AD patients with apathy only and patients with neither apathy nor depression had similar scores on the Hamilton depression scale, suggesting that apathy does not artificially increase depression scores in this population.

The European Psychiatric Association Task Force on apathy has recently published standardized diagnostic criteria for apathy in AD [25]. These criteria

Table 3 Diagnostic criteria for apathy (adapted from [24])

A. Lack of motivation relative to the patient's previous level of functioning or the standards of his or her age and culture as indicated either by subjective account or observation by others.

B. Presence *for at least 4 weeks, during most of the day*, of at least one symptom belonging to each of the following three domains:

Diminished goal-directed behavior

(1) Lack of effort or energy to perform everyday activities

(2) Dependency on prompts from others to structure everyday activities

Diminished goal-directed cognition

(3) Lack of interest in learning new things, or in new experiences

(4) Lack of concern about one's personal problems

Diminished concomitants of goal-directed behavior

(5) Unchanging or flat affect

(6) Lack of emotional responsivity to positive or negative events

C. The symptoms cause clinically significant distress or impairment in social, occupational, or other important areas of functioning.

D. The symptoms are not caused by diminished level of consciousness or the direct physiological effects of a substance.

follow the same general structure as the standardized criteria published by Starkstein and Leentjens, but were made more sensitive by requiring symptoms on two of the three domains rather than symptoms in each of the three domains. Regardless of which criteria are used, it is important to note the suggestion by Marin and Wilkosz [26] that apathy should be diagnosed only after a comprehensive mental state examination, which should include assessments of the individual's social and physical environment, variability in human goals, interests, emotional displays, and activities, as well as their level of education, social status, age cohort, and other cultural factors.

Several instruments are currently used to measure the severity of apathy in AD. Marin and coworkers were the first to develop a specific scale to measure the severity of apathy. The apathy evaluation scale (AES) [27] has three versions: a self-rated scale, a caregiver version, and a clinician version. Starkstein and coworkers developed the apathy scale [28], an abridged and modified version of Marin's scale. This scale has been validated for use in AD, Parkinson's disease, and stroke. Cummings and coworkers developed the NPI [29], an instrument administered to caregivers that includes a specific module on apathy. The dementia apathy interview and rating [30] assesses dementia-related changes in motivation, emotional responsiveness, and engagement. Finally, Robert and coworkers developed the apathy inventory [31], which rates several dimensions of apathy such as emotional blunting, lack of initiative, and loss of interest.

To our knowledge, there is one single structured interview for apathy in AD. Starkstein and coworkers developed the structured clinical interview for apathy (SCIA) to screen for symptoms of apathy into standardized diagnostic criteria [23]. The SCIA includes a series of questions to assess the domains of lack of motivation, lack of effort, dependency on others, lack of interest and concern, and blunted affect. Based on responses to these questions, a diagnosis of apathy may be made using the Starkstein and Leentjens' or the European diagnostic criteria for apathy.

Differential Diagnosis of Apathy in AD

The first differential diagnosis to be considered is abulia, defined by Ribot as a "loss, lack or impairment of the power of the will to execute what is in mind" [32]. Marin considered abulia and apathy to be on a continuum of motivational and emotional deficits, with abulia as the most severe manifestation [20]. Marin defined abulia as poverty of behavior and speech output, lack of initiative, loss of emotional responses, psychomotor slowing, and prolonged speech latency [20]. Akinetic syndromes have been described to range from psychic akinesia (defined as the lack of goal-directed activities among patients who are fully responsive), to akinetic mutism (defined as a state of immutability caused by lack of voluntary movement, mutism, and vigilant gaze) [33]. Laplane and Dubois [34] described the "auto-activation deficit," which is characterized by inertia, mental emptiness, stereotyped activities, flat affect, and blunted emotional responses. A full reversal of the negative state on external stimulation was suggested as the main difference between this syndrome and abulia.

Frequency of Apathy in AD

In a recent study, Starkstein and coworkers [35] examined the frequency of apathy in a series of 319 patients with AD, 117 patients with depression but no dementia, and 36 age-comparable healthy individuals. Apathy was diagnosed in 37% of the AD patients, in 32% of the depressed patients, and in none of the healthy controls. A Latin American study [36] examined 60 AD patients with the NPI, reporting a frequency of apathy of 53%. A similar frequency (59%) was recently reported by an American study [37].

Clinical Correlates of Apathy in AD

In a recent series of longitudinal studies, our group examined the predictive validity of apathy in AD. The first study included a series of patients who were followed for 1–4 years [38]. At baseline, apathy was significantly associated with older age and depression (both major and minor). The frequency of apathy increased from 14% in the stage of very mild AD to 61% in the stage of severe AD. Therefore, cognitive deficits are not sufficient to produce apathy in AD because about half the patients with moderate or severe dementia did not show apathy. Whether cognitive deficits are necessary to produce apathy has not been yet determined, but most studies assessing patients with a variety of neurological conditions such as stroke and Parkinson's disease found a significant association between greater apathy and more severe cognitive impairments [39, 40]. At follow-up, patients with apathy at baseline or patients who developed apathy during follow-up had a significant increase in Hamilton depression scale scores compared to AD patients with no apathy at baseline. Moreover, patients with apathy at baseline or those who developed apathy during follow-up had a significantly greater functional and cognitive decline and more severe parkinsonism than patients without apathy at baseline [41]. Based on these findings, we proposed that apathy may be a behavioral marker of a more "malignant" type of AD, with more severe behavioral problems and a faster cognitive, functional, and motor decline.

Conclusions

Apathy is present in about half of patients with AD and is significantly related to more severe dementia. There is a variety of instruments to rate the severity of apathy in AD, but structured clinical interviews have been developed only recently. There is now a consensus among international researchers on a common set of standardized criteria to diagnose apathy in AD. Apathy is associated with poor prognosis. Patients with apathy and dementia have a faster functional, cognitive, and motor decline than patients without apathy. Future studies should aim at finding successful therapies for apathy in dementia.

Acknowledgments This study was partially supported with grants from the University of Western Australia, and the National Health and Medical Research Council.

References

1. Cohen-Cole SA, Stoudemire A (1987) Major depression and physical illness. Psychiatr Clin North Am 10:1–17
2. Gallo JJ, Rabins PV, Anthony JC (1999) Sadness in older persons: 13-year follow-up of a community sample in Baltimore, Maryland. Psychol Med 29(2):341–350
3. Olin JT, Katz IR, Meyers BS et al (2002) Provisional diagnostic criteria for depression of Alzheimer disease: rationale and background. Am J Geriatr Psychiatry 10(2):129–141
4. Verkaik R, Nuyen J, Schellevis F et al (2007) The relationship between severity of Alzheimer's disease and prevalence of comorbid depressive symptoms and depression: a systematic review. Int J Geriatr Psychiatry 22(11):1063–1086
5. Lyketsos CG, Sheppard JM, Steinberg M et al (2001) Neuropsychiatric disturbance in Alzheimer's disease clusters into three groups: the Cache County study. Int J Geriatr Psychiatry 16(11):1043–1053 (see comment)
6. Olin JT, Schneider LS, Katz IR et al (2002) Provisional diagnostic criteria for depression of Alzheimer disease. Am J Geriatr Psychiatry 10(2):125–128

7. Chemerinski E, Petracca G, Sabe L et al (2001) The specificity of depressive symptoms in patients with Alzheimer's disease. Am J Psychiatry 158(1):68–72
8. Starkstein SE, Jorge R, Mizrahi R et al (2005) The construct of minor and major depression in Alzheimer's disease. Am J Psychiatry 162:2086–2093
9. Starkstein SE, Mizrahi R, Garau LM (2005) Specificity of symptoms of depression in Alzheimer disease: a longitudinal analysis. Am J Geriatr Psychiatry 13:803–807
10. Levy ML, Cummings JL, Fairbanks LA et al (1998) Apathy is not depression. J Neuropsychiatry Clin Neurosci 10(3):314–319
11. Lyketsos CG, Olin J (2002) Depression in Alzheimer's disease: overview and treatment. Biol Psychiatry 52(3):243–252
12. Starkstein SE, Chemerinski E, Sabe L et al (1997) Prospective longitudinal study of depression and anosognosia in Alzheimer's disease. Br J Psychiatry 171:47–52
13. Burns A, Jacoby R, Levy R (1990) Psychiatric phenomena in Alzheimer's disease. III: Disorders of mood. Br J Psychiatry 157:81–86
14. Aalten P, de Vugt ME, Jaspers N et al (2005) The course of neuropsychiatric symptoms in dementia. Part I: Findings from the two-year longitudinal Maasbed study. Int J Geriatr Psychiatry 20(6):523–530
15. Shin IS, Carter M, Masterman D et al (2005) Neuropsychiatric symptoms and quality of life in Alzheimer disease. Am J Geriatr Psychiatry 13(6):469–474
16. Kunik ME, Snow AL, Molinari VA et al (2003) Health care utilization in dementia patients with psychiatric comorbidity. Gerontologist 43(1):86–91
17. Suh GH, Kil Yeon B, Shah A et al (2005) Mortality in Alzheimer's disease: a comparative prospective Korean study in the community and nursing homes. Int J Geriatr Psychiatry 20(1):26–34
18. Lee HB, Lyketsos CG (2003) Depression in Alzheimer's disease: heterogeneity and related issues. Biol Psychiatry 54(3):353–362
19. Cohen CI, Hyland K, Kimhy D (2003) The utility of mandatory depression screening of dementia patients in nursing homes. Am J Psychiatry 160:2012–2017
20. Marin RS (1991) Apathy: a neuropsychiatric syndrome. J Neuropsychiatry Clin Neurosci 3(3):243–254
21. van Reekum R, Stuss DT, Ostrander L (2005) Apathy: why care? J Neuropsychiatry Clin Neurosci 17(1):7–19
22. Levy R, Dubois B (2006) Apathy and the functional anatomy of the prefrontal cortex-basal ganglia circuits. Cereb Cortex 16:916–928
23. Starkstein SE, Ingram L, Garau ML et al (2005) On the overlap between apathy and depression in dementia. J Neurol Neurosurg Psychiatry 76(8):1070–1074
24. Starkstein S, Leentjens AF (2008) The nosological position of apathy in clinical practice. J Neurol Neurosurg Psychiatry 79:1088–1092
25. Robert P, Onyike CU, Leentjens AF et al (2009) Proposed diagnostic criteria for apathy in Alzheimer's disease and other neuropsychiatric disorders. Eur Psychiatry 24(2):98–104
26. Marin RS, Wilkosz PA (2005) Disorders of diminished motivation. J Head Trauma Rehabil 20(4):377–388
27. Marin RS, Biedrzycki RC, Firinciogullari S (1991) Reliability and validity of the apathy evaluation scale. Psychiatry Res 38(2):143–162
28. Starkstein SE, Mayberg HS, Preziosi TJ et al (1992) Reliability, validity, and clinical correlates of apathy in Parkinson's disease. J Neuropsychiatry Clin Neurosci 4(2):134–139
29. Cummings JL (1997) The neuropsychiatric inventory: assessing psychopathology in dementia patients. Neurology 48(suppl 6):S10–S16
30. Strauss ME, Sperry SD (2002) An informant-based assessment of apathy in Alzheimer disease. Neuropsychiatry Neuropsychol Behav Neurol 15(3):176–183
31. Robert PH, Clairet S, Benoit M et al (2002) The apathy inventory: assessment of apathy and awareness in Alzheimer's disease, Parkinson's disease and mild cognitive impairment. Int J Geriatr Psychiatry 17(12):1099–1105
32. Berrios GE, Gili M (1995) Abulia and impulsiveness revisited: a conceptual history. Acta Psychiatr Scand 92(3):161–167

33. Sims A (2003) Symptoms in the mind. Saunders, Philadelphia
34. Laplane D, Dubois B (2001) Auto-activation deficit: a basal ganglia related syndrome. Mov Disord 16(5):810–814
35. Starkstein SE, Petracca G, Chemerinski E et al (2001) Syndromic validity of apathy in Alzheimer's disease. Am J Psychiatry 158(6):872–877
36. Tatsch MF, Bottino CM, Azevedo D et al (2006) Neuropsychiatric symptoms in Alzheimer disease and cognitively impaired, nondemented elderly from a community-based sample in Brazil: prevalence and relationship with dementia severity. Am J Geriatr Psychiatry 14(5):438–445
37. Landes AM, Sperry SD, Strauss ME (2005) Prevalence of apathy, dysphoria, and depression in relation to dementia severity in Alzheimer's disease. J Neuropsychiatry Clin Neurosci 17(3):342–349
38. Starkstein SE, Jorge R, Mizrahi R et al (2006) A prospective longitudinal study of apathy in Alzheimer's disease. J Neurol Neurosurg Psychiatry 77:8–11
39. Starkstein SE, Fedoroff JP, Price TR et al (1993) Apathy following cerebrovascular lesions. Stroke 24(11):1625–1630
40. Starkstein S, Merello M, Jorge R et al (2009) The syndromal validity and nosological position of apathy in Parkinson's disease. Mov Disord 15:1211–1216
41. Starkstein SE, Merello M, Brockman S et al (2009) Apathy predicts more severe parkinsonism in Alzheimer's disease. Am J Geriatr Psychiatry 17(4):291–298

Cognitive Decline and Treatment of Alzheimer's Disease

Luis Ignacio Brusco

Abstract Alzheimer's disease (DTA) constitutes the most common cause of dementia. Its prevalence is about 2–4% at the age of 70 and between 30% and 50% in persons over the age of 85.

The prevalence doubles every 5 years, being even more prevalent in women, which probably reflects their greater longevity. With the increase of life expectancy, the impact of this disease will keep growing significantly unless prevention and/or treatment actions are developed.

Many efforts in diagnostic methodology as well as trials used to stop the progression in this preclinical stage of investigation have been made and still continue, although at present there are not worldwide agreed or approved treatments for it.

Nowadays, there are five drugs that were approved by the FDA for probable DTA treatment; only four of them are used regularly.

Differential diagnosis of Alzheimer's disease constitutes one of the most complex challenges in medicine.

We could say that we can found five possible variables for the differential diagnosis.

1. Clinical interpretation
2. Neuroimaging
3. Differential blood check for cognitive disorders
4. Genetic biomarkers (or data in lifetime clinical record, LCR)
5. Neurocognitive evaluation

L.I. Brusco (✉)
School of Medicine, Buenos Aires University, Buenos Aires, Argentina
e-mail: infoinear@fibertel.com
and
Alzheimer Argentina, www.alzheimer.org.ar
and
Argentine Neuropsychiatric Association, Buenos Aires, Argentina

K. Miyoshi et al. (eds.), *Neuropsychiatric Disorders*,
DOI 10.1007/978-4-431-53871-4_15, © Springer 2010

These items must be studied by a qualified stuff at specialized centers, if possible, to arrive at the closest diagnosis to reality. Finally, biomarkers and genetics constitute substantial progress that will lead to a sensitive and specific diagnosis at the same time.

Keywords Alzheimer disease • Early diagnosis • Genetic biomarkers • Treatment

As longevity increases, aging-related diseases become more and more prominent. Cognition disorders increase with the growing number of elderly individuals in societies, turning the insanity syndrome into one of the main concerns of the elderly populations.

Within dementia, Alzheimer's disease (AD) is the most common cause of dementia associated with age, with a frequency of presentation that increases dramatically at 70 years of age. In 2000, it was estimated that there were approximately 4.5 million individuals with AD in the United States, and that that number is projected to become 14 million by 2050. This alarming statistic has led to the identification and search for markers of early disease as well as redefining the concept of minimal cognitive impairment and its potential conversion to AD. Many efforts in diagnostic methods as well as trials aimed at halting the progression of this preclinical research stage have been conducted and continue to this day.

AD is a neurodegenerative disorder that produces progressive intellectual decline, as well as a variety of neuropsychiatric and behavioral disorders.

This disease is one of the most important health, social, and cultural problems of the new century, given the severity of the symptoms and their evolution, but mainly its association with old age and the fact that our society, with the increasing age of the population, is heading toward aging.

In the clinical framework of AD, we can recognize the effect on the following areas:

1. Cognitive
2. Behavioral
3. Daily rhythms and sleep–wake cycles

Neuropsychological alterations of AD include abnormalities in memory (recent and remote), aphasia, visuo-spatial and visuo-constructive disorders, calculation defects, praxis, gnosias, difficulty in abstraction, and judgment.

The neuropsychiatric alterations include personality disorders, delusions and confusion, hallucinations and depression, sleep, appetite, and sexuality disorders, and abnormal motor behavior. Typically, the most severe and earliest AD symptoms are the insidious problems and progressive memory loss in recalling the most recent learning situations; this stage is followed by language disturbances, compromise of visuo-spatial abilities, praxis, and attention impairment. A number of behavioral symptoms that significantly affect the life quality of patients and cohabitants usually appear in the intermediate and late stages of the disease.

Changes in the biological rhythms involve quantitative and qualitative alterations of sleep, increase of evening symptoms when the sun sets (sundowning), and flattening of biological rhythms, including plane body rhythm with a decline of the patient's daytime mobility and increased activity at night, thus affecting their environment.

The diagnosis of AD is mainly clinical and, to date, we lack a biological marker or diagnostic test that could positively and selectively identify the disease, beyond the final anatomopathological assessment.

Accordingly, the clinical assessment remains the most important tool in the diagnostic process, but neuropsychology and some complementary methods of diagnosis also collaborate [1].

The distinction between the cognitive and noncognitive aspects (also called primary and secondary) will be used with an organizational and didactic criterion because the coexistence and overlapping of these phenomena is normal in the clinical field and is beyond this dichotomy.

Current diagnostic criteria allow for high sensitivity and diagnostic efficiency in close to 85% of cases. Standardizations propose a consensus of diagnostic standards to be used in our environment, thus minimizing disputes arising from the use of the different proposals.

The most commonly used criteria for disease diagnosis are based on the Diagnostic and Statistical Manual, Fourth Revision (DSM IV TR), or the National Institute of Neurologic, Communicative Disorders and Stroke/ Alzheimer's Disease and Related Disorders Association (NINCDS–ADRDA). The American Academy of Neurology has evaluated these criteria and considered them reliable. However, there are several points of evidence indicating the need to update the current criteria for definition, such as inadequate diagnostic specificity: the criteria of DSM IV TR and NINCDS–ADRDA have been validated using neuropathological gold standards, showing a diagnostic accuracy that ranges between 65% and 96%. When the diagnosis was for other dementias and not AD, it was only between 23% and 88%.

The patient's medical history is a key element in the diagnosis of dementia syndromes. Input from informants (not just the story of the patient) is also important. A number of tools are available that can be used to obtain information about the everyday activities and performance of these patients, although none has been able to demonstrate superior efficacy over another; therefore, the doctor's careful inquiry about this item is crucial.

The differential diagnosis of AD is one of the most complex challenges of medicine: not only because it is a disease that compromises the person's thought and behavior, dissocializing them and generating a substantial change in their integrity, but also because it is based on a complex set of diagnostic premises through which we reach a diagnosis that can only be confirmed by analyzing the patient's brain neuropathology, something that is generally not done.

Also, the observational, supplementary, and semiological variables are increasingly complex and difficult to correlate if you do not have the experience and logical criteria that enable us to combine a thought that reaches a possible or probable diagnosis with that which would enable us to establish an adequate treatment for the cognitive patient's diagnostic and evolutional situation.

We could say then that there are five possible variables for the differential diagnosis:

1. Clinical assessment (observation of a case history, etc.)
2. Neuroimaging
3. Differential blood screening for cognitive impairment
4. Genetic biomarkers and/or cerebrospinal fluid (CSF)
5. Neurocognitive assessment

These items should be examined by qualified staff and, if possible, at specialized centers to reach a diagnostic certainty as close to reality as possible. Finally, biomarkers and genetics are a significant advancement that will enable a sensitive and specific diagnosis.

Genetic study currently enables a greater approach, particularly of the study of the apolipoprotein-E (APO-E) gene, which in some cases enables us to take the diagnosis to even more than 85% of certainty [2].

The approach to AD therapy implies recognizing the different types of symptoms present: basically cognitive, noncognitive, and behavioral. The term "noncognitive" is used to include behavioral, mood, and perception (illusions and hallucinations) alterations, alterations in the course and content of thought, and changes in level of activity (both motor and verbal) [3]. Verbal and physical aggression, apathy, social withdrawal, depression, distrust, sleep disorders, increased or reduced sexual activity, and negativism or resistance to treatment should be considered as noncognitive symptoms [4].

The term "noncognitive" has been chosen to differentiate these symptoms from those that are cognitive in their origin, that is, symptoms that are a direct result of the impairment of the memory, judgment, visuo-spatial function, math abilities, object manipulation when the motor function is intact (praxia), and language, among others. Although the distribution of noncognitive and cognitive symptoms is clear in theory, it is not that clear in practice. For instance, if a patient falsely accuses his relatives of stealing things from him, this could be described as a paranoid-like idea. However, the patient's cognitive impairment may be the origin of the symptom, having himself forgotten where he leaves his belongings. The noncognitive symptom is his accusation against his relatives, but the cognitive symptom of origin is fixation hypomnesia.

The clearest symptom of AD is the impairment of cognitive capacity as a result of neuronal destruction. However, noncognitive symptoms occur frequently and are a source of difficulty both for the patient and for the caretakers. Some authors consider these are the real core symptoms of the dementia syndrome. Even though we can admit that noncognitive symptoms do not appear in all AD patients, they are often the main reason why a patient seeks medical attention. It is therefore obvious that a correct treatment of the behavioral changes of an AD patient not only generates an improvement of the behavioral performance of the subject but also an increase of their intellectual possibilities [5]. Also, these disorders limit the patient at a social level and may be the most frequent cause for an early hospitalization, which undoubtedly changes the future situation and clearly increases the costs generated by this disease.

Treatment of AD

The approach to AD therapy implies recognizing the different types of symptoms present: basically cognitive, noncognitive, and behavioral.

The term "noncognitive" has been chosen to differentiate these symptoms from those that are cognitive in their origin, that is, symptoms which are a direct result of the impairment of the memory, judgment, visuo-spatial function, math abilities, object manipulation when the motor function is intact (praxia), and language, among others. Although the distinction of noncognitive and cognitive symptoms is clear in theory, it is not that clear in practice. For instance, if a patient falsely accuses his relatives of stealing things from him, this could be described as a paranoid-like idea. However, the patient's cognitive impairment may be the origin of the symptom, having himself forgotten where he leaves his belongings. The noncognitive symptom is his accusation against his relatives, but the cognitive symptom of origin is fixation hypomnesia.

The clearest symptom of AD is the impairment of the cognitive capacity as a result of neuronal destruction. However, noncognitive symptoms occur frequently and are a source of difficulty both for the patient and for the caretakers. Some authors consider these are the real core symptoms of the dementia syndrome. Even though we can admit that noncognitive symptoms do not appear in all AD patients, they are often the main reason why a patient seeks medical attention. It is therefore obvious that correct treatment of the behavioral changes of an AD patient not only generates an improvement of the behavioral performance of the subject but also an increase of their intellectual possibilities. Also, these disorders limit the patient at a social level and may be the most frequent cause for an early hospitalization, which undoubtedly changes the future situation and clearly increases the costs generated by this disease.

Five drugs are currently approved by the U.S. Food and Drug Administration (FDA) for the treatment of possible AD, of which only four are used regularly [6]. Three of these commonly used drugs are acetylcholinesterase inhibitors, the rational use of which is based on the literature evidence stating that AD patients suffer from a cholinergic deficit [7]. These anticholinesterase drugs are used in an independent manner; that is, only one is administered.

The other drug used in combination with the aforementioned ones is memantine, a partial antagonist of glutamate used in combination therapy with cholinergic therapy [8].

Specific Goals of Treatment

Restoring Neuronal Function

It is generally accepted that the clinical course of neuropsychiatric and behavioral symptoms of AD arises as a result of alterations in the complex intracellular and intercellular communication system. It is currently known that some of the AD symptoms result from the dysfunction of specific neuronal systems caused by alterations in the transmission of signals and/or cell death. The initial effect leading to the cascade of events that produce transmission alterations is not yet known, and we cannot accurately state whether single or multiple genetic factors, either in a sequence or in combination, are involved in the degenerative process.

Preventing Synapse and Cell Death

There is evidence indicating that AE is associated with an important loss of synapses, dendritic changes, and cell death. The severity of the dementia is clearly related to the extension of the synaptic loss. Even though the exact cause and the underlying mechanisms of neuronal loss are not clear, there are several possible factors, such as endogenous and exogenous neurotoxins, metabolic alterations, alterations in calcium homeostasis, abnormal processing of the amyloid precursor protein, and changes in the proteins of neurons.

To delay the progression of the degenerative process, it is essential to develop treatments that maintain synaptic stability and ensure the survival of neurons. Some treatments that use neuronal growth factors and genetic therapy techniques could be fruitful in the future [9].

Treatment of the Primary Cognitive Symptoms

The primary symptoms are defined as those that involve memory loss (both fixation and evocation memory) and other cognitive disorders (such as aphasia, apraxia, agnosia, and further impairment of the executive function).

Cholinergic Agents

Multiple data prove the significant role that cholinergic mechanisms play in AD:

1. Anticholinergic agents with core action produce cognitive deficit in humans
2. Cholinergic neurotransmission shapes memory and learning
3. The lesions that affect central cholinergic pathways cause learning and memory impairment, which may be reversed through the administration of cholinomimetics
4. Postmortem studies of AD patients show loss of cholinergic neurons in the septum and basal nucleus of Meynert, reduction of the cholines acetyltransferase and acetylcholinesterase, and correlation between these changes and the level of cognitive impairment

Relative to these points, it was theorized that increasing central cholinergic transmission would be useful in the treatment of AD. This effect may be achieved by using acetylcholine precursors, by inhibiting cholinesterase, the enzyme that reduces it, or by using direct postsynaptic agonists.

Acetylcholine Precursors

At the beginning, the proposal was to increase the availability of acetylcholine precursors, which would increase both its synthesis and neurotransmission. Lecitine or choline was administered for that purpose. However, because the choline absorption system is usually saturated in normal conditions (from 98% to 99%), the increase of extracellular precursors will not increase the synthesis of choline or its release, and would only be useful when there is great cholinergic activity and an increased demand of the precursor (not very probable in regular clinical conditions, which would explain their limited clinical usefulness).

Acetylcholinesterase Inhibitors

Even though acetylcholinesterase inhibitors are not useful for all AD patients, there is a group of subjects who might benefit from treatment with acetylcholinesterase inhibitors; these are patients with late onset of the symptoms, initial stages of the disease, and lack of a related organic disease.

Donepezil is a benzyl methyl piperidine, mixed inhibitor (competitive-noncompetitive) of the enzyme, which shows a therapeutic profile similar to that of the prototype drug, tacrine, although it is much more powerful [10]. It presents a prolonged half-life, more than 80 h, which facilitates its administration in just one daily intake, 5 or 10 mg/day being the indicated dose [11]. In contrast to tacrine, it does not show hepatotoxicity or high incidence of digestive intolerance. The most common adverse effects are nausea, vomiting, anorexia, insomnia, cramps, and bradycardia.

Rivastigmine is an acetylcholinesterase inhibitor also approved by the FDA. It is a pseudo-irreversible inhibitor that dissociates the enzyme slowly. It is administered twice a day and is also a butyrylcholinesterase inhibitor, which would have certain implications in its adverse effects profile. It starts with a 1.5-mg dose twice a day, and it is possible to increase the dose in 1.5-mg/day phases up to 6 mg twice a day. The adverse effects profile is similar to that of donepezil, although with greater incidence of gastrointestinal effects. To lessen this adverse effects incidence, it is recommended that the dose increases be made every 2–4 weeks. The effect of rivastigmine in the ADAS-Cog and the CIBIC Plus is more or less the same as that of donepezil. The presentation in transdermal absorption patches has been recently approved as a way to minimize the adverse effects of the drug.

Galantamine is an amine tertiary phenantrene used in the treatment of paresis, paralysis, and miasthenia gravis; the recommended dose is between 20 and 60 mg/day. Its half-life is 8 h; among the most common adverse effects are agitation, insomnia, and irritability. Nowadays there exists a form of presentation of prolonged release and one intake per day.

Glutamate Regulators

Memantine is a new therapy that has recently been approved by the FDA for the treatment of moderate to severe AD [12]. It belongs to the family of partial antagonists of the NMDA receptor and can added to the treatment with inhibitors [13]. Its use has been approved both alone and in combination with the mentioned inhibitors. It could also have an effect on the basic physiopathogenic process of the disease through the inhibition of the entrance of calcium at rest, which would exist as a pathological process in neurodegenerative disease. The adverse reactions are milder than those with anticholinesterase drugs: anxiety, akathisia, and mild gastrointestinal pain. There is a new presentation and administration of memantine, based on work that guarantees the use in a single intake of 20 mg, with the same effect and tolerance.

It is the only drug approved for the severe form of the disease: pharmacoeconomic analyses have been conducted in most cases by comparing the drug to non-pharmacological treatment [14].

In general, the different trials have shown that memantine is less costly and more effective than nonpharmacological treatment, although, given the limited number of pharmacoeconomic studies performed, it is still too early to draw conclusions on the drug's cost-effectiveness.

Antioxidants

Within this heterogeneous group we must mention vitamin E, selegiline, and bifemelane.

Vitamin E (tocopherol) has been proved to have protective properties against neuronal damage in animals. This finding inspired the conduction of clinical trials in patients with dementia. It has been used in doses of 2,000 UI/day, showing a 7-month delay in the progression of the disease, but without improving the symptoms.

It has proved to be a safe drug with low incidence of adverse events, among which the most important ones are blood clotting disorders.

Research has shown oxidative damage is present in the brains of AD patients. Consequently, the use of antioxidants in treatment has gained popularity. There are considerable data suggesting that antioxidants are linked to a lower incidence of the disease. A clinical trial in subjects with moderate disease has shown that vitamin E and selegiline were effective in delaying the progression of moderate AD into more severe stages. Doses of vitamin E 1,000 UI twice a day and selegiline 10 mg/day were administered in this study. The results regarding selegiline have not been as convincing; this, associated with its pharmacological interactions and potential toxicity, has led to the preference of vitamin E. There exists theoretical concern regarding the gastrointestinal toxicity and bleeding with the latter, although in general it is well tolerated. These findings have not been argued, nor is there agreement regarding the ideal dose of vitamin E. The American Academy of Neurology (AAN) has indicated that 1,000 UI vitamin E twice a day can be considered in an attempt to reduce the progression of AD. The risk–benefit ratio determined for selegiline appears to be less favorable.

The use of vitamin E should be considered (despite this simple positive study) in the face of a recent meta-analysis that indicates that with doses of 400 UI/day or higher there would be an increased risk of death from cardiovascular conditions. It is still uncertain whether this increased risk appears essentially in patients with premorbid cardiologic conditions or if it is also applicable to patients without significant cardiovascular history.

Selegiline is an irreversible inhibitor of monoaminoxidase B at low doses and of monoaminoxidase A at high doses; used for the treatment of depression and Parkinson's disease, it is believed to act similarly to other antioxidants, that is, by avoiding cell death and thus the progression of the disease [15]. Also, it interferes with the hyperactivity of monoaminoxidase B observed in AD. It is effective at low doses (10 mg/day); its improving effect is not related to the antidepressant effect. The main adverse effects of this drug are nausea, dizziness, abdominal pain, and mouth dryness, being the tyramine syndrome difficult to observe given the doses used. This drug is not recommended for patients who receive tricyclic antidepressants, selective serotonin reuptake inhibitor (SSRI), or mepridine.

Antiinflammatory Drugs

It is clinically observed that patients who received antiinflammatories in a clinical manner, such as populations with rheumatoid arthritis or leprosy, present a much lower incidence of AD; therefore, the prolonged use of antiinflammatories such as indometacine is considered beneficial for this disease.

Research on AD has shown the presence of an inflammatory component involved in the degenerative process. Because this element can influence the progression of the disease and increase its symptoms, some studies have suggested the possibility of using antiinflammatory agents as treatment. Epidemiological studies indicate that the use of nonsteroidal antiinflammatory drugs (NSAIDs) could protect against the development of AD. Some NSAIDs, such as indometacine, were suggested, but in the case of the latter, the abandonment rate by the patients was very high because of the adverse effects.

Trials performed treating patients with glucocorticoids, such as prednisone or NSAIDs, have been negative. One study with mild to moderate AD patients in the course of a year showed no significant difference in the performance of the ADAS-Cog. In fact, the group treated with prednisone showed greater behavioral worsening as compared to the placebo group.

Recently, attention has been drawn to cyclooxygenase 2 (COX-2) inhibitors as they are better tolerated than nonselective antiinflammatories. However, the beneficial effect of these drugs has not been proved. There are currently a few positive studies regarding the use of NSAIDs. There is a long trial still in course that assesses a NSAID and a COX-2 inhibitor in the prevention of the onset of AD, the results of which will be known in the years to come.

There are some recent negative studies in relationship to the use of NSAIDs and steroids in the treatment of AD. Even though some epidemiological studies seem to show a potential benefit in postponing the development of AD, none of the randomized clinical trials has been able to prove these findings. Moreover, some concerns regarding the safety of COX-2 inhibitors and other NSAIDs have emerged. Therefore, none of them is currently recommended to prevent or treat the disease.

In contrast with these studies, there has been recent speculation that some NSAIDs would have a specific property lowering the alpha-beta levels and would therefore be useful in the treatment of AD through an alternative mechanism.

Estrogen Replacement Therapy

Similar to the use of the drugs already described, there has been epidemiological proof that postmenopausal women who have received hormone replacement therapy with estrogens would be more protected against AD. It is likely that estrogens may have a neuroprotective effect in delaying the onset of the disease, but the data on the use of estrogens have not been positive [16].

An open, randomized, double-blind, placebo-controlled trial on mild to moderate AD failed to prove the benefits of hormone replacement after a term of 12 months. There were no changes in the primary measures of efficacy in this trial, and concern was raised regarding deep vein thrombosis as a possible adverse effect. An additional smaller trial of 16 weeks also failed to show benefits with this therapy. Consequently, there are no data supporting the recommendation of the use.

There are longitudinal studies in course regarding a possible prophylactic effect of estrogen in reducing the risk of developing dementia, but the data of this study are still pending.

More recently, the Women's Health Initiative Memory Study has proved that the postmenopause use of estrogens may constitute a risk factor for the development of AD and mild cognitive impairment (MCI) instead of having a protective effect.

Neurotrophic Factors

There is a new medication, Cerebrolysin, that is proposed for the treatment of Alzheimer-like diseases and vascular dementia. This drug is a peptide preparation produced by the standardized, controlled, enzymatic decomposition of purified brain proteins; it consists of low molecular weight peptides (10 kDa) and amino acids.

The drug is provided as a watery solution and administered through intravenous infusion. It has both neurotrophic and neuroprotective effects on the neuron. In animal models with AD, cerebrolysin protects against the degeneration of cholinergic neurons (producers of acetylcholine). Improvement has been shown in the neuropathological and behavioral changes of the animals. There is basic work showing that it directly influences the neuronal and synaptic plasticity, improving neurotransmission [17]. It promotes neuronal sprouting and ramification and induces neuronal repair processes.

Protection against cell death in different experimental animals and cell cultures is also proposed. It has an antiapoptopic effect, in such a way that it promotes neuronal survival.

There are various double-blind clinical trials that show cognitive and behavioral improvement with the intravenous use of cerebrolysin [18–20]. It was proposed for the treatment of Alzheimer-like diseases and vascular dementia in other trials [21].

Treatment of Secondary Noncognitive Symptoms

Although the primary symptoms of AD are memory impairment and loss of other cognitive abilities, patients also develop secondary symptoms, among which are depression, anxiety, agitation, delirium, hallucinations, and insomnia. It is recommendable to manage with caution the use of antipsychotics and anxiolytics, keeping in mind that both have side effects [22]. The first behavior is to wait for the therapeutic effects of memantine and anticholinesterase medication as, besides cognition, both drugs also improve the neuropsychiatric inventory [23].

With antipsychotics it is necessary to avoid the typical ones that cause parkinsonism, given the predisposition of elderly dementia patients to experience extrapyramidal symptoms. However, the atypical drugs have proved an increase in mortality in late-life psychosis. Quetiapine (with the family's informed consent) may be the drug to indicate in the psychotic disorders of dementia, given the low production of extrapyramidal effects in low doses.

These symptoms should not be minimized, as it is estimated that they occur in a large majority of patients (around 60%), being in general the basis of most complications of the disease. Psychoactive drugs are the ones most used for these symptoms, but they carry potential adverse effects such as sedation, disinhibition, depression, falls, incontinence, parkinsonism, and akathisia [24, 25]. Chronobiotics such as melatonin have proved their benefit in the treatment of alterations of the sleep–wake cycle and evening irritability that are typical of these patients.

The use of the antiepileptic drugs carbamacepine and valproic acid has also been brought forward for the psychiatric disorders of these patients, particularly if there are associated epileptic disorders [26, 27].

There are general principles to follow for the treatment of secondary AD symptoms:

1. Define the type of symptoms as clearly as possible to focus the therapy and work with monodrugs (one drug at a time) in combined treatments.
2. Assess the importance of the symptom both for the patient and for the caretakers.
3. Take into account that some symptoms are temporary and typical of the natural evolution of the disease.
4. Look for precipitating events.
5. Consider modifications of the environment and nonpharmacological therapies.
6. Start with low doses of drugs and slowly make necessary increases.
7. After controlling the symptoms, evaluate the possible reduction or withdrawal of the medication, pursuant to each symptom.

New Nonpharmacological Possibilities of Treatment

It is important to consider not only the patient but also his or her caretaker, who in general is a relative and is under chronic stress. Therefore, aid measures through support groups for relatives and caretakers such as those at the Asociación Alzheimer Argentina, that advise, orient, and support relatives and caretakers, are particularly important.

Assistance to the patient involves not only medication, but also the work of psychologists, occupational therapists, voice specialists, and physical therapists in a treatment modality in which multiple stimulation is essential.

It is important to remember that this disease affects the entire family and that interdisciplinary work is essential for the correct approach to the patient and his or her environment.

References

1. American Academy of Neurology (2009) AAN guideline summary for clinicians: detection, diagnosis and management of dementia. http://www.aan.com/professionals/practice/pdfs/dementia_guideline.pdf. Accessed 15 April 2009

2. Small GW, Siddarth P, Burggren AC et al (2009) Influence of cognitive status, age, and APOE-4 genetic risk on brain FDDNP positron-emission tomography imaging in persons without dementia. Arch Gen Psychiatry 66(1):81–87
3. Reisberg B, Auer SR (1996) Behavioral pathology in Alzheimer's disease. Psychogeriatrics 8:301–308
4. Wragg RE, Jeste DV (1989) Overview of depression and psychosis in Alzheimer's disease. Am J Psychiatry 146:577–587
5. Salzman C (1997) Treatment of the elderly agitated patient. J Clin Psychiatry 48(5 suppl):19–22
6. Schatzberg A, Nemeroff C (1998) Textbook of psychopharmacology, 2nd edn. American Psychiatric, Washington, DC
7. American Psychiatric Association (2009) Practice guideline and resources for treatment of patients with Alzheimer´s disease and other dementias, 2nd edn. http://www.psychiatryonline.com/pracGuide/pracGuideTopic_3.aspx. Accessed 15 April 2009
8. APA Work Group on Alzheimer´s Disease and other Dementias, Rabins PN, Blacker D et al (2007) American Psychiatric Association practice guideline for the treatment of patients with Alzheimer´s disease and other dementias. Second edition. Am J Psychiatry 164(12 suppl):5–56
9. Moizeszowicz J (1998) Psicofarmacología psicodinámica IV: estrategias terapéuticas y psiconeurobiológicas, 4th edn. Paidós, Buenos Aires
10. Raskind MA, Sadowsky CH et al (1997) Effect of tacrine on language, praxis and noncognitive behavioral problems in Alzheimer's disease. Arch Neurol 54:836–840
11. Howard RJ, Juszczak E, Ballard CG et al (2007) Donepezil for the treatment of agitation in Alzheimer´s disease. N Engl J Med 357(14):1382–1392
12. Tariot PN, Farlow MR, Grossberg GT et al (2004) Memantine treatment in patients with moderate to severe Alzheimer disease already receiving donepezil: a randomized controlled trial. JAMA 291:317–324
13. Farlow M et al (2003) Memantine/donepezil dual therapy is superior to placebo/donepezil therapy for treatment of moderate to severe Alzheimer´s disease. Neurology 60(suppl 1):A412
14. Reisberg B, Doody R, Söffler A et al (2003) Memantine in moderate to severe Alzheimer's disease. N Engl J Med 348:1333–1341
15. Tolbert SR, Fuller MA (1996) Seleginine in treatment of behavioral and cognitive symptoms of Alzheimer disease. Ann Pharmacother 30:1122–1129
16. Kawas C, Resnik S, Morrison A (1997) A prospective study of estrogen replacement therapy and the risk of developing Alzheimer disease: the Baltimore longitudinal study of aging. Neurology 48:1517–1521
17. Rüther E, Ritter R, Apecechea M, Freytag S, Gmeinbauer R, Windisch M (2000) Sustained improvements in patients with dementia of Alzheimer's type (DAT) 6 months after termination of cerebrolysin therapy. J Neural Transm 107:815–829
18. Ruether E, Alvarez XA, Rainer M, Moessles H (2002) Sustained improvement of cognition and global function in patients with moderately severe Alzheimer's disease: a double-blind, placebo-controlled study with the neurotrophic agent Cerebrolysin®. J Neural Transm Suppl 62:265–275
19. Panisset M et al (2002) Cerebrolysin in Alzheimer's disease: a randomized, double-blind, placebo-controlled trial with a neurotropic agent. J Neural Transm 109:1089–1104
20. Xiao SF et al (2000) Efficacy of FPF 1070 (Cerebrolysin) in patients with Alzheimer's disease: a multicentre, randomized, double-blind placebo-controlled trial. Clin Drug Invest 19:43–53
21. Alvarez XA et al (2006) A 24-week double blind, placebo-controlled study of three dosages of Cerebrolysin in patients with mild to moderate Alzheimer's disease. Eur J Neurol 13:43–54
22. Barnes R, Veith R, Okimoto J et al (1992) Efficacy of antipsychotic medications in behaviorally disturbed dementia patients. Am J Psychiatry 139:1170–1174

23. Qaseem A, Snow V, Cross JT et al (2008) Current pharmacologic treatment of dementia: a clinical practice guideline from the American College of Physicians and the American Academy of Family Physicians. Ann Intern Med 148(5):370–378
24. Stern RG, Duffelmeyer ME et al (1991) The use of benzodiazepines in the management of behavioral symptoms in dementia patients. Psychiatr Clin North Am 14:375–384
25. Tariot PN, Erb R et al (1994) Carbamazepine treatment of agitation in nursing home patients with dementia: a preliminary study. J Am Geriatr Soc 42:1160–1166
26. Gleason RP, Schneider LS (1990) Carbamazepine treatment of agitation in Alzheimer's outpatients refractory to neuroleptics. J Clin Psychiatry 51:115–118
27. Lott AD, Mcelroy SL, Keys MA (1995) Valproate in the treatment of behavioral agitation in elderly patients with dementia. J Neuropsychiatry Clin Neurosci 7:314–319

Alzheimer's Disease in Japan: Current Situation and Issues of the Care for Persons with Dementia

Akira Homma

Abstract It is estimated that the number of persons with dementia in 2005 will double in 2035 in Japan from more than 2 million to 4.5 million. In the wake of the introduction of long-term care insurance in Japan in 2000, there have been particularly marked changes in the awareness and recognition of dementia. However, considering that the aim of the care for persons with dementia is to support their independence or daily life, we envisage many more issues ahead of us. Early detection and diagnosis are important for all diseases, and particularly in the case of dementia. Underdetection of persons with dementia means underdiagnosis and treatment. At present, no data are available on the proportion of persons with dementia diagnosed and treated appropriately. Such a situation clearly indicates the role of primary care physicians to detect persons with dementia in the early stage. Also, "dignity" is emphasized in Article 1 of the Long-term Care Insurance Law revised in 2006. That is, persons with dementia must not be discriminated for the reason of dementia. However, persons with dementia are often discriminated in various situations. Here, I consider some of these issues with a view to establishing a future ideal model.

Keywords Alzheimer's disease • Dementia care • Human right • Management • Persons with dementia

Introduction

Dementia is an umbrella term used to refer to pathology from various causes. According to the estimates made by Awata et al. [1], the number of persons with dementia in 2005 will double in 30 years (in 2035) from more than 2 million to 4.5

A. Homma (✉)
Center for Dementia Care Research and Training in Tokyo, Tokyo, Japan
e-mail: ahomma96@dcnet.gr.jp

K. Miyoshi et al. (eds.), *Neuropsychiatric Disorders*,
DOI 10.1007/978-4-431-53871-4_16, © Springer 2010

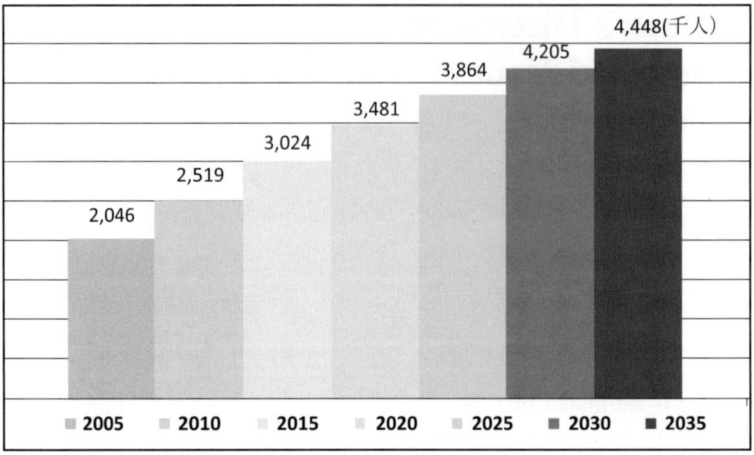

Fig. 1 Projected increase of persons with dementia

million. In Japan, the number of persons with dementia will be increasing most rapidly in Saitama Prefecture (3.2 times). These estimates were obtained from the epidemiological surveys that have been conducted by experts in certain areas throughout Japan. Other estimates have been obtained by estimating the percentage of persons with dementia among those designated for the long-term care insurance [2]. According to these, approximately half (48%) of those designated for long-term care insurance are suspected of having dementia. Furthermore, a tentative report on the long-term care insurance in September 2008 indicated that there were approximately 4.6 million individuals designated for this insurance in Japan. Forty-eight percent of this figure is 2.21 million, which is comparable to the estimate made by Awata et al. Given these numbers, dementia can be regarded as a very familiar condition, as shown in Fig. 1.

In the wake of the introduction of long-term care insurance in Japan in 2000, there have been particularly marked changes in the awareness and recognition of dementia. However, considering that the aim of the care for persons with dementia is to support their independence or daily life, we envisage many more issues ahead of us. Here, I consider some of these issues with a view to establishing a future ideal model.

Early Detection and Diagnosis

Early detection and diagnosis are important for all diseases, and particularly in the case of dementia, because persons with dementia are less likely to complain of memory impairment and visit medical facilities by themselves than those with other diseases such as hypertension and diabetes. Those with very mild dementia may, nevertheless, seek help for their memory loss as a chief complaint. However, most of these individuals rarely visit a hospital, even if their family members, or others, notice forgetfulness. Accordingly, the estimated number of persons with dementia is relatively small compared to, for example, the estimated 16 million persons with diabetes. However, it is critically important to determine the actual percentage of potential persons with dementia who are able to visit a hospital and receive appropriate diagnosis and treatment. Currently, there are no data available on the number of such persons. Relatively old survey results provide several examples demonstrating that early diagnosis in the community is not necessarily sufficient. In an epidemiological survey of the elderly aged 65 and above, conducted throughout Tokyo in 1995, approximately 5,000 persons were randomly sampled from approximately 1.49 million people aged 65 and above [3]. Eventually, 123 persons were diagnosed as having dementia. Of these 123 individuals, only 26.5% were diagnosed as having dementia by their primary care physicians. Thus, three-fourths of persons with dementia may not actually be diagnosed as having dementia. The severity of dementia among these patients was classified as mild (18.5%), moderate (12.5%), and severe (46.7%). Severe dementia is accompanied by total disorientation and requires total care in daily life. We should note that half of the elderly with severe dementia were not diagnosed as having dementia. In the results, the diagnoses of dementia by primary care physicians were Alzheimer's dementia (20.8%) and vascular dementia (56.8%). The percentage of those diagnosed as having Alzheimer's dementia was lower than those having vascular dementia. These data seem very important, because primary care physicians were the second person with whom family members taking care of the elderly with dementia consulted at that time.

Further data were obtained from a questionnaire survey conducted to members of the regional medical association in Tokyo before the introduction of the long-term care insurance [4]. The response rate was found to be as low as 50% ($n=56$). However, a relatively high percentage of the physicians replying commented that they took care of symptoms of dementia in their daily practice (73.2%) and that they responded to consultations with patients' families regarding dementia (69.6%). However, only 19.6% of the physicians said that they referred their patients to special medical facilities for diagnoses, etc., or that they used public health centers. This situation is far from satisfactory. At this time, immediately before the enforcement of the long-term care insurance, only 32.1% of physicians were aware of the criteria for determining the independence level of the elderly with dementia, which was an item of attending physicians' written opinion to be submitted to municipalities to determine the eligibility for the long-term care insurance.

I give a third example here. Diagnoses of dementia made by physicians and experts immediately before the enforcement of the long-term care insurance were directly compared [5]. Primary care physicians and experts (four persons) made diagnoses independently for 36 subjects, including healthy individuals, using the NM scale, a behavior rating scale that measures the severity of dementia. The results indicated that there was consistency in the diagnosis of severe dementia between the physicians and specialists. However, of the eight persons diagnosed as having mild dementia by the experts, the primary care physicians diagnosed four as normal and one as having moderate dementia. Further, of the eight persons diagnosed as having suspected dementia by the experts, the primary care physicians diagnosed three as normal, another three as having mild dementia, and two as having moderate dementia. Thus, the diagnoses were inconsistent. Of the eight persons diagnosed with moderate dementia by the experts, six were diagnosed similarly as having moderate dementia by the primary care physicians. Thus, the less severe the disorder, the lower was the consistency rate.

Given these results, we can easily understand that primary care physicians play a key role in early detection of dementia. However, in a paper entitled "Screening for Cognitive Impairment In General Practice: Toward a Consensus" [6], Brodaty, an Australian geriatric psychiatrist specializing in the community care of dementia, considered various expenses, and concluded that it was inappropriate to seek dementia screening from primary care physicians. I completely agree with this view: one should not directly seek diagnosis from a primary care physician. Establishing a network, including experts and health and welfare professionals with whom you can consult at any time, is important. Also, in a model project of total care collaborative system for the elderly with dementia, implemented by the Tokyo Metropolitan Government, capable experts were secured in areas where a counseling system for the elderly with dementia was established [7]. Conversely, experts skilled in clinical practice for dementia are indispensable for facilitating consultation projects, including the early detection of dementia.

Responding to this situation, in 2000 we launched a training model for the early detection and diagnosis of dementia by primary care physicians. On the basis of the results of this model, in 2006 the Ministry of Health, Labour and Welfare commenced education for primary care physicians to improve medical skills for treating persons with dementia. To date, approximately 21,000 primary care physicians have undergone this training. Such training has been reported to improve the diagnostic rate of dementia, including Alzheimer disease, by primary care physicians [8]. Figure 2 shows a conceptual structure for early detection and management of persons with dementia in the community. At present, although not every resource shown in the figure works satisfactorily, it seems that the structure itself is quite valid in the management of persons with dementia. Furthermore, the former Centers for Dementia Disorders were abolished in 2008. Subsequently, Medical Centers for Dementia Disorders have been founded as core organizations responsible for the local management of dementia (Fig. 3). The target is to establish 150 such centers throughout Japan. In addition, since June 2009, a screening test for dementia has been introduced into the training course for driver license renewal at the age of 75. Those suspected of having dementia should undergo diagnosis for the presence or absence of dementia by primary care physicians or experts when they have a history of specific traffic violations within the past year. Thus, in view of the rapidly increasing number of persons with dementia, primary care physicians in local areas will be required to play more important roles, because dementia cannot be handled only by experts.

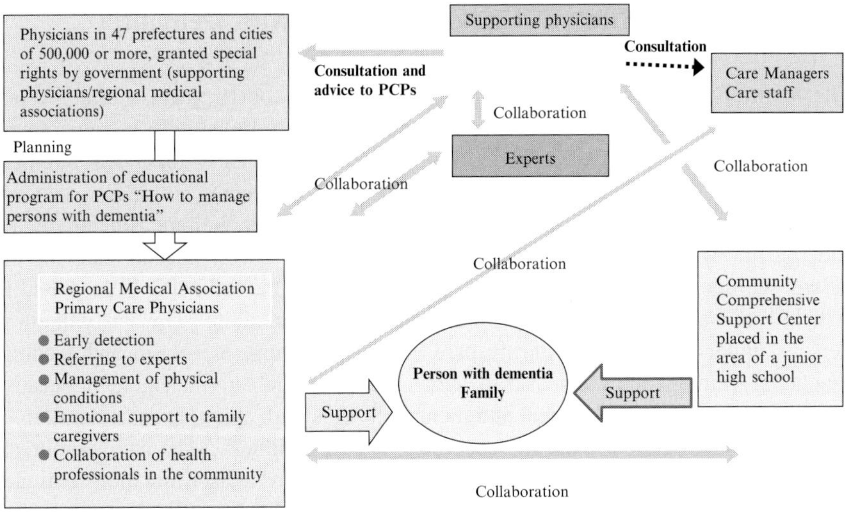

Fig. 2 Supporting system for persons with dementia in the community with the involvement of primary care physicians (PCPs)

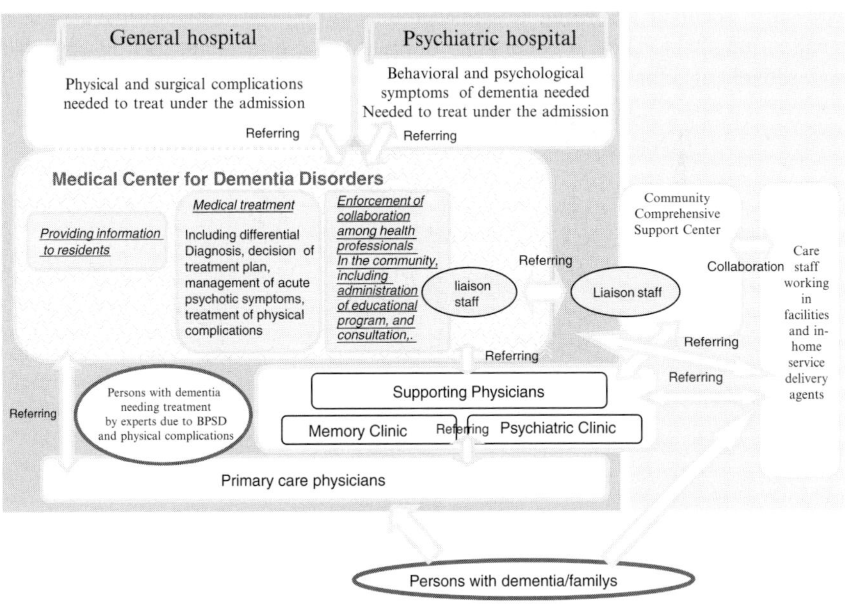

Fig. 3 Medical Center for Dementia Disorders

Supporting the Human Rights of Persons with Dementia

The long-term care insurance has now been in force for 10 years. Certainly, our understanding and recognition of dementia have improved markedly in some areas. With this improvement, medical technology to facilitate early diagnosis has also advanced, and the local network for early detection is also being consolidated. "Care for the Elderly in 2015" [2], proposed by the Health and Welfare Bureau for the Elderly, the Ministry of Health, Labor and Welfare in 2003, presents care for the elderly with dementia as a new care model. In addition, the following is described in Article 1 of the Long-term Care Insurance Law revised in 2006: "This law will allow persons under conditions requiring care, such as bathing, excretion, and feeding, functional training, and medical care, such as nursing and care management because of illness resulting from physical and mental changes with aging, to maintain dignity and lead an independent daily life according to their abilities." (The rest is omitted.) Thus, the term "dignity" was used for the first time. However, discrimination continues to remain in spite of the changes in attitudes toward dementia [9]. A revised adult guardianship law was introduced in April 2000. A total of 24,988 applications associated with the adult guardianship law were filed in the year between April 2007 and March 2008. The long-term care insurance contracts accounted for 6.2% (1,560 persons) of all the motives for the applications (Fig. 4; http://www.courts.go.jp/). In 2007, 2.3 million people were suspected of having dementia [1]. Of these, those who used the adult guardianship law for long-term care insurance contracts accounted for only 0.007%. Not all people suspected of having dementia seem to use the adult guardianship law for long-term care insurance contracts. However, it does not necessarily seem to be wrong to consider that those with dementia have slightly impaired judgment. Thus, it is certainly desirable to use the adult guardianship law more actively also for application for long-term care insurance contracts, because it is

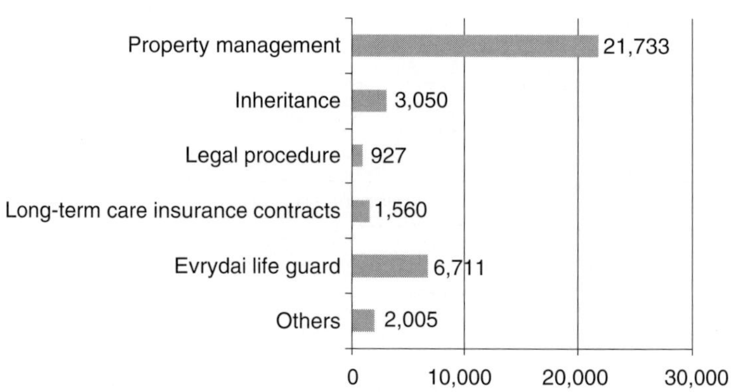

Fig. 4 Number of applicants to the adult guardianship system and its motives: April 2007–March 2008, $n=24{,}988$

a useful means for protecting the human rights of persons with dementia. All persons involved should always consider health, medicine, welfare, care, and family in connection with dementia, thereby supporting the dignity of persons with dementia.

The second issue naturally concerns measures against behavioral and psychological symptoms. According to the results of a questionnaire survey that we conducted among members ($n=1{,}049$) of the Japanese Psychogeriatric Society and the Japanese Association of Psychiatric Hospitals, which has established dementia treatment wards and medical treatment wards [10], among behavioral and psychological symptoms, the drug of first choice for hallucination, delusion, abusive language and violence, and delirium was risperidone, an atypical antipsychotic agent. As yet, no final conclusion has been reached concerning the effectiveness of antipsychotic drugs on the behavioral and psychological symptoms of dementia. However, antipsychotic drugs are indispensable for supporting the lives of the elderly with dementia, either at home or in institutions, as a therapeutic procedure for hallucination and delusion that may cause dangerous situations for persons with dementia and their families when they develop. We should administer such medication with periodic monitoring, comprehensively considering the actual needs and health conditions of the patients and the effectiveness and side effects expected. In the present situation, off-label use of antipsychotic drugs is inevitable for the behavioral and psychological symptoms of dementia. Experts are expected to be skilled in the use of these drugs. However, the most serious issue in the surveillance is the situation where no informed consent has been obtained in the more than half of patients who are administered antipsychotic drugs. Although no stratified analysis has been conducted on this data, regardless of use status, informed consent should be obtained appropriately for any treatment using an antipsychotic drug. Furthermore, the concept of informed consent should be examined for persons with dementia with notably impaired mental capacity. This is one of the serious issues regarding the current adult guardianship law and requires immediate revision.

The third issue is the response to caregivers and families. In recent years, many outpatients with milder dementia have visited a hospital for diagnosis. In less severe cases, disclosing to persons with dementia the proper name of their disease is more important. Next, the circumstances of caregivers and families, as well as those of the persons with dementia, should be accurately evaluated. Caregivers often find it difficult to recognize the facts. Naturally, they may be unwilling to accept or want to deny the reality, and may therefore be confused for a while. In such situations, it is impossible for a caregiver to properly take in the variety of information that they may be provided. As a matter of priority, caregivers' feelings should be acknowledged with sympathy. Such responses are required from all persons concerned, including physicians.

Issues for the Future

Early detection, precise diagnoses, and management are essential requirements for persons with dementia. Simultaneously, support is needed to allow those with dementia to live in the community. To meet these requirements, we should maintain close communication with those involved in health, medicine, welfare, and care based on appropriate diagnoses. This activity will greatly influence the therapeutic effects, course, and prognosis. However, in view of the present educational curriculum described above, we cannot deny the bias of its contents toward diagnostics. In contrast to diagnosis or treatment skills, it is certainly difficult to evaluate these roles to support persons with dementia in the community. Currently, five dementia-associated academic societies (the Japan Psychogeriatric Society, the Japan Society for Dementia Research, the Japanese Society of Neurology, the Japan Geriatrics Society, and the Japanese Society of Neurological Therapeutics) are jointly drawing up a guideline for the diagnoses and treatment of dementia. In this guideline, emphasizing their philosophy for diagnoses, treatment, and care of persons with dementia is extremely important.

In addition, we should continuously construct a structure to maintain the quality of care for dementia and simultaneously conduct positively educational and enlightening activities, including familiarizing such care to the public.

References

1. Awata S et al (2000) Model of integrated emergency care for dementia; Grants-in-Aid for Scientific Research, Ministry of Health, Labour and Welfare, 2007; The Health Science Research of Heart, Psychiatric Emergency Care; Study report on treatment of physical disorders and complications of dementia, pp 135–156
2. Elderly Care Study Group (2003) Elderly Care in 2015 – for the establishment of care to support dignity of the elderly – Elderly Care Study Group. Houken, Tokyo
3. Bureau of Social Welfare and Public Health, Tokyo Metropolitan Government: Special investigation report on daily life and health of the elderly in 1995; 1995, Bureau of Social Welfare and Public Health, Tokyo Metropolitan Government, 1995
4. Homma A (2000) Geriatric psychiatry: millennium. Jpn J Geriatr Psychiatry 11:68–69
5. Office for the Promotion of Measures for the Elderly, Tokyo Metropolitan Government: Summary of the interim report from the Committee for Establishment of Service Organization for the Elderly, Tokyo Metropolitan Government in 1998; 1999, Office for the Promotion of Measures for the Elderly, Tokyo Metropolitan Government, 1999
6. Brodaty H et al (1998) Screening for cognitive impairment in general practice: toward a consensus. Alzheimer Dis Assoc Disord 12:1–13
7. Office for the Promotion of Measures for the Elderly, Tokyo Metropolitan Government: Report from the Committee for Evaluation of Total Care Collaboration System for the Elderly with Dementia, Tokyo Metropolitan Government 2000, Office for the Promotion of Measures for the Elderly, Tokyo Metropolitan Government, 2000
8. Homma A, Awata S, Ikeda M, Ueki A, Urakami K, Kitamura S, Shigeta M, Nakamura Y, Nakamura M, Ohta K (2006) Local collaboration for the elderly with dementia: model project to improve diagnostic skills of dementia by primary care physicians. Jpn J Geriatr Psychiatry 17:483–489
9. Homma A (2007) Issues of the adult guardianship law concerning informed consent for treatment of the elderly with dementia. In: Arai M (ed) Adult guardianship and medical practice. Nippon Hyoronsha, Tokyo, pp 19–31
10. Homma A (2006) Questionnaire survey about use status of antipsychotic drugs for behavioral and psychological symptoms of dementia (BPSD). Jpn J Geriatr Psychiatry 17:799–783

AD-FTLD Spectrum: New Understanding of the Neurodegenerative Process from the Study of Risk Genes

Masatoshi Takeda, Takashi Kudo, Toshihisa Tanaka, Masayasu Okochi, Ryota Hashimoto, Takashi Morihara, and Shinji Tagami

Abstract Typical cases of primary neurodegenerative diseases causing dementia, such as Alzheimer's disease (AD), diffuse Lewy body disease, frontotemporal lobar degeneration (FTLD), and corticobasal degeneration, show characteristic clinical signs and symptoms, but there are some cases in which the differential diagnosis among neurodegenerative dementias is difficult because of their atypical clinical presentation. Considering recent findings in molecular genetics of familial cases of AD and FTLD, the relationship between causative genes and clinical signs is becoming more complicated, and the concept of an AD-FTLD spectrum is proposed. Protein fragments derived from amyloid precursor proteins, tau and TDP-43, are deposited in the cerebral tissue of patients with AD and FLTD in different degrees. In familial cases, these deposited protein fragments are caused by mutations in the precursor protein genes. The majority of cases of AD and FTLD are sporadic, wherein loss of function of presenilin and progranulin increases the risk of these neurodegenerative disorders. Under the concept of AD-FTLD, it is more helpful to elucidate the common neurodegenerative pathway in which aggregated protein fragments are deposited after partial proteolysis, phosphorylation, and ubiquitination, leading to the formation of amyloid angiopathy, senile plaque, neurofibrillary tangles, and the inclusion body of FTLD.

Keywords Alzheimer's disease • Frontotemporal lobar degeneration • Progranulin • Tau • TDP-43

Introduction

Dementia is a neurodegenerative disease causing severe dysfunction in daily and social life as a result of impairment in memory and cognitive function. Because of the large number of patients, severity of dysfunction, long duration of the course,

---

M. Takeda (✉), T. Kudo, T. Tanaka, M. Okochi, R. Hashimoto, T. Morihara, and S. Tagami
Department of Psychiatry, Osaka University Medical School, Suita, Japan
e-mail: mtakeda@psy.med.osaka-u.ac.jp

K. Miyoshi et al. (eds.), *Neuropsychiatric Disorders*,
DOI 10.1007/978-4-431-53871-4_17, © Springer 2010

and burden to caregivers, dementia is regarded one of the most malignant diseases in this century. There are 24.3 million dementia patients in the world, and 4.6 million people are newly diagnosed every year [1]. In Japan alone there are now 1.5 million dementia patients, and the number of dementia patients is steadily increasing for reasons of the extension of the average lifespan. It is expected there will be 3.5 million dementia patients in Japan by the year 2035.

Alzheimer's disease (AD) is the most frequent primary neurodegenerative disease, accounting for 50–70% of all dementia patients. Higher age, female gender, family history of dementia, head injury, and lower education are reported to be the risks for AD, among which higher age is the most significant. The prevalence rate of AD increases age after 65, almost doubling by every 5 years, and reaching more than 40% prevalence in the elderly over 85 years old [2].

Primary neurodegenerative diseases causing dementia include AD, diffuse Lewy body disease (DLB), frontotemporal lobar degeneration (FTLD), and corticobasal degeneration (CBD). Each disease shows characteristic clinical signs and symptoms. The initial sign of AD is memory impairment, and later impairment in cognitive function follows, such as aphasia, apraxia, agnosia, and executive dysfunction. Those impaired cognitive functions together result in dysfunction in judgment. DLB is the second most common disease among the elderly more than 75 years old, characterized by varying levels of cognitive function, visual hallucination, and parkinsonism. The neuropathological feature of DLB is abundant Lewy bodies in the cerebral cortical neurons. In persons of younger age, less than 65 years old, FTLD is the second predominant dementing disease [3]; it is characterized by personality change, dysinhibition, abnormal behavior, and language disability. In the early phase of FTLD, memory can be preserved despite the deteriorating daily life of the patients. The classification of frontotemporal dementia has been discussed for many years, and FTLD is the broadest concept, which includes Pick's disease and other diseases characterized by progressive lobar atrophy of frontal and temporal lobe. FTLD is classified into three types: (1) frontotemporal dementia (FTD), (2) progressive aphasia, and (3) semantic dementia. FTD is further divided into frontal lobar degeneration, Pick's type, and motor neuron disease type (Fig. 1).

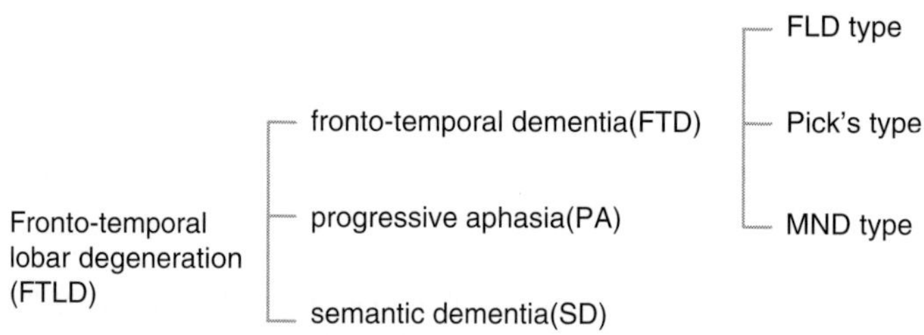

Fig. 1 Classification of frontotemporal lobar degeneration (FTLD) [4]

Genes for AD and FTLD

AD is genetically heterogeneous and complex (Fig. 2). About 10% of AD is early-onset AD, and about 60% of the early-onset type is inherited in an autosomal dominant manner. Mutations in the amyloid precursor protein (APP) gene [5], presenilin1 (PSEN1) gene [6], and presenilin 2 (PSEN2) gene [7] are identified as causative genes of familial AD (Fig. 3).

Even though the pathological process of AD has not yet been fully elucidated, the amyloid cascade hypothesis has been widely accepted [8], in which beta amyloid (A beta) is produced by consecutive cutting by beta-secretase (BACE 1) and gamma-secretase (PSEN complex). The presenilin complex is composed of presenilin, nicastrin, Aph-1, and Pen-2, in which the presenilin molecule carries the catalytical site of gamma-secretase in its molecular structure [9], whereas the other three molecules are functioning in stabilizing the structure of gamma-secretase complex. Gamma-secretase produces several different species of beta amyloid with different C-terminal sites between 37 and 43 amino acids long. Beta amyloid with 40 amino acids is the most abundant, and beta amyloid with 42 amino acids is the form most toxic to neurons.

The amyloid cascade hypothesis is supported by the finding that mutations in APP, PSEN1, or PSEN2, which are found in some familial AD patients, are all relevant key players in processing of APP, in which the core pathogenic process is the increase in beta amyloid, caused by either overproduction, abnormal processing, or delayed secretion of beta amyloid. Increased beta amyloid will be aggregated and deposited, and it is believed to cause neurofibrillary tangle (NFT) formation, or neuronal degeneration, resulting in the symptomatology of AD.

More than 75% of the late-onset AD is sporadic, but there are also some late-onset cases showing familial aggregation [10]. Apolipoprotein E4 (APOε) is involved in the familial cases of late-onset type AD [11]. An individual with one APOε4 allele has 3–5 times higher risk and those with two APOε4 alleles have 10–15 times higher risk for AD [12]. In addition to the higher risk of AD, the APOε4 allele causes the earlier onset of AD [13], and also makes the response to the intervention much worse than in those without e4 [14].

Cause	% of Cases
Chromosomal (Down syndrome)	<1%
Familial	~25%
Late-onset familial (AD2)	15% -25%
Early-onset familial AD (AD1,AD3, AD4)	<2%
Unknown (includes genetic/environment interactions)	~75%

Fig. 2 Causes of Alzheimer disease

Early-onset familial Alzheimer disease (EOFAD)

Locus name	Proportion of EOFAD	Gene symbol	Chromosomal locus	Protein name	Test availability
AD3	20%-70%	*PSEN1*	14q24.3	Presenilin-1	Clinical
AD1	10%-15%	*APP*	21q21	Amyloid beta A4 protein	Clinical
AD4	Rare	*PSEN2*	1q31-q42	Presenilin-2	Clinical

Late onset familial Alzheimer's disease

Locus name	Gene symbol	Chromosomal locus	Protein name	Test availability
AD2	*APOE*	19q13.2	Apolipoprotein E	Clinical

Fig. 3 Early-onset familial Alzheimer disease (EOFAD)/late-onset familial Alzheimer's disease

Apoε is the protein involved in lipid metabolism; however, the mechanism of AD pathogenesis is not yet elucidated. Apoε is expected to function in cholesterol transport, oxidative stress, neurite extension, tau phosphorylation, beta amyloid aggregation, and beta amyloid metabolism. The APOε4 allele increases amyloid deposition in the AD brain [15], and it is also shown that in human healthy elderly subjects the APOε4 allele causes more amyloid load in the brain [16].

Most FTLD cases occur in the age groups of the fifties and sixties, which is much earlier than those of AD. FTLD also shows more familial aggregation than AD. Even though 40–50% of FTLD is claimed to be familial, no causative gene had been identified despite intensive research endeavors. It was only in 2007 that new genes were discovered that are related to the pathogenesis of FTLD [17]. The first gene is the tau gene (MAPT) on chromosome 17. Mutations in MAPT were originally identified from patients of FTDP-17, a subtype of FTLD showing parkinsonism and genetic correlation with chromosome 17 [18]. It was discovered that tau mutations are involved in the formation of tau-positive inclusion bodies (FTLD-tau) in the FTDP-17 patient brain. This finding had a high impact on understanding of neurodegeneration because neurons of FTDP-17 are degenerated without amyloid cascade. In other words, it is shown that neurodegeneration can be induced without amyloid involvement. A single mutation in MAPT is enough to cause neurodegeneration in the cortical neurons, leading to formation of NFTs and neuron loss.

In the brain tissue of FTLD patients, there are two types of inclusion body: one is the inclusion body that is positive with anti-tau antibody (FTLD-tau) and the other is negative with anti-tau antibody and positive with anti-ubiquitin antibody (FTLD-U). The protein component of FTLD-tau is tau, but the component protein of FTLD-U has been unidentified for many years. In 2004, valosin-containing protein (VCP) was reported as the component of FTLD-U [19], and in 2005 charged multivesicular body protein (CHMP2B) was reported [20] as genes related to FTLD-U inclusion body formation. However, there are only a few cases caused by mutation in VCP or CHMP2B, and further search for the genetic cause of FTLD-U has continued.

Progranulin and TDP-43

Tau is a microtubule-associated protein involved in stabilization and elongation of microtubules. NFT in the AD brain and Pick bodies of the FTLD brain are known to be composed of hyperphosphorylated tau. FTDP-17 is the first example of neurodegenerative dementia caused by mutation of the MAPT gene, and it is well accepted that mutated tau is the cause of the FTLD-tau inclusion body observed in the brain of FTLD patients, including FTDP-17. However, the majority of FTLD patients show tau-negative, ubiquitin-positive inclusion bodies (FTLD-U), and the causative gene of FTLD with FTLD-U is yet to be identified.

Further search for genes causing FTLD with the FTLD-U inclusion body was for long unsuccessful. The newly identified gene causing FTLD is the progranulin (PGRN) gene, which is located in a position only 1.7 Mb apart from MAPT on chromosome 17. PGRN is shown to be the causative gene of many FTLD patients with FTLD-U inclusion bodies [21, 22].

PGRN, called by several other names such as acrogranin, epithelin precursor, or proepithelin, classified in the epitherin family, is secreted protein having 7.5 repeated sequences after the signal peptide sequence. PGRN is cleaved by a protease, resulting in a peptide 6 kDa in size (granulin A-G and para granulin), which functions in differentiation, wound healing, inflammation, and tumor formation. Four peptides of PGRN are known to make up a stable structure through S–S bonds [23, 24]. The function of PGRN in the brain is not yet fully elucidated but it is speculated to be a neuronal growth factor [25].

Sixty-six mutations have been reported with 199 families of FTLD. The mutations are spanning all genomic region of PGRN except exon 13. The types of mutations are nonsense mutations (14 kinds), splice site mutations (11 kinds), and deletion/insertion mutation causing frameshift (24 kinds). Loss of function (LOF) of PGRN is speculated to be the cause of FTLD. A more important finding is that PGRN mutations are observed in many neurodegenerative diseases including AD, amyotrophic lateral sclerosis (ALS), and Parkinson's disease (PD).

Soon after the discovery of PGRN mutations with FTLD, TDP-43 was identified as the major protein component of the FTLD-U inclusion body [26]. In the brain tissue of FTLD caused by mutations in PGRN, TDP-43 is deposited as an intracellular inclusion body after hyperphosphorylation and ubiquitination.

TDP-43 (TAR-DNA-binding protein 43) is an intranucleus protein ubiquitously expressed in all tissue, and it is speculated to be involved in transcription, splicing, and stabilization of mRNA [27]. It is also speculated to be involved in biosynthesis of micro-RNA (miRNA) [28]. TDP-43 is initially found accumulated in the brain of ALS, and further studies have revealed that TOP-43-positive deposits are observed in the brain with AD and DLB [29–31]. So, it is believed that TDP-43 and/or its gene (TARDBP) should be involved in the pathogenesis of AD and DLB in addition to ALS and FTLD. Even though no mutation of TDP-43 has been reported with either FTLD or AD, several mutations of TDP-43 are found with patients with familial as well as sporadic ALS. Considering these findings, TARDBP should be involved with the pathogenesis of neurodegenerative diseases of many different kinds [32, 33].

So far, the three genes have been identified as the causative genes of FTLD, that is, MAPT, PGRN, and TARDBP. Still another gene on chromosome 9 is speculated to be causative for FTLD because there are papers reporting high association with the 9p21–13 region in families with FTLD with motor neuron disease [34, 35].

The study of risk genes of neurodegenerative disease has opened up new understanding of neurodegenerative dementia. Of course, these implications should be taken cautiously to apply to the pathogenesis of sporadic cases; involvement of these genes should be some hint for understanding the pathogenesis of sporadic cases of neurodegenerative dementia.

Copy Number Variation, miRNA, and Neurodegeneration

Copy number variation (CNV) is the repetition of a sequence 1 kb long and more including several genes. CNV is now shown to be the causative factor of many disorders, including chronic neuroimmunological (CND) disease. More than 20,000 CNVs exist in the whole genome, which has more than 7,000 genes. In 2006, CNV including the APP gene was reported with five families of AD [36] whose CNV region covers 0.58–6.37 M, including APP and 5–12 other genes. The phenotype of the cases of this CNV is AD with cerebral amyloid angiopathy (CAA), and it was implied that an increased copy number of APP results in AD pathogenesis [37]. Considering the pathogenesis of Down syndrome, which is caused by the increased copy number of APP that is included in the 21q21region, it is quite reasonable to understand this increased copy number of APP is causing AD pathology in the brain of Down syndrome patients more than 30 years old [38]. CNV of the alpha-cynuclain gene is also reported with familial PD patients [39, 40].

These findings support the notion that increased copy number of a certain gene can lead to the deposition of abnormal protein, causing neurodegenerative dementia. Increased numbers of APP may explain the pathogenesis of AD, and this also supports the validity of the amyloid cascade hypothesis.

Increased expression of APP may be caused by several different mechanisms other than CNV. For example, there might be mutations in promoter regions, which could increase the expression level of APP gene up to 50%. Increased expression of APP may increase the risk of AD. In fact, there are papers reporting that mutations in the promoter region of APP cause a 1.2–1.8 increased expression level of APP in Dutch and Belgium families with AD [41, 42].

In addition to gene replication, several different types of partial or complete deletion of genes are reported with families with AD or FTLD. For example, exon 9 deletion of PSEN1 causes AD with massive deposition of characteristic cotton wool plaques in the brain of the patients [43]. Deletion of PGRN or MAPT are reported with FTLD families [44]. There is a paper reporting partial deletion of exon 6–9 of MAPT gene [45], and the tau protein coded by the deleted MAPT gene shows decreased binding activity with microtubules and shows more binding with MAP1B, which might result in the neurodegeneration caused by defective tau protein.

The importance of miRNA should be mentioned in this context. miRNA is an endogenous small RNA molecule that supposedly stimulates mRNA degradation or regulates gene expression after binding with the target mRNA. There are more than 1,000 different kinds of miRNA in the human genome, which are supposed to be relevant to control of the expression level of more than 30% of genes. Especially, more miRNA exist in brain tissue. Search with miRNA array has revealed the significant reduction of miR-107 in the brain with AD [46], which is correlated with the severity of AD pathology. It was also shown that miR-107 binds with mRNA of BACE1 and speculated that reduction of miR-107 results in the increased expression level of BACE1. It is quite reasonable that reduction in miRNA will cause AD pathology through higher expression of BACE1. Significant increase of miR-146a in the AD brain tissue is reported compared with that of the healthy control brain by pooled RNA sample study [47].

These findings just described show the possibility that the change in expression level of certain genes will increase the risk of neurodegenerative diseases such as AD and FTLD, which may lead to a proposal that explains the common neuropathological process among neurodegenerative dementia.

AD-FTLD Spectrum

In the brain of AD patients, there are abnormal depositions of beta amyloid and tau protein. Beta amyloid deposits in the core of senile plaque as well as in the cerebral vessel wall of CAA. Tau is deposited in the soma of degenerating neurons, in ghost tangles, and in dystrophic neuritis as NFT. On the other hand, in the brain of FTLD, tau protein is deposited in Pick body (FTLD-tau) and TDP-43 is deposited intracellularly and intranuclearly as a ubiquitin-positive inclusion body as inclusion body (FTLD-U).

There are 32 different missense mutations reported with the APP gene. Most of these mutations cause AD pathology, such as KM670/671NL Swedish mutation, V717I,P,G London mutation, V715M France mutation, V715A German mutation, and I716V Florida mutation. However, some APP mutations are observed in hereditary cerebral hemorrhage with angiopathy, such as HCHWA Dutch (E693Q) and CAA Italian (E693K). Flemish-type APP mutation (Flemish A692G) causes CAA as well as AD pathology.

There are 177 different mutations reported with the PSEN gene, most of which cause early-onset type AD. The earliest onset of AD is reported with a subject of 24 years old, implying strong pathogenic effects of PSEN1 gene mutation. It should be noticed that there are PSEN1 mutations whose phenotype is FTLD symptoms (L113P, G183V, insArg352).

There are 44 different mutations reported with MAPT, most of which are concentrated in 9–13 exons and an intron between exon 10 and 11. The major phenotype of MAPT mutations is FTLD with typical Pick body and FTLD-tau inclusion body in the intracellular and intranuclear space. The characteristics of MAPT mutations is the fact that they show a wide range of symptoms of FTLD, whose major symptom is parkinsonism (i.e., FTDP-17), or with behavioral abnormalities, or aphasia. There are also tau mutations whose symptoms are very similar to those of AD. For example, patients with the MAPT R406W mutation show memory impairment in the initial stage and then gradually show FTLD symptoms.

FTLD-tau inclusion is observed in 25% of FTLD patients, and the majority of FTLD patients show a tau-negative, ubiquitin-positive inclusion (FTLD-U), which is composed of TDP-43. LOF of PGRN is closely related with pathogenesis of FTLKD-U formation. Mutation of PGRN explains about 25% of familial FTLD, which coincides with the frequency of the MAPT mutation among FTLD cases. There is a wide variety of onset age with FTLD patients with MAPT or PGRN mutations: 20–70 years for MAPT mutations and 30–80 years for PRGN mutations. When the average onset age is compared between patients with PGRN mutation (61 ± 9 years old) and those with MAPT mutations (48 ± 10 years old), the PGRN mutation causes FTLD with later-onset age.

Furthermore, there are cases with AD phenotypes and ALS phenotypes among the patients with PGRN mutations.

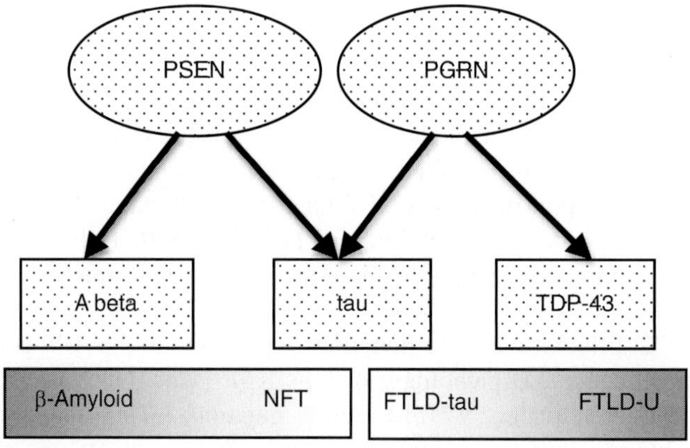

Fig. 4 AD-FTLD Spectrum

It is reasonable to speculate that there is a common pathogenic process among different neurodegenerative dementia disorders (Fig. 4). APP is cleaved by consecutive proteolysis by beta-secretase and gamma-secretase to produce beta amyloid, which deposits in the core of senile plaques and the vascular walls of CAA. Tau protein is phosphorylated and partially cleaved and deposited in NFT and in dystrophic neurites. TDP-43 is also partially cleaved, phosphorylated, and ubiquitinated, and then deposited in the FTLD-U inclusion body in the intracellular and intranuclear space.

Many types of mutations in the PSEN gene (177 kinds) and in the PGRN gene (68 kinds) are distributed through a wide area of the molecule, which is characterized by LOF of the protein. It can be proposed that LOF mutations of PSEN induces beta amyloid and NFT deposition, whereas the LOF mutations of PGRN causes the deposition of FTLD-tau and FTLD-U. However, it should be noted that there are intermediate phenotypes between AD and FTLD, implying that both pathological processes share a common path, which can be characterized by each extreme case of pathogenesis.

References

1. Ferri CP, Prince M, Brayne C et al (2005) Global prevalence of dementia: a Delphi consensus study. Lancet 366:2112–2117
2. Breteler MM, Claus JJ, van Duijn CM et al (1992) Epidemiology of Alzheimer's disease. Epidemiol Rev 14:59–82
3. Graff-Radford NR, Woodruff BK (2007) Frontotemporal dementia. Semin Neurol 27:48–57
4. Neary D, Snowden JS, Gustafson L et al (1998) Frontotemporal lobar degeneration: a consensus on clinical diagnostic criteria. Neurology 51(6):1546–1554
5. Goate A, Chartier-Harlin MC, Mullan M et al (1991) Segregation of a missense mutation in the amyloid precursor protein gene with familial Alzheimer's disease. Nature (Lond) 349:704–706
6. Sherrington R, Rogaev EI, Liang Y et al (1995) Cloning of a gene bearing missense mutations in early-onset familial Alzheimer's disease. Nature (Lond) 375:754–760
7. Levy-Lahad E, Wasco W, Poorkaj P et al (1995) Candidate gene for the chromosome 1 familial Alzheimer's disease locus. Science 269:973–977
8. Hardy J (1997) Amyloid, the presenilins and Alzheimer's disease. Trends Neurosci 20:154–159
9. De Strooper B (2003) Aph-1, Pen-2, and nicastrin with presenilin generate an active gamma-secretase complex. Neuron 38:9–12
10. Bird TD (2008) Genetic aspects of Alzheimer disease. Genet Med 10:231–239
11. Strittmatter WJ, Saunders AM, Schmechel D et al (1993) Apolipoprotein E: high-avidity binding to beta-amyloid and increased frequency of type 4 allele in late-onset familial Alzheimer disease. Proc Natl Acad Sci USA 90:1977–1981
12. Farrer LA, Cupples LA, Haines JL et al (1997) Effects of age, sex, and ethnicity on the association between apolipoprotein E genotype and Alzheimer disease. A meta-analysis. APOε and Alzheimer disease meta analysis consortium. JAMA 278:1349–1356
13. Corder EH, Saunders AM, Strittmatter WJ et al (1993) Gene dose of apolipoprotein E type 4 allele and the risk of Alzheimer's disease in late onset families. Science 261:921–923
14. Mahley RW, Weisgraber KH, Huang Y (2006) Apolipoprotein E4: a causative factor and therapeutic target in neuropathology, including Alzheimer's disease. Proc Natl Acad Sci USA 103:5644–5651

15. Drzezga A, Grimmer T, Henriksen G et al (2009) Effect of APOε genotype on amyloid plaque load and gray matter volume in Alzheimer disease. Neurology 72:1487–1494
16. Reiman EM, Chen K, Liu X et al (2009) Fibrillar amyloid-beta burden in cognitively normal people at 3 levels of genetic risk for Alzheimer's disease. Proc Natl Acad Sci USA 106:6820–6825
17. Rademakers R, Hutton M (2007) The genetics of frontotemporal lobar degeneration. Curr Neurol Neurosci Rep 7:434–442
18. Hutton M, Lendon CL, Rizzu P et al (1998) Association of missense and 5′-splice-site mutations in tau with the inherited dementia FTDP-17. Nature (Lond) 393:702–705
19. Watts GD, Wymer J, Kovach MJ et al (2004) Inclusion body myopathy associated with Paget disease of bone and frontotemporal dementia is caused by mutant valosin-containing protein. Nat Genet 36:377–381
20. Skibinski G, Parkinson NJ, Brown JM et al (2005) Mutations in the endosomal ESCRTIII complex subunit CHMP2B in frontotemporal dementia. Nat Genet 37:806–808
21. Baker M, MacKenzie IR, Pickering-Brown SM et al (2006) Mutations in progranulin cause tau-negative frontotemporal dementia linked to chromosome 17. Nature (Lond) 442:916–919
22. Cruts M, Gijselinck I, van der Zee J et al (2006) Null mutations in progranulin cause ubiquitin-positive frontotemporal dementia linked to chromosome 17q21. Nature (Lond) 442:920–924
23. He Z, Bateman A (2003) Progranulin (granulin–epithelin precursor, PC-cell-derived growth factor, acrogranin) mediates tissue repair and tumorigenesis. J Mol Med 81:600–612
24. He Z, Ong CH, Halper J et al (2003) Progranulin is a mediator of the wound response. Nat Med 9:225–229
25. Van Damme P, Van Hoecke A, Lambrechts D et al (2008) Progranulin functions as a neurotrophic factor to regulate neurite outgrowth and enhance neuronal survival. J Cell Biol 181:37–41
26. Neumann M, Sampathu DM, Kwong LK et al (2006) Ubiquitinated TDP-43 in frontotemporal lobar degeneration and amyotrophic lateral sclerosis. Science 314:130–133
27. Buratti E, Baralle FE (2008) Multiple roles of TDP-43 in gene expression, splicing regulation, and human disease. Front Biosci 13:867–878
28. Gregory RI, Yan KP, Amuthan G et al (2004) The microprocessor complex mediates the genesis of microRNAs. Nature (Lond) 432:235–240
29. Amador-Ortiz C, Lin WL, Ahmed Z et al (2007) TDP-43 immunoreactivity in hippocampal sclerosis and Alzheimer's disease. Ann Neurol 61:435–445
30. Higashi S, Iseki E, Yamamoto R et al (2007) Concurrence of TDP-43, tau and alpha-synuclein pathology in brains of Alzheimer's disease and dementia with Lewy bodies. Brain Res 1184:284–294
31. Nakashima-Yasuda H, Uryu K, Robinson J et al (2007) Co-morbidity of TDP-43 proteinopathy in Lewy body related diseases. Acta Neuropathol 114:221–229
32. Kabashi E, Valdmanis PN, Dion P et al (2008) TARDBP mutations in individuals with sporadic and familial amyotrophic lateral sclerosis. Nat Genet 40:572–574
33. Sreedharan J, Blair IP, Tripathi VB et al (2008) TDP-43 mutations in familial and sporadic amyotrophic lateral sclerosis. Science 319:1668–1672
34. Morita M, Al-Chalabi A, Andersen PM et al (2006) A locus on chromosome 9p confers susceptibility to ALS and frontotemporal dementia. Neurology 66:839–844
35. Vance C, Al-Chalabi A, Ruddy D et al (2006) Familial amyotrophic lateral sclerosis with frontotemporal dementia is linked to a locus on chromosome 9p13.2–21.3. Brain 129:868–876
36. Rovelet-Lecrux A, Hannequin D, Raux G et al (2006) APP locus duplication causes autosomal dominant early-onset Alzheimer disease with cerebral amyloid angiopathy. Nat Genet 38:24–26
37. Sleegers K, Brouwers N, Gijselinck I et al (2006) APP duplication is sufficient to cause early onset Alzheimer's dementia with cerebral amyloid angiopathy. Brain 129:2977–2983

38. Wisniewski KE, Dalton AJ, McLachlan C et al (1985) Alzheimer's disease in Down's syndrome: clinicopathologic studies. Neurology 35:957–961
39. Singleton AB, Farrer M, Johnson J et al (2003) Alpha-synuclein locus triplication causes Parkinson's disease. Science 302:841
40. Chartier-Harlin MC, Kachrgus J, Roumier C et al (2004) Alpha-synuclein locus duplication as a cause of familial Parkinson's disease. Lancet 364:1167–1169
41. Brouwers N, Sleegers K, Engelborghs S et al (2006) Genetic risk and transcriptional variability of amyloid precursor protein in Alzheimer's disease. Brain 129:2984–2991
42. Theuns J, Brouwers N, Engelborghs S et al (2006) Promoter mutations that increase amyloid precursor-protein expression are associated with Alzheimer disease. Am J Hum Genet 78:936–946
43. Crook R, Verkkoniemi A, Perez-Tur J et al (1998) A variant of Alzheimer's disease with spastic paraparesis and unusual plaques due to deletion of exon 9 of presenilin 1. Nat Med 4:452–455
44. Rovelet-Lecrux A, Deramecourt V, Legallic S et al (2008) Deletion of the progranulin gene in patients with frontotemporal lobar degeneration or Parkinson disease. Neurobiol Dis 31:41–45
45. Rovelet-Lecrux A (2009) Partial deletion of the MAPT gene: a novel mechanism of FTDP-17. Hum Mutat 30:E591–E602
46. Wang WX, Rajeev BW, Stromberg AJ et al (2008) The expression of microRNA miR-107 decreases early in Alzheimer's disease and may accelerate disease progression through regulation of beta-site amyloid precursor protein-cleaving enzyme 1. J Neurosci 28:1213–1223
47. Lukiw WJ, Zhao Y, Cui JG (2008) An NF-kB-sensitive micro RNA-146amediated inflammatory circuit in Alzheimer disease and in stressed human brain cells. J Biol Chem 283:31315–31322

Dementia with Lewy Bodies

Ian Grant McKeith

Abstract Dementia with Lewy bodies (DLB) has over the last two decades become recognised as a common dementia subtype in older people. Since it shares clinical and pathological features with both Alzheimer's disease and Parkinson's disease, knowledge of DLB is essential not only in its own right, but also to obtain a full understanding of its two prototypical boundary disorders. This chapter reviews what is currently known about the clinical, pathological and management aspects of DLB.

Keywords Alpha-synuclein • Dementia • Diagnosis • Lewy body • Parkinson's

Introduction

Dementia with Lewy bodies (DLB), which is now thought to be the second most prevalent cause of degenerative dementia in older people [1] has previously carried a variety of diagnostic labels, including diffuse Lewy body (LB) disease [2], LB dementia [3], the LB variant of Alzheimer's disease [4], senile dementia of LB type [5], and dementia associated with cortical Lewy bodies [6]. The latest International Consensus criteria describe a spectrum of LB disorders with DLB and Parkinson's disease (PD) dementia as two operationally defined phenotypes which are now in widespread clinical use [7]. Primary autonomic failure, rapid eye movement sleep disorder, and PD itself are other syndromes considered to lie along the same continuum. and debate continues about the nature of their interrelationships. The importance of recognizing DLB relates particularly to its pharmacological management, with reports of good responsiveness to acetylcholinesterase inhibitors (AChEIs)[8], extreme sensitivity to the side effects of neuroleptics [9, 10], and limited responsiveness to levo-dopa [11].

I.G. McKeith (✉)
Wolfson Research Centre, Institute for Ageing and Health, Campus for Ageing and Vitality, Newcastle University, Newcastle upon Tyne NE4 5PL, UK
e-mail: i.g.mckeith@ncl.ac.uk

K. Miyoshi et al. (eds.), *Neuropsychiatric Disorders*,
DOI 10.1007/978-4-431-53871-4_18, © Springer 2010

Epidemiology

There is very little systematically collected information about the prevalence, incidence, and associated risk factors for dementia with Lewy bodies (DLB). A community study of individuals 85 and older found 5% met consensus criteria for DLB, representing 22% of all demented cases [12]. This finding is similar to other clinical estimates in research studies [13, 14] and consistent with estimates of Lewy body (LB) prevalence (15%) in a dementia case register followed to autopsy [1]. In routine clinical practice, it is likely, however, that DLB diagnosis rates are significantly lower than this. Risk factors for DLB are unclear as prevalence studies have been too small. It has however been suggested that APO-E4 status reduces survival rate in DLB (as with AD), although its presence has little effect on disease onset or duration [16].

Pathology and Etiology

Alpha (α)-synuclein-positive LBs and Lewy neurites (LNs) are the characteristic autopsy lesions of DLB. Up to a quarter of LB disease cases show a pathological distribution that has extensive neocortical and limbic involvement with relative sparing of midbrain and subcortical structures, that is, not conforming to typical "Braak-like" Parkinson's disease (PD) spread. There is often also abundant Alzheimer-type pathology, predominantly in the form of amyloid plaques. Tau-positive inclusions and neocortical neurofibrillary tangles sufficient to qualify for a diagnosis of concomitant AD (Braak stages V or VI) occur in only 10–25% of cases. Alzheimer pathology is not needed for dementia to occur because a small number of "pure" DLB cases are seen with typical cognitive impairment and neuropsychiatric features. Cortical LB and LN density is not robustly correlated with either the severity or duration of dementia [17, 18], and in some community-based series, Lewy-type pathologies are frequently seen in nondemented, neurologically normal individuals [19, 20]. This finding raises the intriguing possibility that LBs are a neurprotective response to the generation of low molecular weight species of α-synuclein that are located in synaptosomes and impair synaptic function [21]. Synaptic dysregulation and neurotransmitter deficits may therefore be turn out to be better correlates of the fluctuating clinical picture [22] and provide the best drug targets. α-Synuclein immunoreactive deposits with many of the characteristics of LB have also been reported in a high proportion of AD cases usually occurring exclusively in the amygdala [23]. In this context they may simply reflect end-stage aggregation of α-synuclein in severely dysfunctional neurons that are already heavily damaged by plaque and tangle pathology [24, 25]. Triplication of the α-synuclein gene (SNCA) can cause DLB, PD, and Parkinson's disease dementia (PDD), whereas gene duplication is associated only with motor PD, suggesting a gene dose effect [26]. However, SNCA multiplication is not found in most LB disease patients [27]. Mutations in the glucocebebrosidase (GBA) gene, previously associated with the lipid storage disorder Gaucher's disease, have also recently been reported in PD and DLB [28] although the mechanism of this association remains speculative [29].

Clinical Features

DLB is recognized by progressive signs and symptoms of dementia, with marked impairments in visuo-spatial, attentional, and executive functions. Episodic recall can be relatively preserved in the early stages, in contrast to Alzheimer's disease (AD), in which memory failure is often the presenting complaint. The course is generally progressive, with cognitive test scores declining about 10% per annum, similar to AD [30]. Survival times from onset until death are generally similar to AD [31], although DLB patients are at greater risk of hospital admission because of fall-related injuries and bronchopneumonia [32] and sometimes have a very rapid disease course [33]. Fluctuating cognition, recurrent visual hallucinations, and extrapyramidal motor symptoms are the core features distinguishing DLB clinically, although these features are now known to be absent in a significant minority of cases [10], leading to difficulties in diagnosis. The onset tends to be insidious, although reports of a period of increased confusion or prominent hallucinations may give the impression of a sudden onset. Extrapyramidal symptoms (EPS) are reported in 25–50% of DLB cases at diagnosis, and 75–80%, that is, not all cases, develop some EPS during the natural course. The profile of EPS in DLB is generally similar to that in age-matched, nondemented PD patients [34], with greater postural instability and facial impassivity but less tremor [35]. Rate of motor deterioration is about 10% per annum, similar to PD [36], but levo-dopa responsiveness is reduced, possibly because of additional intrinsic striatal pathology and dysfunction [37].

Fluctuations in cognitive function, which may vary over minutes, hours, or days, occur in 50–75% of patients and are associated with shifting levels of attention and alertness. The assessment of fluctuating cognitive impairment poses considerable difficulty to most clinicians and has repeatedly been cited as a reason for low clinical ascertainment of DLB. The use of caregiver- and observer-rated scales may be particularly helpful in this regard [38]. Questions such as, "Are there episodes when his or her thinking seems quite clear and then becomes muddled?" were originally thought to be useful probes [39], until two studies [40, 41] found that most caregivers responded positively to such questions regardless of whether the patient had AD or DLB. More reliable predictors of DLB diagnosis are objective questions about daytime sleepiness, episodes of staring blankly or incoherent speech, and qualitative assessment of the range of fluctuation (e.g., best versus worst).

Persistent visual hallucinations in a patient with dementia are a strong predictor of a DLB diagnosis, occurring in up to 80% of cases. Patients with mild to moderate dementia can usually give a good account of these symptoms, but in the later stages the clinician needs to use caregiver reports, and as with

References

1. McKeith IG, Galasko D, Kosaka K et al (1996) Consensus guidelines for the clinical and pathologic diagnosis of dementia with Lewy bodies (DLB): report of the Consortium on DLB International Workshop. Neurology 47:1113–1124
2. Kosaka K, Yoshimura IK et al (1984) Diffuse type of Lewy body disease: progressive dementia with abundant cortical Lewy bodies and senile changes of varying degree – a new disease? Clin Neuropathol 3(5):185–192
3. Gibb WRG, Esiri MM, Lees AJ (1987) Clinical and pathological features of diffuse cortical Lewy body disease (Lewy body dementia). Brain 110:1131–1153
4. Hansen L, Salmon D, Galasko D et al (1990) The Lewy body variant of Alzheimer's disease: a clinical and pathologic entity. Neurology 40:1–8
5. Perry RH, Irving D, Blessed G et al (1990) Senile dementia of Lewy body type. A clinically and neuropathologically distinct form of Lewy body dementia in the elderly. J Neurol Sci 95:119–139
6. Byrne EJ, Lennox G, Godwin-Austen LB et al (1991) Dementia associated with cortical Lewy bodies. Proposed diagnostic criteria. Dementia 2:283–284
7. McKeith IG, Dickson DW, Lowe J et al (2005) Diagnosis and management of dementia with Lewy bodies. Third report of the DLB consortium. Neurology 65:1863–1872
8. McKeith I, Del Ser T, Spano P et al (2000) Efficacy of rivastigmine in dementia with Lewy bodies: a randomised, double-blind, placebo-controlled international study. Lancet 356:2031–2036
9. McKeith I, Fairbairn A, Perry R et al (1992) Neuroleptic sensitivity in patients with senile dementia of Lewy body type. Br Med J 305:673–678
10. Ballard C, Grace J, McKeith I et al (1998) Neuroleptic sensitivity in dementia with Lewy bodies and Alzheimer's disease. Lancet 351:1032–1033
11. Molloy S, McKeith IG, O'Brien JT et al (2005) The role of levodopa in the management of dementia with Lewy bodies. J Neurol Neurosurg Psychiatry 76:1200–1203
12. Rahkonen T, Eloniemi-Sulkava U, Rissanen S et al (2003) Dementia with Lewy bodies according to the consensus criteria in a general population aged 75 years or older. J Neurol Neurosurg Psychiatry 74(6):720–724
13. Shergill S, Mullen E, D'Ath P et al (1994) What is the clinical prevalence of Lewy body dementia? Int J Geriatr Psychiatry 9:907–912
14. Stevens T, Livingston G, Kitchen G et al (2002) Islington study of dementia subtypes in the community. Br J Psychiatry 180:270–276
15. Holmes C, Cairns N, Lantos P et al (1999) Validity of current clinical criteria for Alzheimer's disease, vascular dementia and dementia with Lewy bodies. Br J Psychiatry 174:45–51
16. Singleton AB, Wharton A, O'Brien KK et al (2002) Clinical and neuropathological correlates of apolipoprotein E genotype in dementia with Lewy bodies. Dement Geriatr Cogn Disord 14:167–175
17. Harding AJ, Halliday GM (2001) Cortical Lewy body pathology in the diagnosis of dementia. Acta Neuropathol 102:355–363
18. Gómez-Tortosa E, Newall K, lrizarry MC et al (1999) Clinical and quantitative pathological correlates of dementia with Lewy bodies. Neurology 53:1284–1291
19. Parkkinen L, Kauppinen T, Pirttilä T et al (2005) Alpha-synuclein pathology does not predict extrapyramidal symptoms or dementia. Ann Neurol 57:82–91
20. Zaccai J, Brayne C, McKeith I et al (2008) Patterns and stages of alpha-synucleinopathy: relevance in a population-based cohort. Neurology 70:1042–1048
21. Kramer ML, Schulz-Schaeffer WJ (2007) Presynaptic alpha-synuclein aggregates, not Lewy bodies, cause neurodegeneration in dementia with Lewy bodies. J Neurosci 27:1405–1410
22. Perry EK, Piggott MA, Johnson M et al (2003) Neurotransmitter correlates of neuropsychiatric symptoms in dementia with Lewy bodies. In: Bedard M-A, Agid Y, Chouinard S et al (eds) Mental and behavioral dysfunction in movement disorders. Humana, Totowa, NJ, pp. 285–294
23. Hamilton RL (2000) Lewy bodies in Alzheimer's disease: a neuropathological review of 145 cases using alpha-synuclein immunohistochemistry. Brain Pathol 10:378–384

24. Lippa CF, McKeith I (2003) Dementia with Lewy bodies: improving diagnostic criteria. Neurology 60:1571–1572
25. Uchikado H, Lin WL, DeLucia M et al (2006) Alzheimer disease with amygdala Lewy bodies: a distinct form of alpha-synucleinopathy. J Neuropathol Exp Neurol 65:685–697
26. Singleton A, Gwinn-Hardy K (2004) Parkinson's disease and dementia with Lewy bodies: a difference in dose? Lancet 364(9440):1105–1107
27. Johnson J, Hague SM, Hanson M et al (2004) SNCA multiplication is not a common cause of Parkinson disease or dementia with Lewy bodies. Neurology 63(3):554–556
28. Clark LN, Kartsaklis LA, Wolf Gilbert R et al (2009) Association of glucocerebrosidase mutations with dementia with Lewy bodies. Arch Neurol 66:578–583
29. Hardy J, Lewis P, Revesz T et al (2009) The genetics of Parkinson's syndromes: a critical review. Curr Opin Genet Dev 19:254–265
30. Ballard C, O'Brien J, Morris CM et al (2001) The progression of cognitive impairment in dementia with Lewy bodies, vascular dementia and Alzheimer's disease. Int J Geriatr Psychiatry 16(5):499–503
31. Walker Z, Allen RL, Shergill S et al (2000) Three years survival in patients with a clinical diagnosis of dementia with Lewy bodies. Int J Geriatr Psychiatry 15:267–273
32. Hanyu H, Sato T, Hirao K et al (2009) Differences in clinical course between dementia with Lewy bodies and Alzheimer's disease. Eur J Neurol 16:212–217
33. Armstrong TP, Hansen LA, Salmon DP et al (1991) Rapidly progressive dementia in a patient with the Lewy body variant of Alzheimer's disease. Neurology 41:1178–1180
34. Aarsland D, Ballard C, McKeith I et al (2001) Comparison of extrapyramidal signs in dementia with Lewy bodies and Parkinson's disease. J Neuropsychiatry Clin Neurosci 13:374–379
35. Burn DJ, Rowan EN, Minett T et al (2003) Extrapyramidal features in Parkinson's disease with and without dementia and dementia with Lewy bodies: a cross-sectional comparative study. Mov Disord 18(8):884–889
36. Ballard C, O'Brien J, Swann A et al (2000) One year follow-up of parkinsonism in dementia with Lewy bodies. Dement Geriatr Cogn Disord 11:219–222
37. Duda JE, Giasson BI, Mabon ME et al (2002) Novel antibodies to synuclein show abundant striatal pathology in Lewy body diseases. Ann Neurol 52(2):205–210
38. Walker MP, Ayre GA, Cummings JL et al (2000) The Clinician Assessment of Fluctuation and the One Day Fluctuation Assessment Scale. Two methods to assess fluctuating confusion in dementia. Br J Psychiatry 177:252–256
39. Ballard CG, Mohan RNC, Patel A et al (1993) Idiopathic clouding of consciousness – do the patients have cortical Lewy body disease? Int J Geriatr Psychiatry 8:571–576
40. Bradshaw J, Saling M, Hopwood M et al (2004) Fluctuating cognition in dementia with Lewy bodies and Alzheimer's disease is qualitatively distinct. J Neurol Neurosurg Psychiatry 75:382–387
41. Ferman T, Smith GE, Boeve BF et al (2004) DLB fluctuations: specific features that reliably differentiate from AD and normal aging. Neurology 62(2):181–187
42. Mosimann UP, Rowan EN, Partington CE et al (2006) Characteristics of visual hallucinations in Parkinson disease dementia and dementia with Lewy bodies. Am J Geriatr Psychiatry 14(2):153–60
43. Birkett DP, Desouky A, Han L et al (1992) Lewy bodies in psychiatric patients. Int J Geriatr Psychiatry 7:235–240
44. Boeve BF, Silber MH, Ferman TJ (2004) REM sleep behavior disorder in Parkinson's disease and dementia with Lewy bodies. J Geriatr Psychiatry Neurol 17(3):146–157
45. Klatka LA, Louis ED, Schiffer RB (1996) Psychiatric features in diffuse Lewy body disease: findings in 28 pathologically diagnosed cases. Neurology 46:A180
46. Ballard C, Shaw F, McKeith I et al (1998) High prevalence of neurovascular instability in neurodegenerative dementias. Neurology 51:1760–1762
47. Del-Ser T, Munoz DG, Hachinski V (1996) Temporal pattern of cognitive decline and incontinence is different in Alzheimer's disease and diffuse Lewy body disease. Neurology 46:682–686
48. McKeith I, Mintzer J, Aarsland D et al (2004) Dementia with Lewy bodies. Lancet Neurol 3:19–28

49. Mollenhauer B, Cullen V, Kahn I et al (2008) Direct quantification of CSF alpha-synuclein by ELISA and first cross-sectional study in patients with neurodegeneration. Exp Neurol 213(2):315–25
50. Burton EJ, Barber R, Mukaetova-Ladinska et al (2009) Medial temporal lobe atrophy on MRI differentiates Alzheimer's disease from in dementia with Lewy bodies and vascular cognitive impairment. Brain 132:195–203
51. Lobotesis K, Fenwick JD, Phipps A et al (2001) Occipital hypoperfusion on SPECT in dementia with Lewy bodies but not AD. Neurology 56:643–649
52. O'Brien JT, Paling S, Barber R et al (2001) Progressive brain atrophy on serial MRI in dementia with Lewy bodies, AD, and vascular dementia. Neurology 56(10):1386–1388
53. Walker Z, Costa DC, Ince P et al (1999) In-vivo demonstration of dopaminergic degeneration in dementia with Lewy bodies. Lancet 354:646–647
54. McKeith I, O'Brien J, Walker Z et al (2007) Sensitivity and specificity of dopamine transporter imaging with ^{123}I-FP-CIT SPECT in dementia with Lewy bodies: a phase III, multicentre study. Lancet Neurol 6:305–313
55. O'Brien JT, McKeith IG, Walker Z et al (2009) Diagnostic accuracy of ^{123}I-FP-CIT SPECT in possible dementia with Lewy bodies. Br J Psychiatry 194:34–39
56. Emre M (2003) Dementia associated with Parkinson's disease. Lancet Neurol 2(4):229–237
57. Aarsland D, Andersen K, Larsen JP et al (2003) Prevalence and characteristics of dementia in Parkinson disease: an 8-year prospective study. Arch Neurol 60(3):387–392
58. Emre M, Aarsland D, Brown R et al (2007) Clinical diagnostic criteria for dementia associated with Parkinson's disease. Mov Disord 22:1689–1707
59. Ballard CG, Aarsland D, McKeith I et al (2002) Fluctuations in attention: PD dementia vs DLB with parkinsonism. Neurology 59(11):1714–1720
60. Aarsland D, Ballard C, Larsen JP et al (2001) A comparative study of psychiatric symptoms in dementia with Lewy bodies and Parkinson's disease with and without dementia. Int J Geriatr Psychiatry 16:528–536
61. McKeith I (2007) Dementia with Lewy bodies and Parkinson's disease with dementia: where two worlds collide. Pract Neurol 7:374–382
62. McKeith I (2009) Commentary: DLB and PDD: the same or different? Is there a debate? Int Psychogeriatr 21:220–224
63. McKeith IG (2004) Dementia with Lewy bodies (DLB) and other difficult diagnoses. Int Psychogeriatr 16(2):123–127

Dementia with Lewy Bodies and Parkinson Disease with Dementia Within the Spectrum of Lewy Body Disease

Kenji Kosaka

Abstract The history of Parkinson disease (PD) and dementia with Lewy bodies (DLB) is briefly presented. Since Lewy reported Lewy bodies in the brainstem nuclei of the PD brain in 1912, Lewy bodies had been considered an essential pathological finding for the diagnosis of PD. It had been, however, considered that there were almost no Lewy bodies occurring in the cerebral cortex. In 1976, we reported our first autopsied case showing numerous Lewy bodies in the cerebral cortex. In 1978, we reported the detailed characteristics and distribution pattern of cortical Lewy bodies, based on three autopsied cases showing diffuse Lewy body disease (DLBD), a term that we proposed in 1984. We also reported two German autopsied cases showing DLBD in 1979, which were the first DLBD cases reported in Europe. In 1980, we also proposed the term Lewy body disease and classified it into three types: brainstem type, transitional type, and diffuse type. The brainstem type is the same as PD, and the diffuse type was later designated DLBD. In 1990, we reviewed all the 37 DLBD cases reported in Japan and classified DLBD into two forms: a common form with more or less Alzheimer pathology and a pure form without such pathology. Since then, we have reported many papers concerning DLBD. The term dementia with Lewy bodies (DLB) was proposed at the first international workshop held in 1995. CDLB guidelines were published in 1996, and the CDLB guidelines–revised were reported in 2005. In the revised guidelines the term Lewy body disease was used as a generic term that included DLB, PD, and PDD, as we had insisted since 1980.

Keywords Dementia with Lewy bodies (DLB) • Diffuse Lewy body disease • Lewy body disease • Parkinson disease • Parkinson disease with dementia (PDD)

K. Kosaka (✉)
Yokohama Houyuu Hospital, Yokohama, Japan
e-mail: kenji@memosync.com

K. Miyoshi et al. (eds.), *Neuropsychiatric Disorders*,
DOI 10.1007/978-4-431-53871-4_19, © Springer 2010

Introduction

Dementia with Lewy bodies (DLB) is now the second most frequent dementing illness in the elderly, following Alzheimer-type dementia (ATD). The term DLB was proposed at the first International Workshop [1], which was held in Newcastle upon Tyne in 1995. Lewy bodies are essential for the neuropathological diagnosis of Parkinson's disease (PD). PD patients frequently show dementia, and such patients are diagnosed as having PD with dementia (PDD). Recently, it has usually been considered that DLB and PDD are almost the same disease not only clinically but also neuropathologically.

In this chapter, the author briefly introduces the history of PD and DLB, and insists that DLB and PDD should be understood within the spectrum of Lewy body disease, a term that we proposed in 1980 [2].

History of PD and DLB

James Parkinson [3] published the first report detailing the clinical features of "shaking palsy" in 1817. Then, he described that cognition remained intact in this disease. Charcot [4] proposed the term "Parkinson disease" in 1968, and described cognitive disturbance in PD. In 1912, Lewy [5] reported eosinophilic round intraneuronal inclusions in the substantia innominata and dorsal vagal nuclei of PD brain. Tretiakoff [6] nominated these inclusions "Lewy bodies" and indicated the importance of the substantia nigra in PD in 1919. Thereafter, the difference of PD and postencephalitic parkinsonism was discussed for a long time. Hassler [7] reported the difference in the distribution of neuronal loss in the substantia nigra between these two diseases in 1938. In 1953, Greenfield and Bosanquet [8] pointed out for the first time that the presence of Lewy bodies is the essential pathological finding for the diagnosis of PD whereas the presence of neurofibrillary tangles is essential for the diagnosis of postencephalitic parkinsonism. Furthermore, den Hartog Jager and Bethlem [9] described the detailed distribution of Lewy bodies in the brainstem of PD brain in 1960. Thus, the pathological basis of PD was established about one and a half centuries after the first report of Parkinson in 1817. It had been, however, considered that there were almost no Lewy bodies occurring in the cerebral cortex. In 1976, we [10] reported our first autopsied case showing numerous Lewy bodies in the cerebral cortex as well as in the brainstem nuclei. In 1978, we [11] reported the detailed characteristics and distribution pattern of cortical Lewy bodies, based on our own three autopsied cases with "diffuse Lewy body disease (DLBD)," a term that we [12] proposed in 1984. We [13] also reported two German autopsied cases showing DLBD in 1979, which were the first DLBD cases reported in Europe. In 1980, we [2] proposed the term "Lewy body disease" and classified it into three types: brainstem type, transitional type, and diffuse type. The brainstem type is the same as PD, and the diffuse type was later designated DLBD

[12]. Furthermore, we [14] reviewed all 37 DLBD cases reported in Japan and classified DLBD into two forms: a common form with more or less Alzheimer pathology and a pure form without such findings. Since then, we have published several papers concerning DLBD. The term "dementia with Lewy bodies" (DLB) was proposed at the first international workshop in 1995 [1]. The CDLB guidelines were published in 1996 [15], and the CDLB guidelines–revised were reported in 2005 [16].

The most important recent findings in this field were (1) alpha-synuclein gene mutation in familial PD [17] and (2) alpha-synuclein as the main component of Lewy bodies [18]. Thereafter, alpha-synuclein has received considerable attention in the research on Lewy body disease.

DLB and PDD Within the Spectrum of Lewy Body Disease

At the first international workshop held in 1995, the difference between DLB and PDD was discussed. In the CDLB guidelines [15], the "1-year rule" was adapted. According to these guidelines, PDD is differentiated from DLB by the appearance of dementia at least 1 year after the onset of PD symptoms. At the third international workshop held in 2003, not a few researchers insisted that this 1-year rule should be abolished. This rule was, however, maintained even in the CDLB guidelines–revised reported in 2005 [16]. Considerable evidence has been reported that DLB and PDD are almost the same not only clinically but also neuropathologically. Therefore, in the revised guidelines, the term "Lewy body disease" was used as a generic term that includes DLB, PD, and PDD [16]. In the report of the DLB and PDD working group in 2007 [19], a similar description was also introduced.

Since our proposal of Lewy body disease in 1980 [2], we have insisted that Lewy body disease is a generic term that includes PD, PDD, and DLBD [12, 14, 20–22].

Lewy body disease is now defined as follows: "Lewy body disease is a chronic neuropsychiatric disease characterized clinically by idiopathic parkinsonism of early- or late-onset, frequently followed by progressive dementia. In many cases, progressive dementia is the main symptom, followed frequently by idiopathic parkinsonism. It is neuropathologically characterized by the presence of numerous Lewy bodies and Lewy neurites in the central and sympathetic nervous systems."

As indicated above, we classified DLBD into two forms: a common form with more or less ATD pathology and a pure form without it [14]. Then, we described differences in the clinical features between the common form and the pure form. In the common form, most cases showed later onset, and the initial symptom was memory disturbance followed by progressive dementia, and about 70% of patients later developed parkinsonism. However, the pure form was characterized by younger onset, idiopathic parkinsonism as the initial symptom and later followed by progressive dementia. Therefore, the pure form can be diagnosed as PDD. In 1992, when the 150th anniversary congress of the German Psychiatry Association was held in Koeln, I was invited to a symposium and reported the differences in clinical features between Japanese and European-American DLBD cases [23]. The features of the common form do not show any differences between the two regions, while the pure form showed marked differences between regions: most Japanese cases were characterized, as indicated above, by younger onset and initial parkinsonism followed by dementia, whereas most European-American cases demonstrated later onset and progressive dementia followed by parkinsonism, as in the common form. In 2003, when I was invited as a symposist at the annual meeting of the Japan Neurology Association, I [24] reported a neuropathological study of 24 PDD cases. The findings showed that all our 24 PDD cases were pathologically diagnosed as DLB. Thus, PDD did not show neuropathological differences from DLB.

In 1996, we [21] proposed the term "cerebral type" of Lewy body disease. In the cerebral type, the main symptom is progressive dementia without parkinsonism. Neuropathologically, numerous Lewy bodies appeared in the cerebral cortex as in DLBD, but only rare Lewy bodies were found in the brainstem nuclei. Braak's theory [25] insisted that Lewy bodies occur from the medulla oblongata through the pons and midbrain to the cerebral cortex in PD. This cerebral type means suggests that Lewy bodies occur at first in the cerebral cortex and then migrate down to the brainstem nuclei . Therefore, the cerebral type of Lewy body disease should receive more attention.

In conclusion, Lewy body disease is a generic term that includes PD, PDD, and DLB. It is neuropathologically classified into four types: brainstem type, transitional or limbic type, diffuse type, and cerebral type.

References

1. Perry R, McKeith I, Perry E (1996) Dementia with Lewy bodies. Cambridge University Press, Cambridge
2. Kosaka K, Matsushita M, Oyanagi S, Mehraein P (1980) A clinicopathological study of Lewy body disease. Psychiat Neurol Jap 82:292–311
3. Parkinson J (1817) An essay on the shaking palsy. Sherwood, Neely and Jones, Wittingham and Rowland, London
4. Charcot JM (1892) De la paralysie agitante Euvures completes, 6th edn. Progres Medicale, Paris
5. Lewy FH (1912) Paralysis agitans. I. Pathologische anatomie. In: Lewandowsky M (ed) Handbuch der neurologie, vol 3. Berlin, Springer, pp 920–958
6. Tretiakoff C (1919) Contribution a l'etude de l'Anatomie pathologique du Locus Niger de Soemmerung avec quelques deductions relatives a la pathogenie des troubles du tonus musculaire et de la Parkinson. These de Paris
7. Hassler R (1938) Zur pathologie der paralysis agitans und des postenzephalitischen parkinsonismus. J Psychol Neurol 48:387–476
8. Greenfield JG, Bosanquet FD (1953) The brain-stem lesions in Parkinsonism. J Neurol Neurosurg Psychiatry 16:213–226
9. Den Hartog Jager WA, Bethlem JU (1960) The distribution of Lewy bodies in the central and autonomic nervous systems in idiopathic paralysis agitans. J Neurol Neurosurg Psychiatry 23:283–290
10. Kosaka K, Oyanagi S, Matsushita M et al (1976) Presenile dementia with Alzheimer-, Pick- and Lewy body changes. Acta Neuropathol 36:221–233

11. Kosaka K (1978) Lewy bodies in cerebral cortex; report of three cases. Acta Neuropathol 42:127–134
12. Kosaka K, Yoshimura M, Ikeda K, Budka H (1984) Diffuse type of Lewy body disease. A progressive dementia with numerous cortical Lewy bodies and senile changes of various degree. A new disease? Clin Neuropathol 3:185–192
13. Kosaka K, Mehraein P (1979) Dementia-Parkinsonism syndrome with numerous Lewy bodies and senile plaques in cerebral cortex. Arch Psychiatr Nervenkr 226:241–250
14. Kosaka K (1990) Diffuse Lewy body disease in Japan. J Neurol 237:197–204
15. McKeith I, Galasko D, Kosaka K et al (1996) Consensus guidelines for the clinical and pathological diagnosis of dementia with Lewy bodies (DLB). Neurology 47:1113–1124
16. McKeith IG, Dickson DW, Lowe J et al (2005) Diagnosis and management of dementia with Lewy bodies: third report of the DLB consortium. Neurology 65:1863–1872
17. Polymeropoulos MH, Lavedan C, Leroy E et al (1997) Mutation in the α-synuclein gene identified in families with Parkinson's disease. Science 276:2045–2047
18. Spillantini MG, Schmidt ML, Lee VMY et al (1997) α-Synuclein in Lewy bodies. Nature (Lond) 388:839–840
19. Lippa CF, Duda JE, Grossman M et al (2007) DLB and PDD boundary issues. Diagnosis, treatment, molecular pathology, and biomarkers. Neurology 68:812–818
20. Kosaka K, Iseki E (1996) Diffuse Lewy body disease within the spectrum of Lewy body disease. In: Peery E, McKeith E, Perry E (eds) Dementia with Lewy bodies. Cambridge University Press, Cambridge
21. Kosaka K, Iseki E, Odawara T et al (1996) Cerebral type of Lewy body disease. Neuropathology 17:32–35
22. Kosaka K (2000) Diffuse Lewy body disease. Neuropathology 20 (suppl):73–78
23. Kosaka K (1992) Diffuse Lewy Koerperchen: vergleich klinisch- pathologischer Daten zwischen Japanischen und Europaeischen/Amerikanischen Faellen. 150. Jahren Psychiatrie in Deutschland, Koeln
24. Kosaka K (2004) Dementia with Lewy bodies and Parkinson's disease with dementia. Do most of the demented PD patients have DLBD? The 45th Annual Meeting of Japan Neurology Association, Tokyo (panel discussion)
25. Braak H, Del Trediel K, Rub U et al (2003) Staging of brain pathology related to sporadic Parkinson's disease. Neurobiol Aging 24:197–211

Clinicopathological Characterization of Frontotemporal Lobar Degeneration

Yoshio Mitsuyama

Abstract Frontotemporal lobar degeneration (FTLD) is a clinically, genetically, and pathologically heterogeneous group of diseases, including Pick disease, frontotemporal lobar dementia with lacking distinctive histology (FTLD-LDH), and FTLD with motor neuron disease (FTLD-MND). Pick disease is essentially taupathy. FTLD-LDH has inconsistent clinicopathological findings with different immunohistochemical characterization.

FTLD-MND shows characteristic combinations with FTLD and MND. FTLD and FTLD-MND represent distinct clinicopathological entities. The relationship between FTLD-MND and amyotrophic lateral sclerosis is uncertain.

Keywords Frontotemporal lobar dementia • Motor neuron disease • Pick disease

Introduction

Frontotemporal lobar degeneration (FTLD) is one of the most common neurodegenerative disorders among aging societies. FTLD accounts for approximately 20% of neurodegenerative dementias [1, 2]. FTLD is the third most common cause of neurodegenerative dementia syndrome after Alzheimer's disease and dementia with Lewy bodies. FTLD occurs primarily between the age of 35 and 75 years, and it is rare to have the onset after age of 75. The disease affects both sexes approximately equally. Some cases may carry a diagnosis of Alzheimer's disease or rapidly dementing illness. Pathologically, it includes a heterogeneous group of sporadic and familial neuropsychiatric diseases.

Y. Mitsuyama (✉)
Psychogeriatric Center of Daigo Hospital, 1270 Nagata, Mimata-cho, Miyazaki 889-1911, Japan
e-mail: mitsuyama@fujimoto.or.jp

K. Miyoshi et al. (eds.), *Neuropsychiatric Disorders*,
DOI 10.1007/978-4-431-53871-4_20, © Springer 2010

In the 1980s and 1990s, several research groups recognized that there were many patients with clinical features similar to those of patients with Pick disease who had neither the classical lobar atrophy nor characteristic neuronal changes. These disorders came to be known by several different names, including FTLD-LDH, which consists of frontotemporal lobar degeneration lacking distinct histology, Pick disease, and FTLD with motor neuron disease (FTLD-MND), primary progressive aphasia (PPA), and semantic dementia (SD) [3–10]. As expected, all variants of FTLD have neuronal loss and gliosis affecting the frontal and temporal cortices in keeping with a diagnosis of FTLD. The research criteria have been focused on the need to have subgroups of patients for study during life and accurate pathological diagnosis on autopsy.

Clinical criteria for diagnosing FTLD include the Lund and Manchester Criteria and the more recent consensus criteria [2, 11, 12]. Patients with FTLD present gradual and progressive changes in behavior, or gradual and progressive language dysfunctions. The most common psychiatric symptom of FTLD is an early change in social and personal conduct, characterized by difficulty in modulating behavior to the social demands of a situation. FTLD patients are impaired in the regulation of conduct. This dysfunction is often associated with a lack of inhibition, resembling in impulsive or inappropriate behavior. Progression of the disease may lead to poor financial judgement, and compulsive-like behaviors are common presenting symptoms among FTLD patients [12, 13]. Complex compulsive acts may result from temporal lobe involvement [14]. In some individuals, inappropriate sexual behavior occurs. Perseverative and stereotyped behaviors encompass simple repetitive acts and verbal expression or stereotypies such as lip smacking, habitual hand rubbing or clapping, and humming that may result from frontostriatal circuit dysfunction or involvement of the caudate nuclei. Psychotic symptoms such as delusions and hallucinations are uncommon in FTLD. Nevertheless, there have been patients with an initial schizophrenia-like psychosis or a psychotic affective disorder such as a sign of FTLD [15, 16]. Dietary habits and personal hygiene may also change. Patients become inactive with decreased behavioral motivation and spontaneity, loss of interest in personal hygiene with failure to wash, bathe, groom, and so on. In FTLD, fragments of the Klüver–Bucy syndrome can occur, particularly the hyperorality that manifests as cramming and bingeing, altered food performance especially for sweets or food fads. They may attempt to eat inedible items. FTLD patients can be so hyperoral that require restraint to prevent suffocation or aspiration. There is a loss of concern for one's personal appearance, and patients may be increasingly unkempt early in the disease. Patients show loss of personal concern for their actions.

FTLD patients tend toward decreased verbal output progressively to complete mutism. Early language disturbances of FTLD are empty speech, nonfluent anomia, especially for words connecting action, and semantic anomia where the word loses its meaning. They usually do not have a true amnestic syndrome. In the FTLD, spatial difficulties are seen in patients with mild or moderate impairments. Many of these patients present with troubles in the expression of language, problems using the correct words, including the naming of persons and things, or expressing oneself. Some patients with FTLD have a progressive aphasia several years before other clinical manifestations; in such cases, speech and language changes predominate (PPA and SD) [17].

FTLD patients have relatively preserved visuo-spatial abilities such as spatial localization and orientation in familiar surroundings. FTLD patients lack sympathy, empathy, emotional warmth, or awareness of the needs of others and appear emotionally shallow and indifferent. FTLD patients have deficits of insight, abstraction, planning, and problem solving, in keeping with a frontal "dysexecutive" syndrome. Judgement is abnormal. FTLD patients are often very concrete on proverb interpretation and tests assessing comprehension of similarities and differences. On neuropsychological testing, frontal-executive functions are compromised early in FTLD, and most memory and occipitoparietal functions are compromised early in most Alzheimer patients.

In the early and middle stages, neurological signs are usually absent or confined to the presence of primitive reflexes such as grasp, snout, and sucking reflexes. Dystonia, ideomotor apraxia, dysphagia, or fasciculations and muscle wasting are occasionally observed.

There are no laboratory findings pathognomonic of FTLD. Routine investigations of blood and urine yield unremarkable results. Conventional EEGs tends to remain normal until late in the course, when they show diffuse slowing and occasional focal frontal or temporal slow wave activity. Structural neuroimaging, particularly magnetic resonance imaging (MRI), can help confirmation in the presence of FTLD. Most FTLD patients show frontal (and anterior temporal) atrophy, enlargement of the Sylvius fissures, anterior callosal atrophy, and eventual hippocampal and entorhinal volume loss. Computed tomography (CT)/MRI may show atrophy of the anterior temporal and frontal lobes. Some FTLD patients may have additional MRI evidence of bilateral caudate nuclear atrophy. Functional imaging is more sensitive than structural imaging for the diagnosis of FTLD. Single-photon emission computed tomography/^{18}F-fluorodeoxyglucose-positron emission tomography (SPECT/FDG-PET) typically demonstrates decreased perfusion and metabolism of the frontal and temporal lobes.

The usual clinical duration of FTLD is about 8–11 years. The clinical course of FTLD can be divided into three stages. In the initial stages, there are prominent personality changes, emotional alterations, and impaired insight and judgement. Speech and language changes also may occur. In the second stage, aphasia and other cognitive changes become pronounced, but there is at least partial preservation of memory, visuo-spatial skills, and computational ability. The third and final stage of the disease is often dominated by progressive muteness, and the patients become profoundly demented.

At autopsy, the brains of patients with FTLD show a lobar distribution of atrophy involving the frontal lobes, temporal lobes, or both. Coronal sections reveal deep sulci and may show knife-edged gyri in the atrophic area, especially in Pick disease. The orbitofrontal cortex and the anterior and medial temporal areas show the most severe atrophic changes. The predominant neuropathological abnormalities are frontotemporal neuronal loss and gliosis with ubiquitin-positive, tau-negative inclusions and without detectable amounts of insoluble tau, with MND or without

MND. The cortical degeneration involves mainly the grey matter, including the insula and the anterior cingulate gyrus. In the past, clinicians have referred to FTLD patients as having "Pick bodies," but on neuropathological examination, most FTLD patients lack the pathognomonic Pick bodies. There has been continuing controversy concerning whether identifiable cellular changes of Pick bodies and ballooned neurons are a requirement for diagnosis. Smaller number of FTLD patients have involvement of substantia nigra, striato-pallidum, parietal cortex, thalamus, and other structures [18, 19]. Most FTLD patients do not have senile plaques or neurofibrillary tangles, although some have amyloid beta deposition, particularly late in the course and in patients with an APO-E epsilon 4-allele [20]. In FTLD, about one-third of patients have tau pathology and about 10% have a tau gene mutation [21, 22]. Pathological findings have, to date, not been associated with specific clinical manifestations.

Pick Disease

Arnold Pick [23–25], in a series of articles based on gross examination of the brain, reported cases of dementia with severe circumscribed atrophy of the frontotemporal regions. The definition of the clinical entity of what became known as Pick disease was presented in a series of articles in the 1920s [26–28]. The initial stage is characterized by prominent personality changes and emotional alterations. Judgment is impaired early, and insight is compromised. Social behavior deteriorates, and language abnormalities are among the earliest intellectual alterations to occur. In the second stage of disease, deterioration of mental status becomes evident and aphasia is more prominent. Cognitive changes are more pronounced, but memory and visuo-spatial skills may remain relatively intact. In the final stage of the disease, progressive extrapyramidal syndrome usually appears and the patient becomes mute and incontinent. Pick disease has a longer illness duration (more than 10 years). CT/MRI may provide supportive evidence for the diagnosis.

Neuropathology shows severe frontotemporal atrophy, often with "knife-edged" gyri (Fig. 1), and extensive neuronal loss with gliosis. An abrupt transition is sometimes evident between involved and uninvolved cortical regions. There is a tendency for selective sparing of the precentral gyrus and the posterior one-third of the superior temporal gyrus. The concept of Pick disease emphasized the importance of Pick bodies and ballooned neurons in the pathological diagnosis and the clinical distinction of this disorder from Alzheimer disease. The diagnosis of Pick disease occurs when there are Pick bodies with or without Pick cells. Pick bodies are spherical, silver-staining (argyrophilic), ubiquitin- and tau-positive intraneuronal inclusions. Pick bodies are concentrated in frontotemporal neocortical layers II–VI, and the hippocampal formation in the granular layer of the dentate gyrus and sector CA1. Pick bodies do not occur in normal aging. There are pathognomonic microscopic findings showing ballooned neurons or Pick cells and definite positive tau and ubiquitin bodies in neurons of the

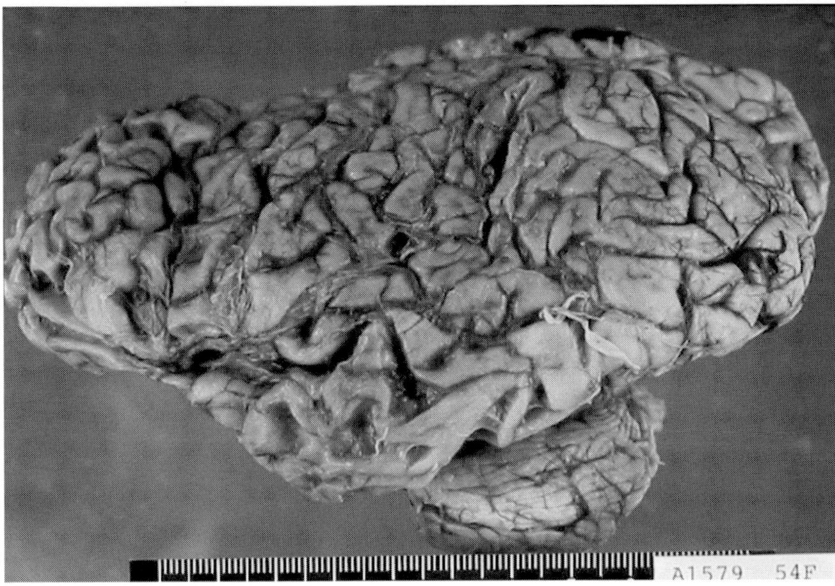

Fig. 1 "Knife-edged" atrophy of the brain

frontotemporal cortex and granule cells of dentate gyrus of the hippocampus (Pick bodies). Pick disease is essentially taupathy, similar to corticobasal degeneration and progressive supranuclear palsy. The volume of the substantia nigra is decreased, but the concentration of neurons is slightly reduced, and there is no clinical parkinsonism until the terminal stages.

FTLD-LDH

FTLD is a clinical term applied to patients who present with progressive dementia with an insidious onset, prominent behavioral or language dysfunction, or both. We have recognized that this term includes groups of patients whose pathological conditions and genetic mechanisms are heterogeneous. The clinical characteristics of FTLD-LDH are almost similar to those of Pick disease. However, the severity of intellectual and personality deterioration is less than those seen in Pick disease. MRI shows frontotemporal atrophy, and SPECT shows selective hypoperfusion of frontotemporal lobes. The most common pathology of FTLD-LDH is a nonspecific frontotemporal atrophy, and FTLD-LDH is the usual FTLD pathology.

Microscopic study shows mild to slight neuronal loss and astrogliosis with sponginess (minute cavities or microvacuolation) of the outer supragranular (II–III) layers of the frontotemporal cortex with ubiquitin- and TDP-43-positive inclusions

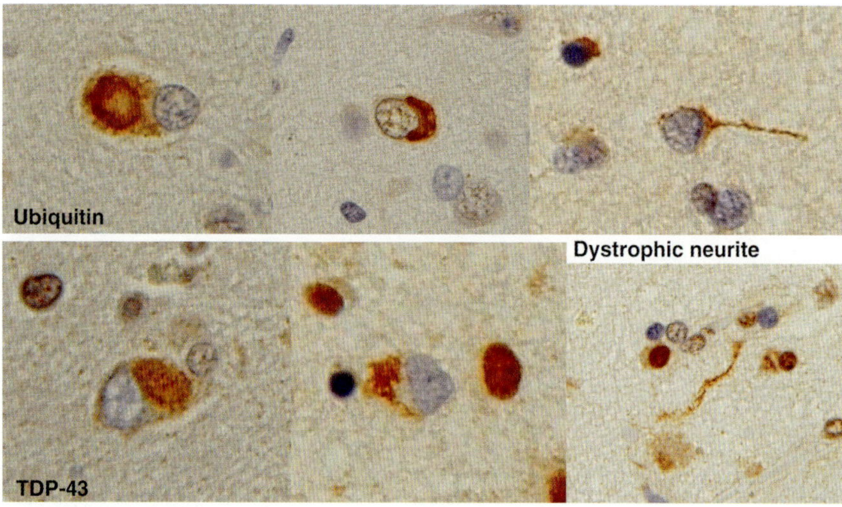

Fig. 2 Ubiquitin- and TDP-43-positive inclusions of the cerebral cortex

(Fig. 2). There is also variable involvement of subcortical and limbic structures. The anterior hippocampal regions are also affected. FTLD-LDH has no Pick bodies, plus depigmentation in the substantia nigra and striato-pallidum.

FTLD-MND

A subset of patients with FTLD develops symptoms suggestive of MND. The mean age at onset and disease duration are 52 years and 2.3 years, respectively. FTLD-MND is a clinicopathological entity characterized by the combination of FTLD and MND. The link between FTLD and MND was suggested by the autopsy in 1984 [29], and the term FTLD-MND was subsequently proposed [30]. The development of MND in patients presenting with a progressive behavioral disorder would strongly support a clinical diagnosis of FTLD-MND. MND is also a clinical term, but it is applied to patients with clinical evidence of corticospinal tract involvement, evidence of brainstem or spinal cord anterior horn cell involvement, or both. FTLD-MND have symptoms of mild forgetfulness and language output impairment, in addition to the more prominent behavioral disorders. These symptoms include weakness and muscle wasting. Symptoms of parkinsonism, such as rigidity, are occasionally seen. Signs of MND may not always be present early. Most of the cases of MND developed approximately 6–24 months after the onset of symptoms of FTLD [29, 31]. Only features of dementia are noted early in the disease course, and both initially carried a diagnosis of FTLD. MRI/SPECT reveals slight to moderate atrophy and selective hypoperfusion in the frontotemporal regions. The patient shows a relatively rapid clinical course, less than 5 years.

The pathological features of FTLD-MND are variable. Neuropathology of FTLD-MND shows slight frontotemporal lobe atrophy and more characteristic features of mild neuronal loss with cortical sponginess and subcortical gliosis, affecting the frontal and temporal cortices in keeping with a diagnosis of FTLD. In addition, all cases have pathological evidence of degeneration of lower motor neurons that contain eosinophilic and ubiquitin-positive inclusions. There are also ubiquitin-positive, tau-negative (nonargyrophilic) inclusions in the neurons of the frontotemporal cortex and granule cells in the dentate fascia of the hippocampus, which are characteristic of MND. Ubiquitin-positive and tau-negative inclusions may be present in FTLD with or without MND. Ubiquitin- and TDP-43-positive inclusions are present in the dentate fascia and neocortex in FTLD-MND. Some cases have a mixture of lower motor neuron degeneration and corticospinal tract degeneration (similar to amyotrophic lateral sclerosis, ALS) and the majority have Bunina bodies, which are a histological hallmark of ALS. The severity of motor neuron degeneration is variable, ranging from absent to severe. Some cases have a predominance of corticospinal tract degeneration, but others have no corticospinal tract degeneration. At the present time, there is no way to distinguish between cases on the basis of extramotor ubiquitin-positive pathological features or on the basis of predominant involvement of upper or lower motor neurons. A large sample size would be needed to address possible clinically useful subtypes. FTLD-MND with pathological changes in the hippocampus seems strikingly similar to other FTLD and some evidence of MND, whereas FTLD-MND without hippocampal pathology seems strikingly similar to ALS with some evidence of FTLD.

FTLD-MND should be taught as a spectrum of diseases and include FTLD-MND with hippocampal pathology and FTLD-MND without hippocampal pathology. Detection of signs of clinical MNDs is difficult when motor neuron degeneration is mild. FTLD-MND is diagnosed if there is evidence of brainstem or spinal cord anterior horn cell degeneration with or without ubiquitin-positive inclusions [32–34], degeneration of the corticospinal tract, or both, in addition to histological evidence of FTLD. Histological evidence of motor neuron degeneration includes loss of large anterior horn cells in the spinal cord or hypoglossal neurons plus (1) shrunken residual motor neurons, (2) evidence of neuronophagia, (3) Bunina bodies, or (4) ubiquitin-immunoreactive intraneuronal inclusions. Evidence of FTLD includes the presence of superficial sponginess, neuronal loss, and astrogliosis affecting predominantly layer II of the cortex, with or without the presence of ubiquitin immunoreactive neuronal cytoplasmic inclusions. Neuronal intranuclear inclusions such as Pick bodies are not detected. The ubiquitin-positive inclusions are negative for tau, alpha-synuclein, and neurofilament. Extramotor ubiquitin-positive neuronal inclusions are present in all cases, in the dentate fascia, neocortex, or both regions. Skeletal muscle has evidence of group atrophy with small acutely angulated fibers consistent with neurogenic atrophy.

Neuronal loss and gliosis of the hypoglossal nucleus and spinal anterior horn cells are variable and ranged from absent to severe. The severity of motor neuron involvement tend to correlate with clinical evidence of MND. Corticospinal tract degeneration also ranged from absent to severe. Severity of corticospinal tract degeneration does not correlate with clinical signs of MND or with severity of neuronal loss and gliosis in the hypoglossal nucleus and spinal anterior horn cells. Extramotor ubiquitin-positive inclusions are absent to sparse in all cortical regions.

Comments

Large clinicopathological series have been published that have clearly demonstrated an overlap between the clinical syndromes subsumed under the term frontotemporal dementia and the progressive supranuclear palsy syndrome, corticobasal degeneration syndrome, and MND. There have also been significant advancements in brain imaging, neuropathology, and molecular genetics that have led to different approaches to the classification.

FTLD and FTLD-MND represents a distinct clinicopathological entity that shows essentially ubiquitin and TDP-43 proteinopathy. There are some cases of FTLD with TDP-43-positive and ubiquitin-negative pathology. TDP-43 proteinopathy has been reported in many neurodegenerative diseases (filament inclusion disease). TDP-43 might be more susceptible to neuronal damage. From these findings, different pathoetiologies could lead to the varied clinicopathological presentations of FTLD.

The pathological features of FTLD-MND are variable. Most cases have a mixture of lower motor neuron degeneration, occasionally associated with corticospinal tract degeneration, similar to progressive spinal muscular atrophy or ALS, and the majority have Bunina bodies, which are a histological hallmark of ALS.

The field is complicated by a barrage of overlapping clinical syndromes, and neuropathological diagnosis that does not always respond to clinical presentations and underlying neuropathology.

It is difficult to distinguish between cases on the basis of extramotor ubiquitin-positive pathological features or on the basis of predominant involvement of upper or lower motor neurons. Hippocampal sclerosis with ubiquitin-positive inclusions in the dentate fascia is a common feature of FTLD with ubiquitin-only immunoreactive changes.

Lower motor neuron involvement including spinal cord anterior horn cell and hypoglossal nucleus degeneration is of the utmost importance for future clinicopathological studies with combined dementia and MND.

It is unclear how neurodegenerative diseases cause dysfunction and death of brain cells or specific neuropsychiatric symptoms. Clinical manifestations of the FTLD cannot accurately predict the nature of the underlying neurodegenerative disease. The neuropathological findings alone cannot establish that a patient had FTLD in the absence of documented clinical information. Although there is no specific treatment for FTLD, many symptomatic therapies can be very helpful. Many of the behavioral psychological symptoms of FTLD may respond to selective serotonin uptake inhibitors (SSRI) [35]. Marked disinhibition, aggressive behavior, or verbal outbursts may respond to small doses of major tranquilizers such as risperidone, olanzapine, or quetiapine. FTLD is very stressful to the caregiver, and support of the family is critically important.

References

1. Pasquier F, Delacourte A (1998) Non-Alzheimer degenerative dementias. Curr Opin Neurol 11:417–427
2. The Lund and Manchester Group (1994) Clinical and neuropathological criteria for frontotemporal dementia. The Lund and Manchester Groups. J Neurol Neurosurg Psychiatry 57:416–418
3. Neary D, Snowden JS, Bowen DM et al (1986) Neuropsychological syndromes in presenile dementia due to cerebral atrophy. J Neurol Neurosurg Psychiatry 49:163–174
4. Neary D, Snowden JS, Northen B et al (1988) Dementia of frontal lobe type. J Neurol Neurosurg Psychiatry 51:353–361
5. Brun A (1987) Frontal lobe degeneration of non-Alzheimer type. I. Neuropathology. Arch Gerontol Geriatr 6:193–208
6. Brun A (1993) Frontal lobe degeneration of non-Alzheimer type revised. Dementia 4:126–131
7. Gustafson L (1987) Frontal lobe degeneration of non-Alzheiemr type II. Clinical picture and differential diagnosis. Arch Gerontol Geriatr 6:209–223
8. Gustafson L (1993) Clinical picture of frontal lobe degeneration of non-Alzheimer type. Dementia 4:143–148
9. Snowden JS, Neary D, Mann DM (1996) Frontotemporal lobar degeneration: frontotemporal dementia. Progressive aphasia, semantic dementia. Churchill-Livingston, London
10. Knopman DS (1993) Overview of dementia lacking distinctive histology: pathological designation of a progressive dementia. Dementia 4:132–136
11. Neary D, Snowden JS, Gustafson L et al (1998) Frontotemporal lobar degeneration: a consensus on clinical diagnostic criteria. Neurology 51:1546–1554
12. Mendez MF, Perryman KM, Milker BL et al (1997) Comprehensive behaviours as presenting symptoms of frontotemporal dementia. J Geriatr Psychiatry Neurol 10:154–157
13. Tonkonogy JM, Smith TW, Barreira PJ (1994) Obsessive-compulsive disorders in Pick's disease. J Neuropsychiatry Clin Neurosci 6:176–180
14. Rosso SM, Roks G, Stevens M et al (1998) Complex compulsive behaviour in the temporal variant of frontotemporal dementia. Ned Tijdschr Geneeskd 142:1962–1965
15. Waddington JL, Youssef HA, Farrell MA et al (1995) Initial "schizophrenia-like" psychosis in Pick's disease: case study with neuroimaging and neuropathology and implications for frontotemporal dysfunction in schizophrenia. Schizophr Res 18:79–82
16. Gregory CA (1999) Frontal variant of frontotemporal dementia: a cross-sectioned and longitudinal study of neuropsychiatric features. Psychol Med 29:1205–1217
17. Ostberg P, Bogdanovic N, Fernaeus SE et al (2001) Jargon aphasia in a case of frontotemporal dementia. Brain Lang 79:333–339
18. Neary D, Snowden JS, Mann DM (1993) Familial progressive aphasia: its relationship of other forms of lobar atrophy. J Neurol Neurosurg Psychiatry 56:1122–1125
19. Sam M, Gutmann L, Schochet SS et al (1991) Pick's disease: a case clinically resembling amyotrophic lateral sclerosis. Neurology 41:1831–1833
20. Gustafson L, Abramason M, Grubb A et al (1997) Apolipoprotein-E genotyping in Alzheimer's disease and frontotemporal dementia. Dement Geriatr Cogn Disord 8:240–243
21. Adams E, Chang HT, Stopa EG et al (2001) Tau protein expression in frontotemporal dementias. Neurosci Lett 315:21–24
22. Poorkaj P, Grossmann M, Steinbart E et al (2001) Frequency of tau gene mutations in familial and sporadic cases of non-Alzheimer dementia. Arch Neurol 58:383–387
23. Pick A (1882) Über die Beziehungen der senilen Hirnatrophie zur Aphasie. Prager Med Wochenschr 17:165–167
24. Pick A (1901) Senile Hirnatrophie als Grundlage von Herd ersheinungen. Wien Klin Wochenschr 14:403–404

25. Oick A (1905) Zur Symptomatologie der linksseitigen Schlafen-lappenn Atrophie. Monatsschr Psychiatr Neurol 16:378–388
26. Gans A (1922) Betrachtungen über Art und Ausbreitung des krankhaften Prozesses in einem Fall von Pickscher Atrophie des Stirnhirns. Z Gesamte Neurol Psychiatr 80:10–28
27. Onari K, Spatz H (1926) Anatomische Beitrage zur Lehre von Pickschen umschriebenen Grosshirnrinden-Atophie ("Picksche Krankheit"). Z Gesamte Neurol Psychiatr 101:470–511
28. Schneider C (1927) Über Picksche Krankheit. Monatsschr Psychiatr Neurol 65:230–275
29. Mitsuyama Y (1984) Presenile dementia with motor neuron disease in Japan: clinicopathological review of 26 cases. J Neurol Neurosurg Psychiatry 47:53–959
30. Neary D, Snowden JS, Mann DM et al (1990) Frontal lobe dementia and motor neuron disease. J Neurol Neurosurg Psychiatry 53:23–32
31. Mitsuyama Y (2000) Dementia with motor neuron disease. Neuropathology 20(Suppl):S79–S81
32. Mendez MF, Selwood A, Mastri AR et al (1993) Pick's disease versus Alzheimer's disease: a comparison of clinical characteristics. Neurology 43:289–292
33. Schmitt HP, Yang Y, Fortstl H (1995) Frontal lobe degeneration of non-Alzheimer type and Pick's atrophy: lumping or splitting? Eur Arch Psychiatry Clin Neurosci 245:299–305
34. Josephs KA, Parisi JE, Knopman DS et al (2006) Clinically undetected motor neuron disease in pathologically proven frontotemporal lobar degeneration with motor neuron disease. Arch Neurol 63:506–512
35. Swartz JR, Miller BL, Lesser IM et al (2001) Frontotemporal dementia: treatment response to serotonin selective reuptake inhibitors. J Clin Psychiatry 56:41–45

Diffuse Neurofibrillary Tangles with Calcification

Shigetoshi Kuroda, Hideki Ishizu, Seishi Terada, Osamu Yokota, Yasuyuki Tanabe, and Takashi Haraguchi

Abstract Diffuse neurofibrillary tangles with calcification (DNTC) is a primary and sporadic presenile dementia that is characterized by temporal and/or frontal atrophy with diffuse neurofibrillary tangles (NFTs) and Fahr-type calcification without senile plaques (SPs).

We reviewed clinical symptoms in 21 autopsy-proven DNTC cases in Japan. It is characterized by slowly progressive cortical dementia mimicking Alzheimer's disease (AD) because of the appearance of memory disturbance and disorientation in the early stages, or simulating Pick's disease as a result of the presence of personality changes in the early to middle clinical stages, followed by various psychiatric and neurological symptoms such as Parkinson's symptoms, aphasia, and apraxia.

In terms of neuropathology, DNTC is characterized by the appearance of massive NFTs in the cerebral cortex and in Meynert's nucleus and the locus ceruleus/raphe nuclei as well. These sites are similar to those with AD. Differing from AD, SPs were absent, or only a small number were detected. Ultrastructural and immunohistochemical study revealed that NFTs with DNTC were morphologically and biochemically the same with those in AD. Fahr-type calcification is also one of the most characteristic findings; it was found in the basal ganglia and the cerebellum. We conducted elementary analysis of the calcified sites. In addition to calcium and iron, a higher level of lead was detected in comparison with control groups. The etiology should be further investigated.

S. Kuroda (✉) and H. Ishizu
Zikei Hospital, 100-2 Urayasu-Honmachi, Minami-ku, Okayama 702-8026, Japan
e-mail: kuroda0704@zikei.or.jp

S. Kuroda, S. Terada, and O. Yokota
Department of Neuropsychiatry, Okayama University Graduate School of Medicine, Dentistry and Pharmaceutical Sciences, 2-5-1 Shikata-cho, Kita-ku, Okayama 700-8558, Japan

Y. Tanabe and T. Haraguchi
Department of Neurology, South Okayama Medical Center, 4066 Hayashima, Tsukubo-gun, Okayama 701-0304, Japan

K. Miyoshi et al. (eds.), *Neuropsychiatric Disorders*,
DOI 10.1007/978-4-431-53871-4_21, © Springer 2010

Keywords Dementia • DNTC • Neurofibrillary tangles • Calcification

Introduction

Diffuse neurofibrillary tangles with calcification (DNTC) is a primary and sporadic presenile dementia. Ando et al. initially reported a patient with this disorder at an annual meeting of the Japanese Society of Neuropathology in 1964 [1]. Because atrophy of the temporal lobe was marked, how to differentiate this disorder from Pick's disease was discussed at that time. Thereafter, these cases were reported in the literature as cases of atypical Alzheimer's disease (AD), Pick's disease, or combined Alzheimer/Pick disease. After Shibayama et al. [2] and Kosaka [3] published their manuscripts, interest in DNTC was particularly emphasized in Japan. More than 20 autopsy cases have been reported. Pathologically, DNTC is characterized by localized temporal and/or frontal lobe atrophy, numerous neurofibrillary tangles (NFTs) without senile plaques (SPs), and calcification in the basal ganglia and dentate nucleus of the cerebellum that exceeded the normal physiological level. The term DNTC, which was proposed by Kosaka, has been used, because it represents well these pathological characteristics.

Case Presentation

Case 1. A 75-year-old woman. Her medical history included hypertension. There was no family history of dementia. At the age of 58 years, memory disturbance was noted. At the age of 62 years, she was admitted to the hospital because she was violent toward her husband. In the ward, her attitude was pleasant, but euphoric. She showed a tendency to repeat the same questions. Disorientation regarding places and persons, perseveration, and confabulation were noted. Neither apraxia nor agnosia was observed. There was no neurological sign other than severe dementia. However, hyperreflexia, tremor, and rigidity were noted at the age of 65 years. After the age of 66 years, she was usually cheerful, but became irritable frequently, and she got angry when displeased. Wandering was marked. Verbal output gradually decreased. At 72 years, she became bedridden. Brain computed tomography (CT) at the age of 74 showed cerebral atrophy of temporal and frontal lobes and calcification in the basal ganglia and cerebellum (Fig. 1). At the age of 75, she died of pneumonia. The clinical course was similar to that of AD. However, intracerebral calcification suggested DNTC. Autopsy was performed. The brain weighed 850 g. On the outer surface, there was an enlargement of the bilateral Sylvian fissures, and the temporal lobe showed marked atrophy. The right side of the temporal lobe showed more marked atrophy. The atrophic sites were brown and hard. Atrophy of the frontal, parietal, and occipital gyri was less marked. There were no marked changes in the cerebellum or brainstem. The basilar arteries showed moderate arteriosclerotic

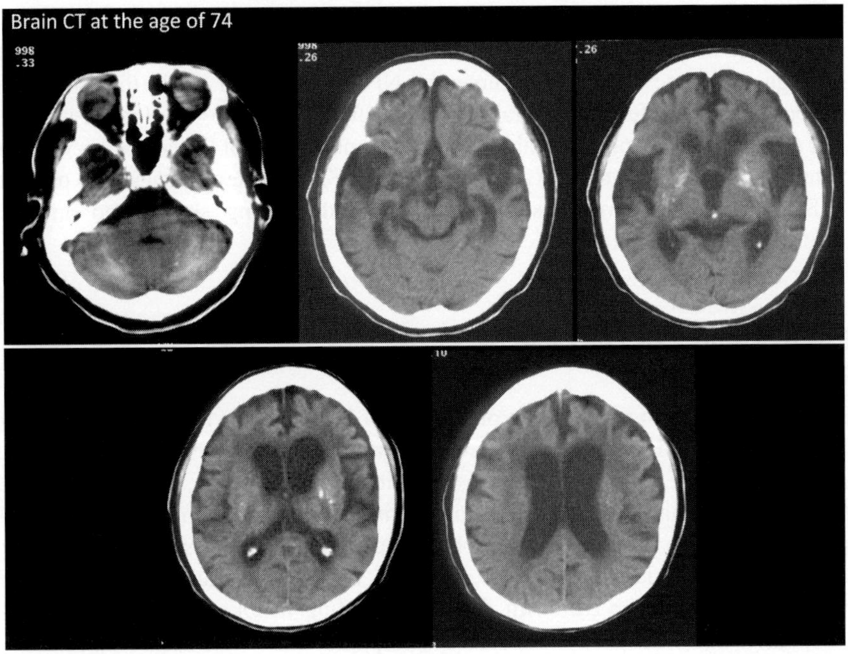

Fig. 1 Brain computed tomography (CT) at the age of 74 (case 21). Cerebral atrophy of temporal and frontal lobes and calcification in the basal ganglia and cerebellum

changes. Microscopically, neuronal loss and gliosis in the atrophic foci of the cortices were observed in the temporal pole in particular. The amygdala, hippocampus, and temporal lobe showed marked gliosis, and the white matter of the frontal and occipital lobed had slight to moderate gliosis. Numerous NFTs were observed in the cerebral cortex involving the frontal to occipital lobes. NFTs contained both 3 repeat and 4 repeat tau. A few SPs were detected in the temporal cortex; however, they were absent in other areas. The caudate nucleus showed atrophy, and there were only a small number of NFTs and neuropil threads. There were a few NFTs in the neurons of the substantia nigra and locus ceruleus. Calcification was present in the pallidum, putamen, granular layer, and the dentate nucleus of the cerebellum.

Case 2. A 48-year-old woman. There was no family history of dementia. At the age of 45, she became unable to do housework. Memory disturbance and disorientation gradually progressed, requiring caregiving for meals and excretion. Neurologically, there were no abnormal findings other than dementia. The blood pressure was normal. Personal contacts were maintained. Euphoria was noted. Neither aggression nor negativism was observed. Wandering and yelling made keeping her at home difficult, and the patient was admitted to a psychiatric hospital. Dementia progressed, and she died of pneumonia, with a dementia follow-up of 3 years. Autopsy was performed. The brain weighed 1,000 g. The frontal lobes showed atrophy bilaterally. On the cut surface, temporal lobe atrophy was noted. In the temporal lobe, the myelin sheath was markedly lightened, and gliosis was observed at the same site. In the frontal lobe, similar changes were also noted, although the grade was lower. Numerous NFTs were observed in the amygdala, hippocampus and inferior temporal gyrus. Calcification was observed in the vascular wall and parenchyma of the basal ganglia and granular layer of the cerebellar vermian cortex. In the substantia nigra, a small number of NFTs and Lewy bodies were present. A SP-like structure was observed, but amyloid staining showed no amyloid deposition in this structure.

Epidemiology of DNTC

Clinical and pathological reports of more than 30 patients with DNTC have been reported in Japan. However, in Western countries, not much interest in this disorder has been shown. Calcification was observed in the basal ganglia, dentate nucleus of the cerebellum, and cerebral white matter in severe cases (Fahr type). Brain CT scanning facilitates detection of atrophy and calcification at these sites. In our survey using the criteria proposed by Kosaka [4], DNTC was suspected in 4 of 3,053 patients (male:female = 1:2) with dementia residing in Okayama Prefecture. All these cases were female. In one case, autopsy led to a definitive diagnosis of DNTC. The incidence of DNTC was 0.13% in patients with dementia in Okayama. However, it may be lower in the general population. In Japan, several patients have been reported in Tokyo, Nagoya, Okayama, and Kochi, suggesting regional differences. In 21 autopsied patients, the male-to-female ratio was 1:3. Familial DNTC has not been reported. The mean age at onset was 53.1 years. A presenile onset (40–69 years of age) was frequent. The mean time of illness duration was 10.5 years (range, 3–24 years). In patients without complications, the clinical course may be prolonged. Generally speaking, the longer the duration, the lower the brain weight. The brain weight had decreased to approximately 800 g in patients with a prolonged course. In some patients, however, cerebral atrophy was evident even in the early stage.

Characteristics of Clinical Symptoms

We reviewed clinical symptoms in 21 patients whose pathological findings led to a definitive diagnosis of DNTC in Japan (Fig. 2).

The most common primary symptoms were memory disturbance and disorientation. In the early stage, they were observed in 80% of the 21 patients. With a slow course, personal contacts were maintained in the initial phase, and neurological symptoms were absent. Therefore, most patients were diagnosed with AD. However, personality changes such as irritability, aggression, euphoria, and disinhibition were noted in the initial phase, suggesting Pick's disease. Some patients showed a loss of spontaneity, depression, and apathy. In the middle phase, memory

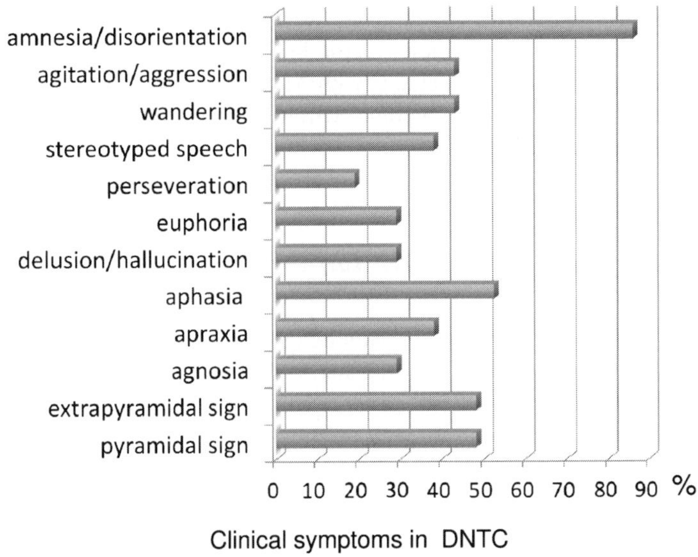

Fig. 2 Clinical symptoms in diffuse neurofibrillary tangles with calcification (DNTC)

disturbance was advanced. During the course, schizophrenia-like symptoms such as auditory hallucination, delusion of persecution, and hypochondriac delusion were observed in some patients. However, no patient showed "delusion of being robbed by a thief," which is very common in patients with AD. Early DNTC did not produce any neurological symptoms, such as Parkinson's symptoms, or focal symptoms, such as apraxia and agnosia. However, these symptoms appeared in approximately 30% to 50% of the patients during the course [5]. When the symptoms were advanced, dysphagia and primitive reflexes were noted, leading to an apallic state. Disease progression varied; memory disturbances and disorientation derived from hippocampal lesions were seen in the early stage, and personality changes derived from frontal/temporal lobe lesions were complicated by extrapyramidal symptoms and cerebrovascular diseases. In 6 of the 21 patients, a diagnosis of schizophrenia was made based on psychiatric symptoms such as hallucination and delusion during the course, and, later, cognitive impairment was observed. In the future, the course of DNTC should be investigated with a large number of cases.

Pathological Characteristics

NFTs

DNTC is characterized by appearance of massive NFTs. A large number of NFTs were observed in the hippocampus and parahippocampal gyrus. They were widely distributed in the cerebral isocortex. They were also found in Meynert's nucleus and the locus ceruleus/raphe nuclei of the brainstem. These sites were similar to those frequently observed in patients with AD. On the other hand, there were no NFTs in the basal ganglia or cerebellum. Differing from AD, SPs were absent, or only a small number were detected.

Characteristics of Degenerative Tau Protein

There are six isoforms of tau protein. Among these, tau protein involving exon-10, which exists in the microtubule-binding site, is termed "4-repeat tau protein," and exon-10-free tau protein is called "3-repeat tau protein." In patients with AD, all six isoforms are detected. In those with progressive supranuclear palsy or cortical basal ganglia degeneration, 4-repeat tau protein is found. In those with Pick body disease, 3-repeat tau protein is present. In patients with DNTC, 60-, 64-, and 68-kDa major and 72-kDa minor bands were recognized in the presence of various anti-tau antibodies. On Western blotting of sarkosyl-insoluble tau protein after dephosphorylation, six isoforms of tau protein were observed [6], indicating that the biochemical features of degenerative tau protein in patients with DNTC were similar to those in AD.

Electron Microscopy Findings

Electron microscopy examination was done with negative staining of sarkosyl-insoluble tau protein. A large number of paired helical filaments (PHFs) measuring 8–20 nm in diameter, with a cycle of approximately 80 nm, and a small number of straight tubules were observed [6]. These results suggest that degenerative tau protein in patients with DNTC is morphologically and biochemically identical to that in AD patients, and that PHFs are formed in the absence of β-protein [6].

Calcification

DNTC is characterized by the presence of calcification in the pallidum, putamen, and dentate nucleus of the cerebellum. Calcification was found in the capillary walls and parenchyma; this refers to false calcification with protein deposition. Calcification is also observed in the cerebral cortex, white matter, and cerebellar cortex in some cases. Neither loss of cells in the basal ganglia with calcification nor functional disturbance is noted [7]. We conducted elementary analysis of the calcified sites. In addition to calcium and iron, a higher level of lead was detected in comparison with control groups. The etiology should be further investigated [8, 9].

Cerebrovascular Lesions

The cases with DNTC have often complications of cerebrovascular disorders. Several studies have indicated the coexistence of cerebrovascular arteriolosclerosis, hypertension, Binswanger's disease-like white matter lesions, and multiple cerebral infarctions [10].

Lewy Body Pathology

We reported that α-synuclein was accumulated in various sites in seven of eight patients with DNTC [11]. α-Synuclein was accumulated in the amygdala, hippocampus, substantia nigra, and temporal/frontal cortex. This pattern was similar to the distribution of Lewy body disease (DLB). Among other types of tauopathy, Lewy body formation has also been reported. However, this finding is the most marked in patients with DNTC [11, 12]. The accumulation of Lewy bodies/neurites may affect nerve cell function. However, it is unclear whether this finding reflected clinical symptoms in DNTC patients. Advanced DNTC cases may have deposition of α-synuclein. DNTC may also be closely associated with DLB as it is in AD patients. Hallucination and Parkinson's symptoms, as observed in DLB patients, may appear in DNTC.

Conclusion

Although the number of patients is small, DNTC is recognized as a disease unit of tauopathy. The pathogenesis remains to be clarified. This refractory disease should be compared with other types of tauopathy to clarify its etiology. In the future, the differentiation of DNTC from Fahr's syndrome, correlation between calcification and NFTs, and involvement of lead should be reviewed. Calcification may initiate before the onset. When Fahr's syndrome is suspected on brain CT, DNTC must be considered. Epidemiologically, few studies have reported DNTC in other countries. Although the reason for this is unclear, an increasing number of patients may be reported in other countries in the future.

References

1. Ando J, Okaniwa T, Tachibana K (1965) An autopsy case of Pick's disease. Shinkei Kenkyu-no-Shinpo 9:181–182 (In Japanese)
2. Shibayama H, Kobayashi H, Nagasawa MI et al (1992) Non-Alzheimer non-Pick dementia with Fahr's syndrome. Clin Neuropathol 11:237–250
3. Kosaka K (1994) Diffuse neurofibrillary tangles with calcification: a new presenile dementia. J Neurol Neurosurg Psychiatry 57:594–596

4. Kosaka K (1997) Non-Alzheimer degenerative dementias. J Senile Dement 11:63–70 (In Japanese)
5. Tsuchiya K, Nakayama H, Haga C et al (2005) Distribution of cerebral cortical lesions in diffuse neurofibrillary tangles with calcification: a clinicopathological study of four autopsy cases showing prominent parietal lobe involvement. Acta Neuropathol 110:57–68
6. Tanabe Y, Ishizu H, Ishiguro K et al (2000) Tau pathology in diffuse neurofibrillary tangles with calcification (DNTC): biochemical and immunohistochemical investigation. Neuroreport 11:2473–2477
7. Ito Y, Kato T, Suzuki T et al (2003) Neuroradiologic and clinical abnormalities in dementia of diffuse neurofibrillary tangles with calcification (Kosaka-Shibayama disease). J Neurol Sci 15(209):105–109
8. Haraguchi T, Ishizu H, Kawai K et al (2001) Diffuse neurofibrillary tangles with calcification (a form of dementia): X-ray spectrometric evidence of lead accumulation in calcified regions. Neuroreport 12:1257–1260
9. Haraguchi T, Ishizu H, Takehisa Y et al (2001) Lead content of brain tissue in diffuse neurofibrillary tangles with calcification (DNTC): the possibility of lead neurotoxicity. Neuroreport 12:3887–3890
10. Terada S, Ishizu H, Tanabe Y et al (2001) Plaque-like structures and arteriosclerotic changes in "diffuse neurofibrillary tangles with calcification" (DNTC). Acta Neuropathol 102:597–603
11. Yokota O, Terada S, Ishizu H et al (2002) NACP/alpha-synuclein immunoreactivity in diffuse neurofibrillary tangles with calcification (DNTC). Acta Neuropathol 104:333–341
12. Hishikawa N, Hashizume Y, Ujihira N et al (2003) Alpha-synuclein-positive structures in association with diffuse neurofibrillary tangles with calcification. Neuropathol Appl Neurobiol 29:280–287

Part VII
Topics of Neuropsychiatric Disorders

Ayahuasca: Current Interest in an Ancient Ritual

Eduardo Gastelumendi

Abstract The amazonic brew *ayahuasca*, with strong psychoactive properties, and which has been used probably for millennia by Amazon tribes as their main "medicine," is currently being used by some groups in cities in Latin America and abroad by people seeking curative effects or transcendent and meaningful experiences. At the same time, research on its effects in treating depression and in neuroimaging is being carried out.

The brew is made of a blend of at least two different plants cooked together that potentiate each other: the stem of a vine, called *ayahuasca* proper (*Banisteropsis caapi*), and the leaves of a bush, *chacruna* (*Psychotria viridis*).

In this chapter, the ritual is described and the pharmacodynamics of the brew are discussed, as well as some of its effects in the brain and in the subjective experience of the self. Two vignettes of patients in analytical psychotherapy are presented to illustrate its effects. Reflections on the risks and benefits of its use are then shared.

Keywords Ayahuasca • Consciousness • Depression • Ethnopsychiatry • Psychotropic

Introduction

Brazil, Bolivia, Colombia, Ecuador, the Guyanas, Peru, and Venezuela share the Amazon rainforest. Hundreds of different tribes inhabit this huge area. At least 70 of those indigenous groups, primarily in the Upper Amazon and Orinoco basins,

E. Gastelumendi (✉)
Peruvian Psychiatric Society, Ave. Angamos Oeste 387/203, Miraflores, Lima 18, Perú
and
Peruvian Psychoanalytic Society, Julio Becerra 235, Miraflores, Lima 18, Perú
and
International Committee of the INA, INA Secretariat Office, Neuropsychiatric Institute, Euroa Centre, The Prince of Wales Hospital, Randwick, NSW 2031, Australia
and
Calle Parque Armendariz 119/4-E, Miraflores, Lima 18, Perú
e-mail: egastel@rcp.net.pe

K. Miyoshi et al. (eds.), *Neuropsychiatric Disorders*,
DOI 10.1007/978-4-431-53871-4_22, © Springer 2010

have used for millennia the blend known as *ayahuasca* for divination, healing, and other cosmogonic and shamanic purposes [1]. In its original milieu, the ritual, which has as its main vehicle the *ayahuasca*, with strong psychotropic activity in virtue of its serotoninergic properties, allows the participants to contact the "other" reality, or the "real aspect of the world," where the spirits of plants, animals, and dead people exist. It is also considered as a preparation for life after death [2]. The shaman of the tribe usually conducts the rite. The ingestion of ayahuasca produces intense visions. At first these are of geometric patterns (which can be seen as part of the Amazon people's crafts, in clothes, paintings, and pottery), and then the visions become gradually more complex, with emotional, cognitive, and somatic components, as we will see later.

The ayahuasca brew is a blend of two different plants cooked together. *Ayahuasca* proper (*Baninsteropsis caapi*) is a vine native to the Amazon – currently it grows in different parts of the world – that contains beta-carbolines such as harmine, harmaline, and tetrahydroharmine, all of which are potent monoamine oxidase (MAO) inhibitors. The other plant is the Chacruna (*Psychoatria viridis*), a bush that contains the tryptamine alkaloid *N,N*-dimethyltriptamine (DMT). DMT is not orally active itself, because it is inactivated by peripheral MAO of the liver and gut.

It is the blend that works: the beta-carbolines present in the ayahuasca vine inhibit the MAO and allows the DMT to enter the internal milieu. The question of how the indigenous people found the right combination remains unanswered, and this is definitely a result of many years of investigation and combinations. Sometimes the brew may include other plants, as tobacco, Toé (*Brugmansia suaveolens*), or coca leaves.

In the last decades, this ceremony has come out from the rainforest and has made its appearance in the main cities of many countries not only of South America but abroad. Conducted also by a leader – a shaman, *Maestro*, or *Curandero* – the aim is to have an inner experience with intense visions, somatic and emotional effects, and occasional key insights. During the ritual, in both Amazon and urban settings, the participants drink the brew from a cup (50–100 ml) and sit in silence waiting for the effects of the substance to occur. In an urban setting, the conductor has previously evaluated the participants, by overt questions or subtle observation, to determine the amount of brew each one will have, if any. This evaluation is important to reduce the risks of a bad experience for the participant for reasons of psychic frailties or other health conditions. In not rare occasions the shaman decides not to give the brew to a participant.

This ritual would be of little importance to our field, or perhaps be taken as a folkloric and curious issue, if it were not that some of our patients in psychotherapy have participated in one or more of these ayahuasca sessions and have talked about their experiences in their psychoanalysis and psychotherapies.

For historical and affective reasons, I would like to mention Carlos Alberto Seguin, who in the decade of 1960 was among the first psychiatrists to study the brew in Peru. These studies vary from a phenomenological approach to ethnographic psychiatry.

At the same time, neuropsychiatric research studies are been made on the effect of ayahuasca in refractory depression [3] and on its effects in visualization, memory, and consciousness [4].

I would like to suggest that the ayahuasca experience, because of its peculiarities, has a unique value for research in both neural and mental fields. Let me share with you a glimpse of what possibilities are open to research and theorization.

Description of an Ayahuasca Ceremony

The ceremony usually takes place at night. The participants and the shaman sit in a circle. The shaman gives a small amount of the brew to each person and then asks all to sit in silence. Shortly, about half an hour later, the visions begin. At first, they are colorful geometric patterns, and then gradually become more complex. Songs sung by the shaman during the session lead the participants to different visions, to changes in mood and in the level and quality of consciousness. The participants describe themselves as entering another state of mind, with keen awareness of the body, thoughts, and inner images. Very elaborate images may also appear.[1]

During the 4 or 5 hours that the experience lasts, old memories may appear, many of them painful and formerly repressed, as well as images of plants, animals, landscapes, and buildings. A numinous feeling or sometimes a feeling of awe may occur. Issues regarding the meaning and direction we give to our lives are not rare.

The shaman closes the ceremony with a brief rite as the participants gradually come back to a "normal" state. The following day there is a feeling of renovation. Insights may still be very clear.

It is interesting to consider that in Brazil there are two organized religions that have the ayahuasca as the core of their inner experience and their beliefs. Medical members of one of these groups, the União do Vegetal (www.udv.org.br; the other one is the "Igreja de Santo Daime"), have participated in research and publication of their data [5]. Also in Brazil, in the University of Ribeirão Preto, research has been conducted on animals as well as in treating refractory depression in humans in a strict medical setting [3]. Brazilian researchers have also published studies on the nature of the visual imagery so vividly enhanced in the participants, using functional magnetic resonance imaging (fMRI) [4].

From the psychodynamic perspective, what our patients bring to their sessions is very impressive and requires an open attitude on our part as therapists to avoid considering the experience as mainly an acting-out or a risk-seeking attitude.

[1] There are many artists that have depicted their visual experiences, with more or less skill. Among the most interesting of them is Pablo Amaringo (Peru, 1943–2009), founder of the Art school Usko-Ayar, in Pucallpa.

Let me share with you two experiences of patients who brought their ayahuasca experience to their psychotherapeutic sessions.

In the first vignette, a woman in her sixties comes to analytical therapy because she still feels somatic and psychic pains after a car accident suffered years ago. In that accident, her teenaged nephew was killed and she was seriously injured. When she came to analytical therapy, 2 years after the accident, she was somewhat recovered, but still felt deep sadness, guilt, and constant pain in her head, side, and legs. One of the issues that appeared during our work was the sadomasochistic bond with her very old but still lucid mother, who lived nearby. It was in the second year of therapy when she decided to participate in an ayahuasca session. Even though some symptoms had become lighter (less guilt and a better disposition toward life), the pain in her body remained, and the relationship with her mother and daughters was still complicated. She talked for some sessions about her interest in drinking the brew and finally decided to participate in one group session with a shaman.

This is a summary of her experience:

> After an hour or so after she drank the brew, the visions started and she entered into a calm mood and heightened sense of awareness. After a while she found herself directing her attention to her body and started exploring every part of it inch by inch. She felt she could distinguish the different kinds of pain and, at the same time, the distinct emotions "tied" to each part. She cried very deeply. After a while a sort of oneiric vision appeared: she saw herself sitting in a chair in a dark room, with her mother behind her, and her grandmother further behind. She could almost guess (or see?) the mother's grandmother further back. In front of her, her daughters were sitting. All these women formed a silent and quiet row. In the same way that my patient had been able to observe every detail of her sore body, now she could see the expressions and emotions of the women of her family. She noticed there was a common pain that passed through all of them, a pain related to a way of being a woman that had been transmitted through generations. Suddenly she had an insight: she recognized the same style of hardening the hearts and controlling the emotions shared by all the women in her family. They had lived doomed, so to say, to live that way.
>
> What happened after her ayahuasca ceremony was a surprise for us. In a very natural way, the next time she approached her mother, some days after the ceremony, her attitude was quite different. When they met, she listened to the querulous old woman with her "heart opened," and then she hugged her with a tenderness she could not remember feeling or having with her. This was the beginning of a new relationship, more kind and affectionate, that lasted until her mother passed away. The relationship with her daughters also gained new life and dimensions, as my patient felt free to express more openly her emotions and to tolerate, and appreciate, the daughters' own characteristics and decisions.

There are also other kinds of insights produced by the experience, as the following vignette can show:

> A man in his late thirties comes for reanalysis. Some years before he had started participating in ayahuasca sessions in Lima and later went to the Amazon. He had his first ayahuasca experience moved by curiosity. He thought he would "enjoy" a psychedelic trip but found something else. Some of the visions he had were in a way similar to the one already described. These visions consisted in seeing himself in relationship with people he

> loved, and he felt he could understand the feelings of each one of them. He also saw himself as a baby and mourned deeply – he felt it was the first time – for the loss of his grandfather, which had occurred when he was 3 years old. He was also able to remember his childhood and adolescent dreams, what he wanted for his life, and could see where he was now professionally and personally. From this perspective he felt he could see what decisions and changes he had to make and take in his present life to redirect it in consistency with his desires, which also became clearer to his eyes. These could be considered important biographical visions and insights.
>
> But during the sessions he also had another kind of experience: he sensed very strongly and deeply something he had known intuitively and by his studies and work: being an ecology activist, he was convinced that the only path to a better life in society passes through the development of a new way of relating to nature and to others. During the most intense part of the experience, between the second and third hour, the patient had a sense of awe of being alive. He felt he could perceive emotionally, not only understand rationally, the interconnectedness of all things. He could feel that the air he inhaled had been just exhaled by the surrounding trees, and that the moon in the sky and his retina receiving that light were intimately connected. And that he shared an intimate "brotherhood" with all forms of existence. He came out from the experience with a sense of profound gratitude.

These insights can be considered not as biographical but having to do with consciousness and awareness. This is a subject to be treated elsewhere. What I can say here is that I have listened to his associations with an open attitude and that an important part of our work has consisted in helping the patient to find and value his own style of searching, thinking, and expressing himself.

There are also risks that have to be taken into consideration. The experience can trigger psychotic symptoms in some participants or enhance narcissistic pathological traits in others. These possibilities are minimized if the shaman who will conduct the session has the experience and skill to detect these structural frailties.

Conclusions

It is thus possible to consider the ayahuasca experience as especially valuable for neuropsychiatric research as well as psychoanalytical investigation. Published papers, as well as conferences on this subject, have become frequent in the past decade. Traditional knowledge can lead us, as mental health professionals, to new insights and ways of understanding health and suffering.

We can also state that the study of the *ayahuasca* experience provides areas of reflection and research:

a. Depression and other mood disorders
b. Visual imagery (and its relationship with dream images)
c. Memory (flashbacks, posttraumatic stress disorders, repression)
d. Consciousness and awareness (meaning of life, ecologically and altruistically driven motivations and acts, etc.)

References

1. Luna LE, White SF (eds) (2000) Ayahuasca reader: encounters with the Amazon's sacred vine. Synergetic, New Mexico
2. Luz P (2004) The American-Indian use of caapi (O uso ameríndio do caapi). In: Labate BC, Araújo WS (eds) The ritual use of ayahuasca (O uso ritual da ayahuasca). Mercado das Letras, Campinas, São Paulo
3. Fortunato J, Réux G, Kirsch T et al (2009) Acute harmine administration induces antidepressive-like effects and increases BDNF levels in the rat hippocampus. Prog Neuropsychopharmacol Biol Psychiatry 33(8):1425–1430
4. De Araujo DB, Ribeiro STG, Cecchi G et al (2009) Neural basis of enhanced visual imagery following Ayahuasca ingestion (Manuscript submitted for publication)
5. Labate BC, Araújo WS (eds) (2004) The ritual use of ayahuasca (O uso ritual da ayahuasca). Mercado das Letras, Campinas, São Paulo

Additional Reading

6. Almendro M (2008) Chamanismo: La vía de la mente nativa. Editorial Kairos, Barcelona
7. Chiappe M (1974) Curanderismo: Psiquiatría folklórica peruana. Tesis para obtener el doctorado en medicina para la Universidad Nacional Mayor de San Marcos, Perú
8. Chiappe M, Lemlij M, Millones L (1985) Alucinógenos y shamanismo en el Perú contemporáteno. Ediciones El Virrey, Lima
9. Gastelumendi E (2001) Madre ayahuasca y Edipo. In: Mabit J (ed) Memoria del Segundo foro sobre Espiritualidad Indígena: ética, mal y transgresion. CISEI, Lima
10. Narby J (1998) The cosmic serpent: DNA and the origins of knowledge. Jeremy P. Tarcher/Putnam, New York
11. Seguín CA (1988) Medicinas tradicionales y medicina folklórica. Fondo editorial del Banco Central de Reserva del Perú, Lima
12. Seguín CA (1979) Psiquiatría folklórica: shamanes y curanderos. Ediciones Ermar, Lima
13. Dobkin de Rios M, Grob Ch (2005) Theme Eds. Ayahuasca Use in Cross-Cultural Perspective. Journal of Psychoactive Drugs 37 (2). Haight-Ashbury Publications. San Francisco
14. Shanon B (2002) The antipodes of the mind: charting the phenomenology of the ayahuasca experience. Oxford University Press, New York

The Molecular Genetics of Suicide

Kiyoshi Maeda, Osamu Shirakawa, Naoki Nishiguchi, and Masaaki Fukutake

Abstract The increasing number of suicidal victims all over the world is a major concern. There are three neurobiological systems involved in the pathophysiology of suicidal behavior: dysfunction of the serotonergic system, hyperactivity of the noradrenergic system, and increased activity of the hypothalamic–pituitary–adrenal (HPA) axis appear to be involved. Increasing evidence points to an overlap between neurobiological and cognitive psychological approaches to understanding suicidal behavior. The authors reviewed the molecular genetics of suicidal behavior. A better understanding of the neurobiology of suicide can help detect at-risk populations and help develop better treatment interventions. Because suicide continues to be a major public health problem, further studies are necessary, including research on the effects of combined medical and psychosocial approaches.

Keywords Dopamine • Molecular genetics • Neurobiology • Noradrenalin • Serotonin • Suicide

Introduction

The number of suicide victims in Japan in the recent 11 years (1998–2008) is more than 30,000 a year, and in the year 2009 this number is 32,753. The suicide rate (number of suicide victims per 100,000 population) in Japan is about 25, and

K. Maeda (✉)
Department of Occupational Therapy, Kobe Gakuin University School of Rehabilitation, Ikawadani-cho 518, Nishi-ku, Kobe 651-2180, Japan
e-mail: maedak@reha.kobegakuin.ac.jp

O. Shirakawa and N. Nishiguchi
Department of Neuropsychiatry, Kinki University School of Medicine, 7-5-2, Kusunoki-Cho, Chuo-Ku, Kobe 651-0017, Japan

M. Fukutake
Department of Psychiatry, Kobe University School of Medicine, 7-5-2, Kusunoki-Cho, Chuo-Ku, Kobe 651-0017, Japan

K. Miyoshi et al. (eds.), *Neuropsychiatric Disorders*,
DOI 10.1007/978-4-431-53871-4_23, © Springer 2010

this number is the fourth highest in the world. Suicide is one of the most important public concerns and a major cause of death among young people throughout the world. No remarkable reduction in the number of suicide victims has yet been achieved, although there has been recent progress in the treatment and management of psychiatric disorders. During the past two decades, there has been a considerable accumulation of findings in the neurobiology of suicide [1].

Although many factors such as biological, psychological, and social factors are involved in suicide behavior, the presence of mental disorder is thought to play an important role in suicide [2]. More than 90% of suicide victims or suicide attempters are diagnosed having mental disorders such as depression, schizophrenia, or alcohol dependence (Fig. 1). However, the underlying mental disorders are diverse, and the severity of the mental disorders does not necessarily correlate with increased risk of suicide.

Even in the psychiatric groups at the highest risk, most patients never attempt suicide. These findings indicate the importance of a diathesis or predisposition to suicidal behavior that is independent of the main psychiatric disorder.

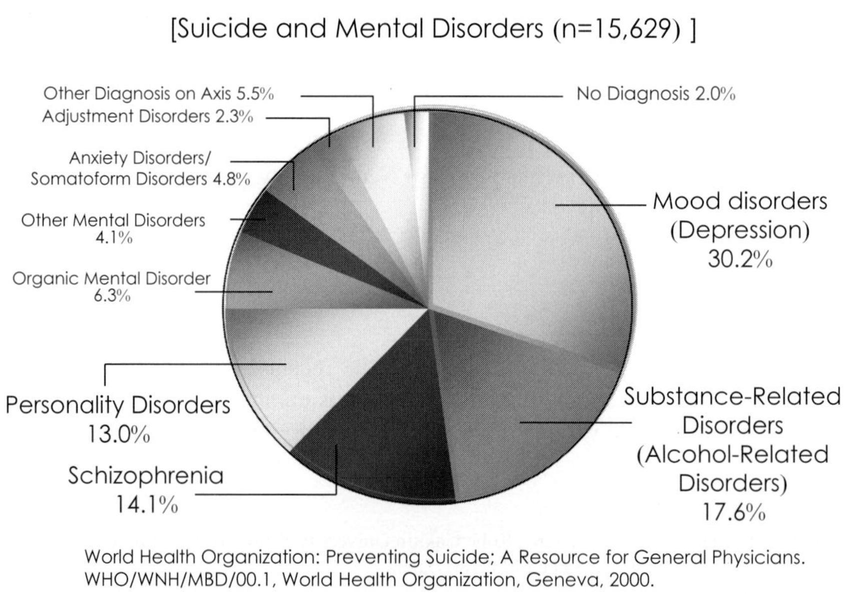

Fig. 1 Mental disorders in suicide. In completed suicide, about 30% of all suicide victims occur in relation to mood disorders, and the rest are related to various other psychiatric disorders, including substance-related disorders, such as substance abuse and alcoholism, schizophrenia and personality disorders. Source: World Health Organization: preventing suicide; a resource for general physicians. WHO/WNH/MBD/00.1, World Health Organization, Geneva, 2000

Molecular Genetics of Suicide

Numerous studies on neurochemical abnormalities have been done; the results obtained from those studies are summarized in Table 1. Recently, studies on the biological aspect of suicide have been shifting from neurochemical to molecular genetic approaches. Genetic studies on suicidal behavior have suggested that the heritability of such behavior is independent of psychiatric diagnosis. Adoption studies have shown a higher rate of suicide in the biological parents of adoptees who commit suicide compared with biological relatives of control adoptees, even after controlling for rates of psychosis and mood disorders (Table 2). Concordance rates for suicide and suicide attempts are higher in monozygotic than dizygotic twins, and the heritability of suicidal behavior was estimated to be approximately 55% based on twin studies in people with serious suicide attempts [3]. People who commit suicide or make suicide attempts are those with a higher rate of familial suicidal acts. These findings suggest the presence of hereditary and biological factors that determine the threshold to commit suicide and which are independent of specific psychiatric disorders. Thus, genetic factors in suicide have been a recent focus, and recognition has been growing that suicide and suicidal behaviors are highly familial and that genetics contributes to suicide and suicidal behaviors (Table 3). In addition, completed suicides are thought to be more homogeneous than suicide attempters in terms of inheritance of suicidal behavior [4].

Table 1 Risk factors for suicide: bio-psycho-social

Biological factors
Mental disorders
Physical disorders
Family history of mental disorders or suicide
Age, sex, race, etc.
Psychological factors
Temperament/character
Coping skills/problem solving skills
Social factors
Economic and livelihood issues
Family problems

Table 2 Genetic studies on suicidal behavior

• Adoption studies: ~sixfold increased risk		
• Twin studies: 38–55% heritability		
No. of twins (%)	Concordant for suicidal behavior	
MZ	DZ	*P*
40/172 (23.0)	2/294 (0.7)	<0.0001
• Family studies: 2- to 12-fold increased risk		

Roy A, Segal NL (2001) [3]

Table 3 Exploration of susceptible genetic variants for completed suicide

Serotonergic system
Suicide-associated personality and cognitive dysfunction (aggressiveness, impulsiveness)
Noradrenergic and hypothalamic–pituitary–adrenal (HPA) system
Stress vulnerability (anxiety/agitation, hopelessness)
The sites of action of mood stabilizers
Antisuicidal effects of lithium
Gene expression analysis in postmortem brains of suicide victims

Table 4 Results of association between polymorphisms of serotonin-related genes and completed suicide

		Suicide		Control				
Gene	Polymorphism	Allele wt	Allele vt	Allele wt	Allele vt	OR	95% CI	*P* value
5-HT1A	Pro16Leu	320	6	322	4	0.66	0.19–2.37	0.524
	Gly272Asp	309	17	311	15	0.88	0.43–1.79	0.717
5-HT1B	G861C	161	165	165	161	0.95	0.70–1.29	0.754
5-HT2A	−1438A/G	157	145	157	169	1.17	0.85–1.59	0.338
5-HT6	u (GCC)2/3	239	87	237	95	1.1	0.78–1.55	0.581
	267C/T	213	113	213	119	1.05	0.76–1.45	0.751
TPH	−6526A/G	220	44	216	48	1.11	0.71–1.74	0.646
	Int 218C/A	138	126	141	123	0.96	0.68–1.34	0.794
5-HTT	Ins/del	148	44	205	61	1	0.64–1.56	0.997
	Int VNTR	331	41	331	29	0.71	0.43–1.17	0.173
MAO-A	u VNTR	107	92	116	98	0.98	0.67–1.48	0.929

On the basis of these findings, we have conducted genetic association analysis of completed suicides to explore the susceptible genetic variants for suicide. Up to the present date, we have found a number of associations for genetic variations with completed suicide. We have been focusing attention on several neurobiological factors including the serotonergic system, noradrenergic and hypothalamic–pituitary–adrenal (HPA) system, and the sites of action of mood stabilizers, especially the antisuicidal effects of lithium.

In addition, for the purpose of identifying new candidate systems and gaining new insight into biological mechanisms mediating suicide, we have conducted gene expression analysis in the postmortem brains of suicide victims [5–11, 13–18]. Recently, molecular genetic studies have been performed intensively to confirm disturbance of serotonergic neurotransmission in suicide. We have performed association studies of polymorphisms and mutations of genes encoding synthesizing and metabolic enzymes, receptors, and transporters involved in serotonergic neurotransmission in suicide [5–11]. However, in our studies, we have not observed any significant association between these polymorphisms and suicide (Table 4).

In addition, many other studies performed to date have not provided strong evidence supporting such an association. The relative risk was small even when association was detected by meta-analysis (Table 5).

Table 5 Summary of meta-analysis of association between serotonergic genes and suicidal behavior

Gene	Polymorphism	No. of studies	Subject origin	OR	95% CI
TPH	Intron 7	16	Inc. Asian	1.14	0.97–1.34
TPH	Intron 7 A218C	7	Caucasian	1.33	1.17–1.50
5-HTT	Ins/del	12	Inc. Asian	1.17	1.04–1.32
5-HT2A	102T/C	9	Inc. Asian	1.09	0.93–1.27

Anguelova M, Benkelfat C, Turecki G (2003) [12]

It has been suggested that noradrenergic system abnormalities are involved in suicide [13, 14]. Recently, we have found that one promoter genetic variant (C-1291G SNP) of the α_{2A}-adrenergic receptor (ADRA2A) gene was significantly associated with suicide in Japanese females ($P=0.043$ and 0.013 for genotypic and allelic comparisons, respectively). One of the common haplotypes, CC of this polymorphism and another variant of the ADRA2A gene (rs3750625C/A), was also associated with suicide in females ($P=0.015$). These associations were also significant in the female violent suicide victims ($P=0.009$ and 0.009 for allelic and CC haplotypic comparisons, respectively; Table 6) [13]. In contrast, neither of these two SNPs showed any association with violent and/or nonviolent suicide in males. The noradrenergic system regulates activation of the HPA axis, dysregulation of which might be involved in the pathogenesis of suicide. Therefore, this promoter variant in the ADRA2A gene might be involved in the pathogenesis of suicide as a result of the noradrenergic dysfunction that destabilizes the HPA system.

The catechol-*O*-methyltransferase (COMT) gene, the catecholamine-degrading enzyme, exhibits a functional common polymorphism (158Met/Val), and this variant is considered to affect the HPA system. Individuals who are homozygous for the low-activity form of COMT (A/A, Met/Met) would exhibit greater HPA-axis activation than those who are either homozygous or heterozygous for the high-activity form of the enzyme. We found that the genotype distribution of the COMT 158Val/Met polymorphism was significantly different between male suicide completers and male controls ($P=0.036$), whereas the frequency of the Val/Val genotype, a high-activity form of the enzyme, was significantly less in male suicide completers than in male controls [odds ratio (OR)=0.52; 95% confidence interval (CI)=0.31–0.89; $P=0.016$] [14]. These findings were not the case in females. We found that this polymorphism was associated with suicide in males, and that high COMT activity could exhibit a protective effect for suicide in males (Table 7) [15].

Table 8 shows the distributions of the four polymorphisms in the μ-opioid receptor (OPRM1) gene. The OPRM1 gene is implicated in stress responses through the HPA system [16]. The substitution of A118G polymorphism in the OPRM1 gene, which results in an Asn to Asp change at amino acid 40, is suggested to influence the HPA axis response in an inhibitory manner and, possibly, decrease the HPA axis response to a social stressor. Therefore, the suicide-protective G allele would be expected to inhibit the HPA axis responses. We genotyped four single-nucleotide polymorphisms, including a

Table 6 Distribution of polymorphisms in the *ADRA2A* gene

Marker	Controls			Minor allele frequency		Suicide victims			Minor allele frequency	Statistics genotype	Statistics allele	
										P value	χ^2	*P* value
Male and female												
C-1291G	CC	CG	GG	C		CC	CG	GG	C			
($n = 185$)	0.086	0.422	0.492	0.297	($n = 171$)	0.117	0.474	0.409	0.354	0.264	2.589	0.108 (0.226)
rs3750625	CC	CA	AA	A		CC	CA	AA	A			
($n = 183$)	0.536	0.404	0.06	0.262	($n = 181$)	0.607	0.343	0.05	0.221	0.397	1.693	0.196 (0.376)
Male												
C-1291G	CC	CG	GG	C		CC	CG	GG	C			
($n = 112$)	0.089	0.446	0.465	0.312	($n = 118$)	0.093	0.458	0.449	0.322	0.98	0.048	0.826 (0.979)
rs3750625	CC	CA	AA	A		CC	CA	AA	A			
($n = 120$)	0.55	0.392	0.058	0.254	($n = 122$)	0.631	0.328	0.041	0.205	0.426	1.66	0.198 (0.386)
Female												
C-1291G	**CC**	**CG**	**GG**	**C**		**CC**	**CG**	**GG**	**C**			
($n = 73$)	**0.082**	**0.384**	**0.534**	**0.274**	**($n = 53$)**	**0.17**	**0.509**	**0.321**	**0.425**	**0.043**	**6.228**	**0.013 (0.027)**
rs3750625	CC	CA	AA	A		CC	CA	AA	A			
($n = 63$)	0.508	0.429	0.063	0.278	($n = 59$)	0.559	0.373	0.068	0.254	0.844	0.173	0.678 (0.977)

Fukutake M, Hishimoto A, Nishiguchi N et al. (2008) [14]

Table 7 Genotype and allele frequencies of the COMT 158Val/Met polymorphism

	Genotype			Allele	
	AA (%)	AG (%)	GG (%)	A (%)	G (%)
Suicides (n = 163)	16 (10)	79 (48)	68 (42)	111 (34)	215 (66)
Controls (n = 169)	18 (11)	61 (36)	90 (53)	97 (29)	241 (71)
Male suicides (n = 112)	**9 (8)**	**60 (54)**	**43 (38)**	78 (35)	146 (65)
Male controls (n = 114)	**10 (9)**	**42 (37)**	**62 (54)**	62 (27)	166 (73)
Female suicides (n = 51)	7 (14)	19 (37)	25 (49)	33 (32)	69 (68)
Female controls (n = 55)	8 (15)	19 (35)	28 (50)	35 (32)	75 (68)

Total: genotype $\chi^2 = 5.4$, $df = 2$, $P = 0.068$; allele $\chi^2 = 2.2$, $df = 1$, $P = 0.14$
Male: genotype $\chi^2 = 6.7$, $df = 2$, $P =$ **0.036**; allele $\chi^2 = 3.1$, $df = 1$, $p =$ **0.080**
Female: genotype $\chi^2 = 0.86$, $df = 2$, $P = 0.96$; allele $\chi^2 = 0.07$, $df = 2$, $P = 0.93$
Ono H, Shirakawa O, Nishiguchi N et al. (2004) [15]

common A118G SNP. The genotypic and allelic distributions of the A118G SNP were significantly different between the completed suicide and control groups ($P = 0.014$ and 0.039, respectively; Table 9). Moreover, the dominant model of genotype (AA vs. AG + GG) analysis showed an enhanced association with suicide ($P = 0.0041$, OR = 0.575). This finding means that individuals with one or two copies of the G allele of the A118G SNP of the OPRM1 gene are less vulnerable to suicide. These results raise the possibility that the A118G SNP of the OPRM1 gene is associated with suicide.

We have conducted another association study examining the functional gene polymorphisms of angiotensin-converting enzyme (insertion/deletion), prostaglandin E receptor subtype EP1 [17], and neuronal nitric oxide synthase (nNOS or NOSI), which affect the HPA system, and demonstrated significant associations with suicide. These findings have suggested that the disturbance of the HPA system plays an important role in suicide (Table 9).

Recently, we found an association between regulators of G-protein signaling (RGS) 2 gene polymorphisms and suicide and observed increased RGS2 immunoreactivity in the postmortem brains of suicide victims (Tables 10, and 11) [18]. RGSs are a family of proteins that negatively regulate intracellular signaling of G protein-coupled receptors (GPCRs), such as the serotonin receptor. RGS2 is thought to play an important role in anxiety and/or aggressive behavior.

To explore the involvement of the RGS2 gene in vulnerability to suicide, we screened Japanese suicide victims for sequence variations in the RGS2 gene and carried out an association study of RGS2 gene polymorphisms with suicide victims. In the eight identified polymorphisms that were identified by mutation screening, we genotyped four common single-nucleotide polymorphisms in the RGS2 gene and found significant differences in the distribution of the SNP3 genotypes and alleles of the SNP2 and the SNP3 between completed suicides and the controls. The distribution of the haplotype was also significantly different between the two groups (Table 11; global < 0.0001). Furthermore, RGS2 immunoreactivity significantly increased in the amygdala and the prefrontal cortex [Brodmann area 9] of the postmortem brain of the suicide subjects (Fig. 2). These findings suggest that RGS2 is genetically involved in the biological susceptibility to suicide in the Japanese population.

Table 8 Distribution of the single-nucleotide polymorphisms (SNPs) in the *OPRM1* gene

Marker	Controls			Minor allele frequency		Completed suicides			Minor allele frequency	Statistics genotype	Statistics allele	
										P value	χ^2	*P* value
rs1074287	AA	AG	GG			AA	AG	GG				
(n=373)	74.8%	23.9%	1.3%	0.132	(n=179)	71.5%	26.8%	1.7%	0.151	0.706	0.666	0.414 (0.927)
rs12205732	GG	GA	AA			GG	GA	AA				
(n=372)	78.0%	21.2%	0.8%	0.114	(n=170)	80.6%	17.6%	1.8%	0.106	0.403	0.127	0.722 (0.998)
A118G	**AA**	**AG**	**GG**			**AA**	**AG**	**GG**				
(n=367)	**26.2%**	**57.2%**	**16.6%**	**0.452**	**(n=181)**	**38.1%**	**46.4%**	**15.5%**	**0.387**	**0.014**	**4.252**	**0.039 (0.198)***
IVS2 +G691C	GG	GC	CC			GG	GC	CC				
(n=370)	4.1%	37.3%	58.6%	0.227	(n=170)	6.4%	37.4%	56.2%	0.251	0.471	0.762	0.383 (0.840)

Hishimoto A, Cui H, Mouri K et al. (2008) [16]

* P <0.05

Table 9 Susceptible polymorphisms for suicide associated with HPA system

Functional variants associated with suicide
COMT Val158Met SNP
OPRM1 Asn40Asp SNP
ACE insertion/deletion polymorphism
ADRA2A promoter C-1291G SNP
Prostaglandin E receptor EP1 gene SNPs
Neuronal nitric oxide synthase SNP
Functional polymorphisms *not associated* with completed suicide
FKBP5 rs1360780 T/C polymorphism
Peripheral benzodiazepine receptor gene polymorphism
Glucocorticoid receptor (*Bcl*IRFLP, N363S, ER22/23EK) polymorphism

Hishimoto A, Shirakawas O, Nishiguchi N et al. (2006) [17]

Table 10 Genotype distributions and allele frequencies of RGS2 gene polymorphisms

	Genotype frequency				Allele frequency			
SNPs	Genotype	Control	Suicide	*P* value	Allele	Control	Suicide	*P* value
SNP 1	A/A	64 (0.30)	39 (0.21)	0.068	A	228 (0.54)	176 (0.47)	**0.0293***
	A/G	100 (0.48)	98 (0.52)	$df=2$				$df=1$
	G/G	46 (0.22)	52 (0.27)	$\chi^2=5.365$	G	192 (0.46)	202 (0.53)	$\chi^2=4.749$
SNP 2	G/G	85 (0.40)	52 (0.28)	**0.0383***	G	260 (0.62)	197 (0.53)	**0.0175***
	C/G	90 (0.43)	93 (0.51)	$df=2$				$df=1$
	C/C	35 (0.17)	39 (0.21)	$\chi^2=6.527$	C	160 (0.38)	171 (0.47)	$\chi^2=5.644$
SNP 3	C/C	68 (0.32)	37 (0.20)	**0.0105***	C	243 (0.58)	179 (0.48)	**0.0048****
	C/G	107 (0.51)	105 (0.56)	$df=2$				$df=1$
	G/G	35 (0.17)	45 (0.24)	$\chi^2=9.119$	G	177 (0.42)	195 (0.52)	$\chi^2=7.939$
SNP 4	T/T	80 (0.38)	47 (0.26)	0.0528	T	257 (0.61)	189 (0.53)	**0.0287***
	C/T	97 (0.46)	95 (0.54)	$df=2$				$df=1$
	C/C	33 (0.16)	35 (0.20)	$\chi^2=5.883$	C	163 (0.39)	165 (0.47)	$\chi^2=4.787$

SNP1: −638 A/G (rs2746071); SNP2: −395 C/G (rs2746072); SNP3: 2,971 C/G (rs4606); SNP4: 3,438 C/T (rs3767488) (db SNP ID)
Cui H, Nishiguchi N, Ivleva E et al. (2008) [18]
* $P < 0.05$, ** $P < 0.01$

Table 11 Haplotype analysis of RGS2 gene SNP 1–4

		Frequency		Global *P* value = 0.000046	
Haplotype of SNP 1–2–3–4		Control	Suicide	χ^2	*P* value
1	A-G-C-T	0.5183	0.4382	4.8671	**0.0274***
2	G-C-G-C	0.3479	0.427	5.0199	**0.0251***
3	G-G-G-T	0.0565	0.0285	3.5473	0.0596
4	G-G-C-T	0.0201	0.0266	0.3563	0.5506
5	G-G-G-C	<0.01	0.0295	12.5573	**<0.01****
6	G-C-G-T	<0.01	0.0144	1.9983	0.1575
7	G-C-C-C	0.0161	<0.01	5.6202	**0.0178***
8	A-C-C-T	<0.01	0.0121	1.2136	0.2706
9	A-G-G-T	<0.01	0.012	1.1609	0.2813
10	G-G-C-C	0.0119	<0.01	4.1444	**0.0418***
…	…	<0.01	<0.01	…	…

SNP1: –638 A/G (rs2746071); SNP2: –395 C/G (rs2746072); SNP3: 2,971 C/G (rs4606); SNP4: 3,438 C/T (rs3767488)
*$P < 0.05$, **$P < 0.01$
Cui H, Nishiguchi N, Ivleva E et al. (2008) [18]

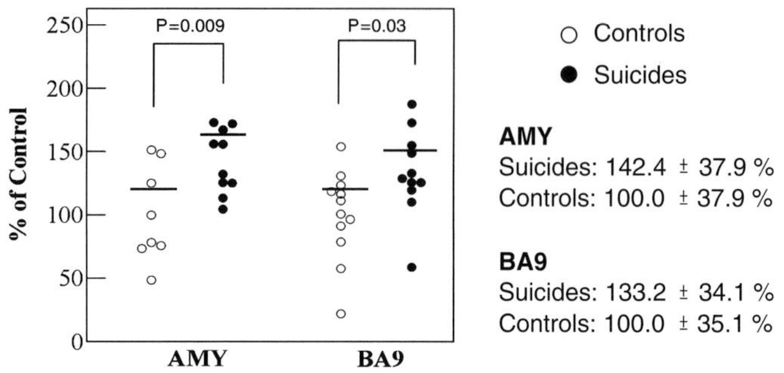

Fig. 2 Increased RGS2 immunoreactivity in suicides. RGS2 immunoreactivity significantly increased in the amygdala and the prefrontal cortex [Brodmann area 9] of the postmortem brain of the suicide subjects. These findings suggest that RGS2 is genetically involved in the biological susceptibility to suicide in the Japanese population. Cui H, Nishiguchi N, Ivleva E et al. (2008) [18]

Conclusion

Taking into consideration the presence of mental disorders as underlying suicide, it is natural that the recent trend tends to link early screening of depression to suicide prevention as a medical approach. It is inadvisable to interpret suicide solely as a symptom or outcome of disease. Expansion of the disease concept and subsequent additional medical intervention may be inappropriate. However, the biological and medical understanding of suicide, that is, interpretation as a condition that allows or requires medical intervention, may encourage people at high risk for suicide to visit psychological counselors and psychiatrists. In addition, although the processes may be indirect or secondary, medical and biological approaches could have considerable influence on individual views and social consciousness of life and death, which may contribute to the prevention of suicide.

References

1. Mann JJ (2003) Neurobiology of suicidal behavior. Nat Rev Neurosci 4:819–828
2. Brent DA, Mann JJ (2005) Family genetic studies, suicide, and suicidal behavior. Am J Med Genet C Semin Med Genet 133:13–24
3. Roy A, Segal NL (2001) Suicidal behavior in twins: a replication. J Affect Disord 66:71–74
4. Bondy B, Buettner A, Zill P (2006) Genetics of suicide. Mol Psychiatry 11:336–351
5. Ono H, Shirakawa O, Nishiguchi N et al (2000) Tryptophan hydroxylase gene polymorphisms are not associated with suicide. Am J Med Genet 96:861–863
6. Ono H, Shirakawa O, Nishiguchi N et al (2001) Serotonin 2A receptor gene polymorphism is not associated with completed suicide. J Psychiatr Res 35:173–176
7. Nishiguchi N, Shirakawa O, Ono H et al (2001) No evidence of an association between 5HT1B receptor gene polymorphism and suicide victims in a Japanese population. Am J Med Genet 105:343–345

8. Ono H, Shirakawa O, Kitamura N et al (2002) Tryptophan hydroxylase immunoreactivity is altered by the genetic variation in postmortem brain samples of both suicide victims and controls. Mol Psychiatry 7:1127–1132
9. Nishiguchi N, Shirakawa O, Ono H et al (2002) Lack of an association between 5-HT1A receptor gene structural polymorphisms and suicide victims. Am J Med Genet 114: 423–425
10. Ono H, Shirakawa O, Nishiguchi N et al (2002) No evidence of an association between a functional monoamine oxidase a gene polymorphism and completed suicides. Am J Med Genet 114:340–342
11. Okamura K, Shirakawa O, Nishiguchi N et al (2005) Lack of an association between 5-HT6 receptor gene polymorphisms and suicide victims. Psychiatry Clin Neurosci 59:345–349
12. Anguelova M, Benkelfat C, Turecki G (2003) A systematic review of association studies investigating genes coding for serotonin receptors and the serotonin transporter: II. Suicidal behavior. Mol Psychiatry 8:646–653
13. Hattori H, Shirakawa O, Nishiguchi N et al (2006) No evidence of an association between tyrosine hydroxylase gene polymorphisms and suicide victims. Kobe J Med Sci 52: 195–200
14. Fukutake M, Hishimoto A, Nishiguchi N et al (2008) Association of α_{2A}-aderenergic receptor gene polymorphism with susceptibility to suicide in Japanese females. Prog Neuropsychopharmacol Biol Psychiatry 32:1428–1433
15. Ono H, Shirakawa O, Nushida H et al (2004) Association between catechol-*O*-methyltransferase functional polymorphism and male suicide completers. Neuropsychopharmacology 29:1374–1377
16. Hishimoto A, Cui H, Mouri K et al (2008) A functional polymorphism of the μ-opioid receptor gene is associated with completed suicides. J Neural Transm 115:531–536
17. Hishimoto A, Shirakawa O, Nishiguchi N et al (2006) Association between a functional polymorphism in the renin-angiotensin system and completed suicide. J Neural Transm 113:1915–1920
18. Cui H, Nishiguchi N, Ivleva E et al (2008) Association of RGS2 gene polymorphisms with suicide and increased RGS2 immunoreactivity in the postmortem brain of suicide victims. Neuropsychopharmacology 33:1537–1544

Part VIII
International Neuropsychiatric Association

Brief History and Current Status of the International Neuropsychiatric Association

Koho Miyoshi

Abstract The International Organization of Neuropsychiatry (ION) was established by Spanish and American neuropsychiatrists in Seville in the year 1996. In conjunction with the second congress in Toronto (1998), the International Neuropsychiatric Association (INA) was established to supersede the ION. Since then, the International Congresses of Neuropsychiatry have been held every 2 years, namely in Kyoto (2000), Buenos Aires (2002), Athens (2004), Sydney (2006), and Cancun (2008). Here, the brief history and topics of the plenary lectures and symposia in the past congresses are reviewed. The current status of the INA, including Mission Statement, Officers, Committees, and Regional Activities, is also mentioned briefly.

Keywords Alwyn Lishman Award • International Neuropsychiatric Association (INA) • Neuropsychiatric disorders • Neuropsychiatry • Ramon y Cajal Award

Introduction

The International Organization of Neuropsychiatry (ION), currently the International Neuropsychiatric Association (INA), was established in 1996. According to the Mission Statement, the INA aims to prevent or reduce the suffering of the patients with neuropsychiatric disorders by studying the psychiatric symptoms or syndromes in cerebral disorders and by investigating neurobiological bases of psychiatric disorders. The INA provides a forum for interaction and exchange of ideas among professionals in neuropsychiatry and endeavors to publicize and disseminate both clinical and academic advances in the field of neuropsychiatry. Here, a brief history of the association and current status are mentioned briefly as an introduction for new INA members.

K. Miyoshi (✉)
Jinmeikai Research Institute for Mental Health Kabutoyama-cho, Nishinomiya, Hyogo, Japan
e-mail: RXI02704@nifty.com

K. Miyoshi et al. (eds.), *Neuropsychiatric Disorders*,
DOI 10.1007/978-4-431-53871-4_24, © Springer 2010

Principal speakers in the First Congress were:

A. Ardila (US), S. Cervera (Spain), J. Cook (US), E. Costa (US), J. Cummings (US), A. David (UK), B. Dubois (France), L. Farrer (US), B. Fogel (US), J. Giner (Spain), P. Gorelick (US), P. Grasby (UK), R. Green (US), J. Guimon (Switzerland), T. Jobe (US), C. Leal (Spain), A. Lishman (UK), H. Markowitsch (Germany), M. Mesulam (US), M. Rasenick (US), S. Rauch (US), J. Vallejo-Ruiloba (Spain), M. Spitzer (Germany), N. Vokow (US), P. Whitehouse (US), and others.

The Reorganization: The Second Congress in Toronto

Soon after the congress in Seville, Dr. Colin Shapiro (Toronto) and Dr. Koho Miyoshi (Kyoto) expressed their intentions to the organizing committee to hold the coming neuropsychiatric congress in their countries. The arrangement of the future congress was discussed in Orlando, Florida, where the Eighth Annual Meeting of American Neuropsychiatric Association was held, in 1997. Dr. Moises Gaviria attended the meeting on behalf of the organizing committee of the First Congress in Seville. It was decided to hold the Second Congress in Toronto.

Dr. Shapiro, Dr. Gaviria, and Dr. Miyoshi gathered to discuss about the financial issues of the INA in Hawaii, where the Ninth Annual Congress of American Neuropsychiatric Association was held in January 1998, and decided to manage the organization temporarily by their financial contributions.

The Second International Congress of Neuropsychiatry, which was called formally the "International Neuropsychiatry Congress (INC) and American Neuropsychiatric Association (ANPA) 1998 Joint Meeting," was held May 31 in Toronto, Canada. The INA sessions and the ANPA sessions were held in the meeting. In conjunction with the Toronto meeting, the INA, dedicated to promoting the study of the brain and behavior from a neuropsychiatric perspective, was established to supersede the ION. Twenty-four countries from Europe, North and South America, Asia, and Australia were represented. It was decided that the association would hold a biennial meeting.

As the first president of the association, Dr. Colin Shapiro (Canada) was elected. Dr. Koho Miyoshi (vice-president) and Dr. Moises Gaviria (secretary-general) were elected as the officers. Drs. R.H. Belmaker (Israel), E.Y.H. Chen (Hong Kong), D.D. Dikeos (Greece), M. Robertson (UK), P. Sachdev (Australia), and P. Sandor (Canada) were elected as the members of the Executive Committee. The office of the INA was decided to be located in the office of the president in Toronto. Dr. Paul Sander (Canada) was elected as a newsletter editor, and Dr. Sharon Chung (Canada) was appointed as the secretariat in the INA office (Fig. 2).

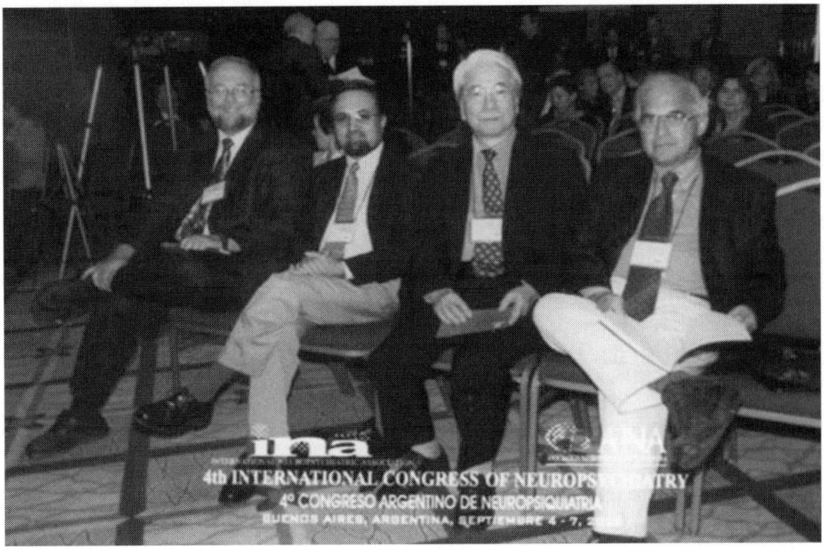

Fig. 2 The Presidents of the INA: Dr. C. Shapiro (1998–2002), Dr. P. Sachdev (2004–2006), Dr. K. Miyoshi (2008–), and Dr. M. Gaviria (2002–2004) in Buenos Aires, 2002 (from *left*)

The Mission Statement was proposed and accepted in the executive committee.

Mission Statement of the International Neuropsychiatric Association (1998)

1. The INA aims to prevent or reduce the suffering of people with brain-behavior disorders by increasing, integrating, and disseminating knowledge and understand the relationships between brain function and human behavior.
2. The INA aims to accomplish this objective by providing a forum for interaction and exchange of ideas among a variety of professionals with an interest in neuropsychiatric issues.
3. The INA endeavors to publicize and disseminate both clinical and academic advances in the field to bring about improved health for people throughout the world. Although rapidly advancing medical technology has greatly expanded the frontiers of neuropsychiatry, the INA will strive to preserve the humanistic values of medicine.
4. The INA endeavors to raise awareness of neuropsychiatry, particularly in those countries where it is not well known or recognized.

The scientific topics and principal speakers in the Second Congress were:

Neuropsychiatry of Tourettes' Syndrome [M. Robertson (UK), E.C. Miquel (Brazil), B.J.M. van de Wetering (the Netherlands)]; The Epidemiology of Hallucinations [M. Ohayon (Canada)], Neuropsychiatry, and Neuroimaging [L. Farde (Sweden), P. Martin (US), R. Dolan (UK)]; Genetics and Psychobiology of Personality (Keynote Lecture) [C.R. Cloninger (US)]; Genetics of Neuropsychiatry [K. Kidd (US), D. Black (US), M. Lepper (US), B. Clementz (US), P. Propping (Germany)], and Art and the Mind [H. Walton (UK)].

The Springboard: The Third Congress in Kyoto

The executive committee was held in New Orleans, where the Tenth Annual Congress of American Neuropsychiatric Association took place, on January 31, 1999. The proposed by-laws of the INA were examined and accepted by the executive committee.

The Third Congress was held in Kyoto, Japan, April 9–13, 2000. The venue of the Congress was The Kyoto International Conference Hall at Takaragaike, Kyoto. At the Kyoto meeting, approximately 700 people participated. Thirty-one countries and districts, including Australia, Belgium, Canada, Croatia, Egypt, France, Germany, Greece, Hong Kong, India, Israel, Italy, Japan, Lithuania, Macedonia, the Netherlands, the Philippines, Poland, Russia, Spain, Sweden, Switzerland, Taiwan, Thailand, Turkey, the United Arab Emirates, the United Kingdom, the United States, Uruguay, and Venezuela, sent delegates.

The topics of the plenary lectures in the Third Congress were:

Dementia with Lewy Body [I. McKeith (UK)]; Tourette Syndrome [M.M. Robertson (UK)]; Neuropsychiatry in the Elderly [J.L. Cummings (US)]; Zen and the Brain [J.H. Austin (US)]; Functional Neuroimaging [H. Shibazaki (Japan)]; Sex Differences in Brain Aging [C.E. Coffey (US)]; Biological Substrate of Late Life Depression [J. Schweitzer (Australia)]; Neuropsychiatry of Stroke [R.G. Robinson (US)]; Neuropsychiatry of Limbic and Subcortical Disorders [S.P. Salloway (US)]; Neuroimaging and Neurobiology of Schizophrenia [N. Andreasen (US)]; Brain Laterality and Psychopathology [G. Gainotti (Italy)]; Behavioral and Psychological Symptoms of Dementia [S.I. Finkel (US)]; Neuropsychiatry in 21st Century [C. Shapiro (Canada)]; Positron Emission Tomography Studies in Schizophrenia [J.J. Lopez-Ibor (Spain)]; Neuropsychiatric Aspects of Sleep Disorders [C. Soldatos (Greece)], Brain Pathology of Dementia [K. Kosaka (Japan)]; Non-Alzheimer Type of Dementia [L. Gustafson (Sweden)]; New Trends of Pharmacological Treatment of Dementia [K. Miyoshi (Japan)]; and Schizophrenia-like Psychoses and Epilepsy [P. Sachdev (Australia)].

The topics of the symposia and workshop in the Third Congress were:

Worldwide Collaborations in Neuropsychiatry, Transcranial Magnetic Stimulation, Advances in Psychooncology and Psychoimmunology, Behavioral Genetics of Personality, Vulnerability Markers of Schizophrenia, Vascular Dementia, Biology of Eating Disorders, Dementia in Asian Countries, Brain and Behavior, Molecular Genetics of Stimulant-Induced Psychosis, Neuropsychiatric Disorders and Related Conditions, Clinical Aspects of Dementing Disorders, Fronto-Temporal Lobe Dementia, Genetics of Schizophrenia and Affective Disorders, Alzheimer's Disease, Neuropharmacology, Neuropsychiatric Aspects of Schizophrenia, Anticonvulsants, Obsessive–Compulsive Disorders and Personality Disorders, Diffuse Lewy Body Disease, Lithium and Signal Transduction, Genetics of Personality, and Post-Mortem Brain Specimens to Study Affective Disorders.

The monograph, *Contemporary Neuropsychiatry*, which consists of selected papers from the Third Congress, was edited by K. Miyoshi, C. Shapiro, M. Gaviria, and Y. Morita, and published by Springer-Verlag Tokyo in 2001.

The Jump: The Fourth Congress in Buenos Aires

The Fourth Congress, chaired by Dr. Marquez (Buenos Aires), was held in Buenos Aires in 2002. The venue was Hotel Crowne Plaza Panamericano in Buenos Aires. Approximately 1,500 people participated in the Congress. The topics of the meeting covered the neuropsychiatric field almost completely. As the Second INA president, Dr. Moises Gavira (US) was elected for a 2-year term. Treasurer [G. Tortora (Argentina)] and the members of Executive Committee [R. Belmaker (Israel), K. Miyoshi (Japan), A. Kanner (US), E.S. Krishnamoorthy (India), M. Marquez (Artentina), S. Shi (China), J. Tellez (Columbia), D. Dikeos (Greece), and C. Soldatos (Greece)] were elected in the Executive Meeting.

Issues of the official journal and committees, such as the education committee and membership committee, were discussed in the Executive Meeting.

The topics of the lectures in the Fourth Congress were:

Psychopathology in Epilepsy [A. Kanner (US)]; G-Protein Signaling in Anti-Depressants [M. Rasenick (US)]; Tau Changes and Deficit in Episodic Memory [L. Binder (US)]; Concussion in Sports [R. Bornstein (US)]; New Trends in the Treatment of Dementia [K. Miyoshi (Japan)]; Cognitive Impairment in Parkinson's Disease [O. Gershanik (Argentine)]; Organic Psychosis as a Model for Schizophrenia [P. Sachdev (Australia)]; Thyroid Hormone and Affective Disorders [R. Bunevicius (Lithuania)]; Neuropsychological and Neuropsychiatric Aspects of Electric Trauma [N. Pliskin (US)]; Mechanism and Action of mu-Opioides [J. Lemos (US)]; Cognitive Therapy [R. Baber (US)]; Towards an Early and Presymptomatic Diagnosis of Primary Degenerative Dementia [C. Mangone (Argentine)]; Prion Disease [A.L. Taratuto (Argentine)], Sleep Disorders [C. Shapiro (Canada)], Cognitive-Motor Disorder in Psychiatric Diseases [R. Leiguarda (Argentine)]; Functional MRI in Neuropsychiatry [G. Stebbens (US)]; Neurogenesis in Adult Hippocampus [A. Schinder (Argentine)]; Current Status and Future Directions in Psychiatric Neurosurgery [K. Slavin (US)]; Music Brain and Culture [M. Gaviria (US)]; A Genetic Approach to the Conceptual Nosological Continuum of Schizophrenia and Mood Disorders [D. Dikeos (Greece)]; Vascular Dementia: an Overview [G. Roman (US)]; Chronobiology and Affective Disorders [D. Cardinali (Argentine)]; Attention Deficit [J. Gutierrez (Mexico)]; Brain Damage and Recovery [M. Gaviria (US)];

ECT in Neuropsychiatric Disorders [C. Campillo (Mexico)]; Neuropsycho Immunology [R. Espaillat (Dominica)]; Neuropsychology of Memory [J. Medina (Argentine)]; Neuronal Networks in OCD [M. Marquez (Argentine)]; and Inflammation Transcription Factors [G. de Erausquin (US)].

The topics of the symposia in the Fourth Congress were:

Neuropsychiatry and Primary Care, Organic Bases of Psychopathology in Epilepsy, Neuroimaging in Neuropsychiatry, Cognitive Assessment Tools for Iberoamerica, Psychic Handicapped Condition, Pharmacological Management of Tourette's Syndrome and Associated Disorders, Alzheimer's Disease, Diagnostic Challenges in Neuropsychiatry, Frontal Lobe and Executive Function, Stress, New Neuropsychiatrics Approaches, New Trends in Depression, Neuropsychiatric Issues of Autism Spectrum, and Spectrum of the Frontotemporal Dementia.

In this conference, the Lishman Award and the Ramon Y. Cajal Award were established. The Lishman Award was established to honor the modern pioneer of Neuropsychiatry, Professor Alwyn Lishman of London. It is presented every 2 years to an individual who has made a notable contribution to clinical neuropsychiatry at the international level. The awardee will be a distinguished clinician and extend practice, teaching, and/or service delivery of neuropsychiatry beyond the boundaries of his or her own country. The Ramon Y. Cajal Award was established to honor the Father of Neuroscience. This award is presented every 2 years to an individual who has made a distinguished contribution to neuroscience with an application to neuropsychiatry. The awardee will be an eminent neuroscientist who has made salient contribution resulting in a paradigm shift or the development of novel diagnostic or management strategies.

Dr. Julio Vellejo Ruiloba (Spain) presented a lecture titled "Issues of Current Neuropsychiatry" as the first awardee of the Ramón y Cajal Award, and Dr. Gustavo Roman (US) gave a lecture on "Vascular Dementia. An Overview" as the first awardee of the Alwyn Lishiman Award.

The Collaborations: The Fifth Congress in Athens

The Fifth International Congress, in conjunction with the First Mediterranean Congress of World Federation of Societies of Biological Psychiatry, was held in Athens, October 14–18, in 2004. The venue of the meeting was the International Conference Center at Megaron. Dr. Constantin Soldatos chaired the Congress. The possibilities to stimulate activities of the INA by collaborating with closely related scientific societies were clearly shown in this meeting.

This was the First Congress in a European country, and approximately 1,000 people participated in this meeting. The scientific topics covered the field of neuropsychiatry very widely as well as biological psychiatry. Since then, the regional INA meeting, named the European Congress of the INA, has been held every 2 years. Dr. Perminder Sachdev (Sydney) was elected as the third INA president, and the INA office was moved to Sydney.

Dr. M Trimble (UK), the awardee of the Alwyn Lishman Award, presented the lecture "The Evolution of the Limbic System and Epilepsy as a Clinical Model of Dissolution," and Dr. V.S. Ramachandran (US), the awardee of the Ramon y Cajal Award, gave a lecture titled "Art and Brain."

The topics of the lectures in the Fifth Congress were:

Vascular Dementia [M. Gaviria (US)]; Schizophrenia as Disorder of Consciousness [C.R. Hojaij (Australia)]; Ethical Issues in Biological Psychiatry Research [A. Okasha (Egypt)]; Long-Term Outcome of Schizophrenia [H.J. Möller (Germany)]; The Psychopathology of Fatigue [C. Shapiro (Canada)]; The Evolution of the Limbic System and Epilepsy [M. Trimble (UK)]; Art and Brain [V.S. Ramachandran (US)]; Bipolar I and II Disorders [L. Judd (US)]; What Causes the Onset of Psychosis? [R.M. Murray (UK)]; Can Stress Cause Depression? [H.M. van Praag (the Netherlands)]; Catatonia [M. Fink (US)]; Neuropsychiatry of Traumatic Brain Injury [R.G. Robinson (US)]; Brain Mechanisms of Cognitive Processes [A. Georgopoulos (US)]; Towards New International Classification and Diagnostic Systems [J.E. Mezzich (US)]; Biological Correlates of Obsessive Compulsive Disorders [J.J. López-Ibor (Spain)]; Genetics of Mood Disorders [J. Mendlewicz (Belgium)]; Agitated Depression in Bipolar Disorder [M. Maj (Italy)]; Biological Perspectives in Psychiatric Prevention [G. Christodoulou (Greece)]; Neuropsychiatric Aspects of Mental Disorders in Old Age [K. Miyoshi (Japan)]; Impulsivity and Aggression [J.L. Ayuso-Gutiérrez (Spain)]; and Whither Neuropsychiatry? [P.S. Sachdev (Australia)].

The topics of the symposia in the Fifth Congress were:

Cognitive Declines and Behavioral Changes in Neuropsychiatric Disorders, Methodological Approaches in Neuropsychiatric Disorders, Psychopharmacology for Children and Adolescents, Basic and Clinical Aspects on Hippocampus in Depression, Management of Post Stroke Depression, ECT, Emerging Pharmacological and Neuroimaging Strategies in the Evaluation and Treatment of Dementia, Neuroimaging, Clinical and Experimental Europsychopharmacology, Clinical Responses and Ethnopsychopharmacology, Neuropathological Vistas in Neuropsychiatry, New Developments in Event-Related Potential Methodology,

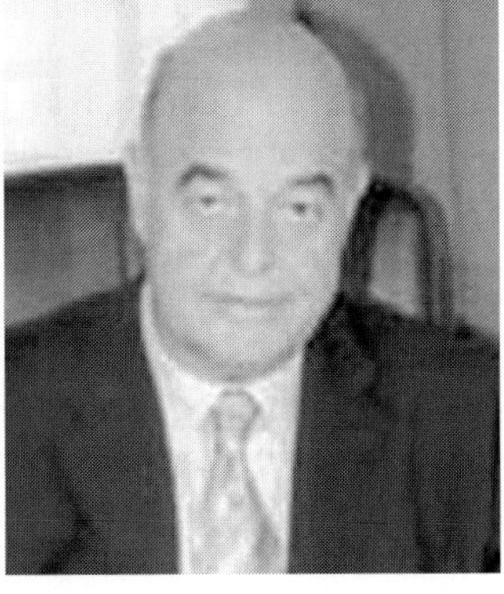

Fig. 3 The INA President Dr. C. Soldatos (2006–2008)

Prise en Charge au long cours dans la schizophrenie (in French), Neuropsychiatry and Beyond, Updates from Clinical Research in Bipolar Disorders, Cognitive Functional and Structural Changes in First-Episode Schizophrenic Children and Adults, The Contribution of New Tools to the Comprehension of Schizophrenia, Nuevos avances en la enfermedad de Alzheimer (in Spanish), Themes and Variations in Neuropsychiatry, The Neuropsychiatry of Epilepsy, Neuroendocrinology of Stress-Related Psychiatric Disorders, Genetics of Cognitive and Eye Tracking Dysfunctions in Major Psychoses, Depression and Aging, Sleep Disorders in Neuropsychiatry and Biological Psychiatry, Neuropsychiatric Disorders in Intellectual and Developmental Disabilities, Alzheimer's Disease and Lewy Body Dementia, Biological Correlates of Learning Disabilities, Research in Neuroscience, Evidence of Schizophrenia as a Systemic Disease, Depression and Late Life Cognitive Disorders, Homocysteine and MTHFR Polymorphism in Psychiatry, Thyroid–Brain Interaction Across the Life Cycle, Continuing Challenges in Bipolar Disorders and Its Treatment, Neurobiology of Eating Disorders, Neuropsychiatric Aspects of Traumatic Brain Injury, Psychopathology in the Era of Neuroscience, Biological Aspects of Suicidal Behaviour, Animal Models of Schizophrenia, Magnetoencephalography in Psychiatry, Cholinesterase Inhibitors in Neuropsychiatry, The Link Between Experimental Studies and Clinical Practice, Neurocognitive Functions in Schizophrenia, Decision-Making Process in Neuropsychiatric Disorders, Utility of Quantitative EEG in Diagnosing and Treating Patients with Psychiatric Disorders, Neuropsychiatric Topics in Mexican Clinical Practice, etc.

The Widening: The Sixth Congress in Sydney

The Sixth Congress was held in Sydney in 2006. Approximately 600 people attended the congress. Neurobiological investigations of the endogenous psychoses as well as the neuropsychiatric disorders were discussed in the congress. In this congress, the realm of the neuropsychiatry was clearly widened by the impressive presentations of the neurobiological bases of endogenous psychoses as well as neuropsychiatric disorders. Dr. Perminder Sachdev, chair of the meeting, publicized the core curriculum for the training of neuropsychiatrists.

In this meeting, Dr. Soldatos was elected the fourth INA president. Professor Alvaro Pascual-Leone had been awarded the Ramon y Cajal award for his outstanding contribution to the understanding of higher cognitive functions and the treatment of neuropsychiatric disorders using transcranial magnetic stimulation. The Lishman Award was awarded to Professor C. Edward Coffey, an accomplished physician and healthcare leader recognized for developing highly successful integrated mental health care systems and for his important contributions to our understanding of brain–behavior relationships. As the Award Lectures, Dr. A. Pascual-Leone presented a lecture entitled "The Right Side in Sigmund Freud," and Dr. C.E. Coffey gave a lecture on "Dramatically Improving the Quality of Care in Neuropsychiatry" (Fig. 3).

Instead of the sessions of the plenary lectures, the symposia and workshops were planned as the main sessions of the congress.

The topics of the symposia in the Sixth Congress were:

Neuropsychiatry as a Discipline for the Future (Presidential Symposium), Transcranial Magnetic Stimulation, Neurophilosophy, Psychiatric Aspects of Epilepsy, Traumatic Brain Injury (TBI), Neurology of Schizophrenia, Newer Antidepressants, Delusional Belief, Developmental Neuropsychiatry, Neuropsychopharmacology, Neuroimaging, Neurobiology of Consciousness, Movement Disorders and Catatonia, Neurobiology of Hallucinations, Neuropsychiatry of Bipolar Disorder, Old Age Psychiatry, Vitamins, Homocysteine and Omega 3 in Neuropsychiatry, Investigative Applications, Genetics of Childhood-Onset Psychiatric Disorders, Brain Stimulation, Neurobiology of Eating Disorders, Neuroimaging, Neurobiology of Melancholia, Unusual and Uncommon Neuropsychiatric Syndromes, New Horizons in Epilepsy and Behaviour, Brain Changes in Early Psychosis, Current Status of Vascular Cognitive Impairment, An Update on ECT, Depression in Old Age, ADHD Across the Lifespan, Catatonia and Cycloid Psychoses, Parkinson's Disease, The Genetics of Neuropsychiatric Disorders, Frontotemporal Dementia, Dementia, Controversies about Mild Cognitive Impairment (MCI), Neuropsychiatry of Sleep, Brain Reserve, and Traumatic Brain Injury.

Principal participants of the meeting in the program of the Sixth Congress were:

R.H. Belmaker (Israel), M. Bennett (Australia), S. Berkovic (Australia), H. Brodaty (Australia), G.A. Broe (Australia), C.E. Coffey (US), D. Copolov (Australia), A. David (UK), M. Gaviria (US), P. Hay (Australia), A. Jablensky (Australia), D. Jeste (US), P. Joyce (New Zealand), E.S. Krishnamoorthy (India), H.S. Mayberg (Canada), R. Meares (Australia), P. Mitchell (Australia), K. Miyoshi (Japan), C. Pantelis (Australia), G. Parker (Australia), A. Pascual-Leone (US), G.C. Román (US), M Ron (US), I. Skoog (Sweden), C. Shapiro (Canada), A. Snyder (US), C.R. Soldatos (Greece), S.E. Starkstein (Australia), M. Trimble (UK), etc.

The Latest: The Seventh Congress in Cancun

The Seventh Congress took place in Hotel Fiesta Americano Condesa, Cancun, Mexico, December 3–5, 2008. As a chairman of the Congress, Professor Ricardo Colin-Piana and his colleagues organized the meeting very nicely. Scientific topics covered the neuropsychiatric field widely. The awardee of Cajal's award, Dr. M Marsel Mesulam, presented a lecture on "Primary Progressive Aphasia." The awardee of Lishman's award, Dr. German E. Berrios, gave a lecture on "Neuropsychiatry–Clinical Epistemology and Hermeneutics".

The topics of the plenary lectures in the Seventh Congress were:

Early Detection of Neurodegenerative and Vascular Dementia [A. Wallin (Sweden)]; Behavioral Disturbances in Dementia [M. Mendez (US)]; Thyroid Axis Functioning and Psychosis [R. Bunevicius (Lithuania)]; Atypical Viral Brain Infections [J. Sotelo (Mexico)]; The Mayan Heritage [J.D. Vos (Mexico)]; Atypical Antipsychotics and

Neuroleptic Malignant Syndrome [J. Trollor (Australia)]; Neuropsychiatry and Humanism [R. Alarcon (US)]; Psychotic Disorders After Temporal Lobectomy [E.S. Krishnamoorthy (India)]; Conversion Disorders [B. Yeong (Singapore)]; Mirrors in the Brain [P. Sachdev (Australia)]; and Dangerous Lives, War and the Emotional Health of Journalists [A. Feinstein (Canada)].

The topics of the symposia in the Seventh Congress were:

Steroid Hormones in Mental Health and Disease, Cognitive Neuroscience, Neuropsychiatry of Frontal Lobes, Neuropsychiatry of Multiple Sclerosis, Neuropsychiatry and Addictions, Neuropsychiatry of Affective Disorders, Traumatic Brain Injury, Brain Stimulation Therapies, Neurointegrative Mechanisms of Psychological Trauma and Chronic Pain, History of Neuropsychiatry, Neurodegeneration, Epidemiology of Vascular and Metabolic Factors in Mental Disorders, and International Health.

Dr. Koho Miyoshi succeeded to the INA presidency, and Dr. I. Skoog (Sweden), Dr. D. Arciniegas (US), Dr. K. Maeda (Japan), and Dr. E. Coffey (US) were elected as the new members of the Executive Committee. Dr. M. Gaviria (Member of the Advisory Council) was re-elected as a member of the Executive Committee.

Regional Activities

The Argentine Neuropsychiatric Association has held the Latin-American Congress of Neuropsychiatry every year since 2003. The Indian Neuropsychiatric Group has held the Indian Symposium of Neuropsychiatry biennially since 2004. The Greek Neuropsychiatric Group hosted the European Congress of the INA every 2 years since 2004. The Japan Neuropsychiatric Association held the Kobe Conference of the INA in Kobe, Japan, September 12–13, 2009.

The Coming INA Meetings

The Eighth International Congress of Neuropsychiatry will be held in Chennai, India, in 2011. Dr. Krishnamoorthy will chair the Congress. The Ninth Congress will be held in Chicago. Dr. Moises Gaviria, one of the founders of the INA, is now organizing the meeting. The Peruvian psychiatrist Dr. Gastelumendi is planning to hold a regional congress of neuropsychiatry in Lima, Peru, June 18–19, 2010. The Third European INA congress will take place in Thessaloniki, Greece, November 18–21, 2010.

Current Status of the INA

Officers and INA Office

Currently, Dr. K. Miyoshi holds the position of INA president. Dr. M. Kopelman will succeed to the presidency in Chennai in the year 2011. Dr. J. Trollor is secretary-general and treasurer until 2013. Ms. Angie Russell is the secretariat in the INA office, located in Sydney. Dr. M. Mula edits the newsletter, and Mr. L. Tortora is the webmaster of INA. The INA Secretariat Office, Neuropsychiatric Institute, The Prince of Wales Hospital, Randwick, NSW 2031, Australia (email: info@inawebsite.org).

Executive Committee

The names of the Members of the Executive Committee are as follows: Ignacio Brusco (Argentina), Robertas Bunevicius (Lithuania), Ricardo Colin-Piana (Mexico), Anthony David (UK), Valsamma Eapen (Australia), Ennapadam S. Krishnamoorthy (India), Robert Belmaker (Israel), Kiyoshi Maeda (Japan), Edward Coffey (US), Moises Gaviria (US), Ingmar Skoog (Sweden), and David Arciniegas (US).

Advisory Council

The past presidents, Colin M. Shapiro (Canada), Moises Gaviria (US), Constantin R. Soldatos (Greece) and Perminder Sachdev (Australia), are the members of the Advisory Council. The core business of this committee is to advise the Executive Committee (EC) on future directions for INA to propose nominations for vacancies of the EC. All members will continue to sit on the Executive.

International Committee

The members of the International Committee are expected to (1) contribute to the life and direction of INA, (2) act as key contacts for local activities of INA, including taking initiative to hold local or regional scientific meetings on behalf of INA, (3) communicate closely and regularly with the INA secretariat, (4) contribute articles regarding neuropsychiatry activities in their country to the newsletter every 2 years, and (5) recruit new INA members in their own countries by sharing e-mail lists of individuals who may have an interest in joining INA.

The members of the International Committee are:

Ahmed Malalia Salah AlAnsari (Bahrain), Celso Arango (Spain), Gilberto Brofman (Brazil), Alexandre Castro Caldas (Portugal), Vytenis Deltuva (Lithuania), Greg Finucane (New Zealand), Simon Fleminger (UK), Eduardo Gastelumendi (Peru), Andres M Kanner (US), Francis Krivoy (Venezuela), Mario Lipez-Gomez (Mexico), Maximiliano Luna (Argentina), Olya Mikova (Bulgaria), Ming-Chyi Pai (Taiwan), Kang Seob Oh (Korea), Ranan Rimon (Finland), Ilya Reznik (Israel), Bernard Saletu (Austria), Surachai Kuasirkul (Thai), Thordur Sigmundsson

(Iceland), Patrick Vuilleumier (Switzerland), Masahito Yamada (Japan), Beng Yeong (Singapore), John Fayyad (Lebanon), Raben Rosenberg (Denmark), Anders Wallin (Sweden), Zoltan Rihmer (Hungary), Xin Yu (China)*, Yongjin Wang (China)* [*rotate-on-duty every 2 years].

Awards

The Lishman Award was established to honor William Alwyn Lishman of London, UK, as the modern pioneer of neuropsychiatry. It is awarded to an individual who has made a notable contribution to clinical neuropsychiatry at an international level. By accepting the award, the recipient presents a lecture at the Biennial Congress.

The Cajal Award was established to honor the "Father of Neuroscience," Santiago Ramon Y Cajal, and is awarded to an individual who has made a distinguished contribution to neuroscience with an application to neuropsychiatry. Similarly to the Lishman award, the recipient presents a lecture at the INA Congress held every 2 years. The inaugural Lishman and Cajal Awards were given at the Congress held in Buenos Aires, Argentina, in 2002.

Journal

The official journal of the INA, *Neuropsychiatric Disease and Treatment*, is an international peer-reviewed journal of clinical therapeutics and pharmacology focusing on concise rapid reporting of clinical or preclinical studies on a range of neuropsychiatric and neurological disorders.

This journal is published by Dove Press, and edited by Dr. Roger Pinder and Dr. David Arciniegas.

Relationships to National Neuropsychiatric Associations

The neuropsychiatric associations in many countries communicate closely with INA. Actually, almost all the presidents of these associations are the members of the executive committee of INA.

The British Neuropsychiatry Association, established in 1987, is the oldest one in the world, and the American Neuropsychiatric Association was established in 1988. There are neuropsychiatric associations in Japan (since 1995) and Argentina (since 2002). The Argentina Neuropsychiatric Association had held the Latin-American Congress of Neuropsychiatry every year since 2003.

In 2006, Slovak neuropsychiatrists established their association. The Indian Neuropsychiatric Group has held the INA Indian Symposium regularly since 2004, and the Greek Neuropsychiatric Group has hosted the European Congress of

Neuropsychiatry biennially since 2006. The Mexican Neuropsychiatric Association held the International Congress of Neuropsychiatry in 2008.

The Chinese Neuropsychiatry Summit (CNS) became active in 2008. Beside these associations, there are many neuropsychiatric groups playing important roles in the INA.

Future Direction

Cerebral disorders almost always cause psychiatric symptoms. Therefore, integration of neurology and psychiatry is necessary for clinical procedures to relieve the distress of patients with brain disorders. In the aged society, the numbers of patients with neuropsychiatric disorders is increasing. There are no doubt that neuropsychiatry will be much more important as society continues to age. In the psychiatric field, neuropsychiatry has been trying to deepen our understanding of psychiatric disorders from the point of view of neurobiology. As you know, recent investigations with current neuroscience have been widening the perspective of neuropsychiatry by revealing the neurobiological bases of so-called functional psychiatric disorders.

The INA welcomes any individuals who are interested in neuropsychiatry and any neuropsychiatric groups to join the INA as regular members and/or affiliated associations.

Core Curriculum in Neuropsychiatry of the International Neuropsychiatric Association*

Perminder Sachdev and The Curriculum Committee of the International Neuropsychiatric Association

Abstract Neuropsychiatry (NP) and behavioral neurology (BN) are rapidly emerging as superspecializations in the fields of psychiatry and neurology, respectively. The International Neuropsychiatric Association (INA) set up a committee to develop a curriculum for reference and guidance in the development of training programs in different countries. The purpose of any training program in NP would be to produce specialists who are competent in the diagnosis and management of common neuropsychiatric disorders, who are able to utilize specialized neuropsychiatric investigations in the evaluation of these disorders, who are able to provide secondary and tertiary level consultations to general physicians, psychiatrists, and neurologists, and who will be involved in teaching and research in relationship to these disorders. It is recognized that this curriculum will need to be adapted to the local needs and available resources in that setting. It is hoped that the curriculum, through the aegis of the INA, will promote NP internationally and help provide the best treatment for patients with neuropsychiatric disorders.

Keywords Behavioral neurology • Curriculum • Neuropsychiatry • Specialization • Training

---

*The Curriculum Committee of the INA was composed of P. Sachdev (chair), M. Gaviria, C. Soldatos, C. Shapiro, J. Trollor, and E.S. Krishnamoorthy.

P. Sachdev (✉)
School of Psychiatry, University of New South Wales,
Sydney, NSW 2052, Australia
and
Neuropsychiatric Institute, Euroa Centre, Prince of Wales Hospital,
Barker Street, Randwick, NSW 2031, Australia
e-mail: p.sachdev@unsw.edu.au

K. Miyoshi et al. (eds.), *Neuropsychiatric Disorders*,
DOI 10.1007/978-4-431-53871-4_25, © Springer 2010

Background

Neuropsychiatry (NP) is an old discipline with its origins in the mid-nineteenth century, or perhaps even earlier to the seventeenth century, much before the birth of modern psychiatry. For many decades, however, neurology and psychiatry developed as separate disciplines, leading to a dearth of dialogue between the disciplines. NP has remerged in the last two decades as a subdiscipline that bridges the two established disciplines of neurology and psychiatry. In its broader role, NP applies the principles of neuroscience to the understanding and treatment of emotional, behavioral, and cognitive disorders. In its narrower and more practical approach, NP is that branch of psychiatry that is concerned with the diagnosis and management of the psychiatric and behavioral consequences of demonstrable brain disturbance. As such, the practice of NP requires skills and knowledge that in part traverse the traditional psychiatry/neurology boundary.

The discipline of NP must be considered in relation to behavioral neurology (BN). In many respects, NP and BN are two slightly different approaches to the same set of disorders and conditions, with the former being biased toward traditional psychiatry and the latter having its route through neurology. The core competencies are similar, with perhaps differences in vemphasis. As this curriculum is being developed under the aegis of the International Neuropsychiatric Association (INA), the term NP is used. An effort is made to identify specific areas that are particularly important to BN so that the curriculum can be readily adapted to it.

Currently there are few training programs worldwide that are exclusive to NP and lead to a specific NP specialist accreditation. In most countries, trainees who gain experience in NP do so within general adult psychiatry, old age psychiatry, child psychiatry, or forensic psychiatry; this is true even for countries in which a number of NP specialist positions exist. Some countries have a dual training in neurology and psychiatry, with a certification in both disciplines. Although this approach meets some of the requirements of training in NP, it is the position of the INA that training in NP specifically, following basic training in psychiatry and neurology, is necessary to meet the requirements of specialist NP training.

Goals of the Training Program

The purpose of a training program in NP is to produce specialists who will be competent in the diagnosis and management of common neuropsychiatric disorders, able to utilize specialized neuropsychiatric investigations in the evaluation of these disorders, able to provide secondary and tertiary level consultations to general physicians, psychiatrists and neurologists, and be involved in teaching and research in relationship to these disorders. Although the range of disorders included in NP is difficult to delineate, an attempt is made in the core competencies section of this chapter to define this territory, with the acknowledgment that this is an evolving process depending upon the knowledge base of the day.

The following are the goals of the training program:

1. To develop a sound knowledge base of the neuroscientific principles underlying neuropsychiatric practice, in relationship to neuroanatomy, neurophysiology, neurochemistry, and neuropharmacology.
2. To gain first-hand experience of common neuropsychiatric disorders and become competent in their diagnosis and management.
3. To develop an expertise in the use and interpretation of specialized neuropsychiatric investigations, in particular, neurophysiology (e.g. electroencephalography), neuroimaging, and neuropsychology.
4. To be competent in the recognition and management of common psychiatric and neurological disorders.
5. To develop specialized skills in the physical treatments in NP, but without ignoring the principles of psychotherapeutic and rehabilitative approaches.
6. To develop skills in the critical evaluation of research evidence in the pathophysiology, phenomenology, and treatment of neuropsychiatric disorders.
7. To conduct research to improve the empirical basis of neuropsychiatric knowledge and practice.
8. To act as advocates for sufferers of neuropsychiatric illnesses, and to contribute to the development of the profession.

Structure of the NP Training Program

There is no one model that will suit all training programs in NP. An attempt is made here to outline the basic tenets of such a program.

1. An NP training program shall endeavor to create specialists in NP who function as secondary and tertiary level specialists. They shall provide consultations to general psychiatrists, neurologists, and general physicians on a range of neuropsychiatric disorders.
2. An NP training program will generally comprise a 2-year fellowship program that focuses on the core competencies detailed below. In some situations, only a 1-year fellowship in NP may be practicable. Full competency should not be assumed after 1 year of training. However, if the trainee works for a further 2 years in a largely or exclusively neuropsychiatric service (but not specifically as a trainee), it would be considered likely that the training requirements would have been met in this period.
3. The NP Fellow will have previously received training in psychiatry and/or neurology. In general, this would have been a 3-year training program in a center that offers training in both specialties. It is expected that the psychiatry trainee would have received at least 6 months training in neurology, but the neurology trainee would have at least 1 year of training in psychiatry. If this is not the case, the Fellowship period would be used to remedy this with a clinical rotation in the appropriate discipline.

4. The NP training will be in a neuropsychiatric center with two or more neuropsychiatrists, one or more clinical neuropsychologists, a neurologist (part-time or full-time), and a working relationship with psychiatric, clinical neurology, and neurosurgical services. The center would be part of a general teaching hospital and have easy access to a neurophysiology service and up-to-date neuroimaging, which would include structural magnetic resonance imaging (MRI) and functional imaging. It would also have a research program.
5. The training program will include a research project, which would preferably be based on empirical research.
6. The training program will have an evaluation component, based on a formal assessment and/or a series of informal assessments by the supervisors.
7. The program will prepare the trainee for a lifelong period of education and professional enhancement.
8. The program will instil by example the highest ethical standards of conduct in clinical practice and scholarly work.

Objectives

Attitude Objectives

NP trainees should develop a positive attitude toward neuropsychiatric patients and their carers. NP trainees will demonstrate this attitude by:

1. Being prepared to advocate for the needs of neuropsychiatric patients and their carers.
2. Recognizing and dealing constructively with biased attitudes toward sufferers of neuropsychiatric illness.
3. Developing an awareness of the impact of illness on carers and the wider community, and striving to balance the needs of neuropsychiatric patients with those of carers and the wider community.

Knowledge Objectives

By the completion of training, NP trainees should be knowledgeable about the following:

1. Normal biological, psychological, and social development of the brain and mind:
   (a) Brain structure at the macroscopic and microscopic levels, in particular the knowledge of neuronal networks, the limbic system, the neuroanatomical substrates of memory, and the frontal executive system;
   (b) Central nervous system (CNS) structure–function correlations;
   (c) Neurochemistry, especially neurotransmitter and receptor function;

(d) A basic grasp of issues related to the mind–brain debate, the biology of consciousness, and other neurophilosophical issues.

2. Basic neuroscience:

(a) The molecular biology of psychiatric disorders;
(b) The biochemical basis of neuropsychopharmacology;
(c) The basic principles of neurophysiology, and their application to diagnosis and treatment of neuropsychiatric disorders;
(d) The basic principles of genetics and immunology as they apply to the CNS;
(e) The basic principles of neuroimaging and their application to diagnosis and assessment of neuropsychiatric disorders.

3. Neuropsychiatric disorders

By the completion of training, NP trainees should be knowledgeable about the epidemiology, etiology, psychopathology, clinical features (including complications), and natural history of neuropsychiatric disorders, including concepts of impairment, disability, and handicap. A sound knowledge of the assessment and care of these conditions is also expected.

(a) The incidence and prevalence of neuropsychiatric illnesses in various populations;
(b) The phenomenology of organic brain syndromes, including nonspecific and atypical presentations of illness such as "pseudodementia," "masked" depression, "conversion" disorders, and behavioral disorders;
(c) The criteria on which neuropsychiatric diagnoses are based, within the framework of one of the widely accepted classification systems;
(d) Possible causative or exacerbating factors in neuropsychiatric disorders;
(e) The natural history of the disease process in neuropsychiatric disorders, which enables identification of (1) the severity of the disease; (2) the urgency of the need for treatment; (3) the stage of the illness; and (4) the prognosis;
(f) The assessment of common neuropsychiatric disorders, including the following:

(i) Cognitive disorders
(ii) Dementias and predementia syndromes
(iii) Nondementing cognitive disorders
(iv) Seizure disorders
(v) Movement disorders
(vi) Traumatic brain injury
(vii) Secondary psychiatric disorders, that is, psychosis, depression, mania, and anxiety disorders secondary to "organic" brain disease
(viii) Substance-induced psychiatric disorders: alcohol, drugs of abuse, etc.
(ix) Attentional disorders [adult attention deficit hyperactivity disorder (ADHD) and related syndromes]
(x) General hospital liaison neuropsychiatry

(xi) Developmental disorders
(xii) Sleep disorders

(g) Appropriate management plans for neuropsychiatric disorders including:

(i) Interpretation of medical, psychological, and neurodiagnostic investigations and assessments
(ii) The use of psychopharmacology, electroconvulsive therapy (ECT), and other physical treatments including the frequency and management of side effects
(iii) Application of psychotherapies, including supportive, cognitive-behavioral, group, and family therapies
(iv) The use of behavior modification, environmental adaptation, and preventive measures
(v) Situations in which referral to, or consultation with, colleagues in psychiatry and other disciplines is appropriate
(vi) Programs involving changes in lifestyle
(vii) Rehabilitation programs
(viii) Management in forensic settings
(ix) Strategies that meet the needs of carers including the role of self-help groups, including Alzheimer's Association, Tourette Syndrome Association, etc.

(h) The influence of specific factors on assessment and care of neuropsychiatric disorders, including:

(i) Age
(ii) Intellectual capacity including intellectual disability
(iii) Medical illness and disability
(iv) Sex
(v) Culture
(vi) Spiritual beliefs
(vii) Socioeconomic status
(viii) Psychiatric comorbidity
(ix) Polypharmacy
(x) Support factors

(i) The influence of factors that affect treatment outcome including other medical illnesses;
(j) The principles underlying the choice and integration of interventions in neuropsychiatry, including the evidence base and relative cost-effectiveness;
(k) The principles of medicolegal aspects to the practice of NP, with particular emphasis on mental health and guardianship legislation, including its local application, testamentary capacity, enduring power of attorney, informed consent, assessment of older offenders, and fitness to plead;
(l) The community care system including the relevant welfare legislation that affects the management of people with neuropsychiatric disorders, especially dementia;

(m) Issues of aging and mental health in older people with intellectual and other disabilities;
(n) Prevention and health promotion in NP;
(o) Issues specific to mental health promotion in relationship to neuropsychiatry;
(p) Risk factors for neuropsychiatric disorders that become apparent earlier in life.

4. Medicine in relationship to NP

   By the completion of training, NP trainees should be knowledgeable about medical and surgical conditions in general. Higher levels of knowledge are expected in those areas of medicine that particularly relate to psychiatric practice, such as neurology, rehabilitation medicine, etc.

5. Research method

   By the completion of training, NP trainees should be knowledgeable about the principles of scientific method in their practice and the use of this knowledge to evaluate developments in neuropsychiatric research.

6. Service issues

   By the completion of training, NP trainees should be knowledgeable about the organization and delivery of mental health care to neuropsychiatric patients, including the ethical, economic, geographic, and political constraints within which it operates.

7. Professional responsibility

   By the completion of training, NP trainees should be knowledgeable about the principles of medical ethics, the development of professional attitudes, and mechanisms for the development and maintenance of clinical competence, acknowledging the need for professional and public accountability.

Skills Objectives

1. Health promotion

   - By the completion of training, the NP trainee should be able to apply specific knowledge of the principles and processes of health promotion and illness prevention:

     – Recognize and address risk factors for common neuropsychiatric problems in the community, in hospitals, and in long-term care, such as falls, confusion, and depression;
     – Recognize and address the needs of carers of neuropsychiatric patients.

2. Assessment of neuropsychiatric patients

   - By the completion of training, trainees should possess the skills necessary for performing a comprehensive neuropsychiatric examination:

– Demonstrate interviewing skills adapted to the needs of neuropsychiatric patients;
– With tact and respect, appropriately use and interpret cognitive tests and document these accurately;
– Appropriately refer people for neuropsychological assessment and effectively utilize the results;
– Conduct assessments in a range of hospital and community settings, including assessment of the environment;
– Perform a functional assessment including activities of daily living and apply it to the determination of the most appropriate form of living arrangements for the individual;
– Recognize and assess relevant features of the family context including the family's role as carers, carer stress, and elder abuse;
– Perform medicolegal assessments with particular emphasis on testamentary capacity, guardianship, enduring power of attorney, competency, and informed consent.

A Survey of Required Competencies in Neuropsychiatry

The curriculum below identifies some core competencies in the skill base and specific modules of the specialist knowledge base; these shall be acquired over 2 years. The competencies are described as modules, but they are not necessarily independent of each other. The importance of the core skills module is highlighted. The aims and objectives of this module will normally be covered within the specific clinical modules undertaken but should represent an additional and specific focus of study within the individual clinical modules. The level of expertise in each of the specific modules will vary, depending upon the facilities available, but a basic level of competence in each module is expected in a 2-year training program.

1. Core skills module
    1.1. Knowledge base in clinical neuroscience
    1.2. Clinical skills in neuropsychiatry
        1.2.1. Neuropsychiatric diagnosis including history and examination, neurophysiological investigations, neuroimaging, neuropsychology, and other investigations;
        1.2.2. Treatment, including pharmacology and other physical treatments [ECT, transcranial magnetic stimulation (TMS), surgical interventions], without neglecting psychotherapeutic and rehabilitative interventions.
    1.3. Critical thinking in neuropsychiatry: research and scholarship
2. Specific modules
    2.1. Cognitive disorders

2.1.1. Dementias and predementia syndromes
2.1.2. Nondementing cognitive disorders

2.2. Seizure disorders
2.3. Movement disorders
2.4. Traumatic brain injury
2.5. Secondary psychiatric disorders, that is, psychosis, depression, mania, and anxiety disorders secondary to "organic" brain disease
2.6. Substance-induced psychiatric disorders: alcohol, drugs of abuse, etc.
2.7. Attentional disorders (adult ADHD and related syndromes)
2.8. General hospital liaison neuropsychiatry
2.9. Developmental neuropsychiatry
2.10. Sleep disorders
2.11. Neuropsychiatric rehabilitation
2.12. Forensic neuropsychiatry

Core Skills Module

Specific Competencies

Knowledge Base in Neuroscience

- Knowledge of brain structure at the macroscopic and microscopic levels, in particular the knowledge of neuronal networks, the limbic system, the neuroanatomical substrates of memory, and the frontal executive system.
- A knowledge of CNS structure–function correlations.
- Knowledge of neurochemistry, especially neurotransmitter and receptor function.
- The biochemical basis of neuropsychopharmacology.
- The basic principles of neurophysiology.
- The basic principles of genetics and immunology as they apply to the CNS.
- A basic grasp of issues related to the mind–brain debate, the biology of consciousness, and other neurophilosophical issues.

Clinical Skills in Neuropsychiatry

1. Undertake clinical assessment of patients with apparent or possible neuropsychiatric problems.

   (a) Take a neuropsychiatric history; this includes all the information routinely gathered as part of a psychiatric and medical history, but with special emphasis on gathering information about:

      - Possible illnesses or injury to the central nervous system.
      - Sudden or gradual changes in intellectual functioning, level of consciousness, personality, and judgment, as well as changes in motor and sensory functions, which might indicate neurological disease.

(b) Perform a neuropsychiatric assessment; this will again involve and encompass all the routine skills required to carry out a psychiatric examination, but in addition will include:

- Demonstration of the ability to elicit information relevant to possible neuropsychiatric disorders and neurological conditions, for example, the ability to list the history of stepwise cognitive decline or psychomotor seizure activity.

(c) Perform a cognitive examination (simple and extended):

- A core skill in NP is the ability to carry out simple tests "at the bedside" to determine a patient's level of orientation, attention, concentration, memory, etc., and to do so in the context of a psychiatric examination.
- A neuropsychiatrist, and in particular one from a neurological background, would be competent in assessing deficits in language, praxis, gnosis, visuo-spatial function, and other cognitive syndromes.
- This competency would not require the ability to administer formal neuropsychological tests, but may involve carrying out paper-and-pencil tests and the use of simple materials such as word lists or pictures.
- A neuropsychiatrist should have competency in interpreting results of such an examination to determine whether the patient is suffering from a dementing illness, a confusional state, or a specific cognitive deficit as well as competency in diagnosing the range of adult psychiatric conditions. Part of the skill would involve placing the results of the examination in the context of the patient's educational and social background and premorbid level of functioning.

(d) Perform a neurological examination:

- The trainee should be able to carry out a full and detailed neurological examination, if necessary, with particular emphasis on the central nervous system and higher cortical functioning.
- The trainee should be able to demonstrate the ability to interpret any abnormal signs elicited and place them in the context of the patient's presentation and a differential diagnosis; this may include eliciting signs, which requires further specialist investigation, either within the realm of NP or neurology or electrophysiology.

(e) Construct a neuropsychiatric differential diagnosis:

- The trainee neuropsychiatrist should be able to demonstrate familiarity with multi-axial forms of classification.
- The trainee should be able to arrange multiple diagnoses into a rational hierarchy and be able to summarize the key elements of the history and examination which support that differential diagnosis.
- The trainee should be able to evaluate the extent to which patterns of psychiatric symptomatology and presentation may be the result of underlying organic brain disease.

- The trainee should be familiar with the range of organic disorders that may account for particular presentations.
- The trainee should be able to communicate this in a clear and concise way to other health professionals as well as to patients and their carers.

2. Undertake and plan investigation of a patient with apparent or possible neuropsychiatric problems:

   (a) Trainees should be familiar with the relevant hematological, metabolic, bacteriological, virological, immunological, and toxicological investigations of relevance to NP. This requirement includes:

   - Demonstrating knowledge and judgment that the relevant parameter is of central importance to the neuropsychiatric presentation.
   - Knowing which investigations need to be pursued with further tests and knowing which may be incidental or within normal limits.
   - Interpretation of examination of cerebrospinal fluid, nerve, muscle, and brain biopsy will also be required, although detailed knowledge is not necessary.

   (b) In contrast to many other specialities within psychiatry, NP requires familiarity with EEG and other neurophysiological investigations and their interpretation:

   - The trainee should be able to discuss the advantages and limitations of the routine EEG, sleep EEG, and longer-term EEG telemetry in patients with possible neuropsychiatric problems.
   - Although the trainee is not expected to be competent in reading EEGs independently, she or he should have a working knowledge of the profiles of normal and abnormal EEGs.
   - In addition, the trainee should understand the use and application of sensory evoked potentials and nerve conduction studies and EMG as they occur in neurological disorders with neuropsychiatric complications, and also as a tool to exclude neurological causes of abnormal function that may in fact have a psychological basis.
   - The trainee should be familiar with the settings in which these investigations are carried out, should be able to query the interpretation with a consultant or experienced technician in the area, and to convey this information to members of the multidiscipline team, carers, and patients alike.

   (c) NP requires sound understanding of the indications for, and interpretations of, the various forms of brain imaging, both structural and functional, including magnetic resonance imaging (MRI), computed tomography (CT), single-photon emission computed tomography (SPECT), and positron emission tomography (PET):

   - The trainee should have sufficient familiarity with these techniques to be able to describe them to a patient and their family/carer and to be able to interpret the results.
   - The trainee should know when such investigations are likely to alter management or treatment decisions and should have some understanding of their theoretical importance.

- The trainee should have sufficient first-hand knowledge of CT and MRI brain scans to be able to detect salient abnormalities and critically assess an expert report.

3. Prescribe and oversee treatment of patients with neuropsychiatric disorders such as those with psychiatric and behavioral symptoms and coexisting neurological disorder. Be familiar with social, psychological, and biological interventions for neuropsychiatric disorders:

   (a) The trainee should have sufficient skill to explain the mode of action, benefits, and side effects of these treatments to fellow health professionals, patients, and their families;
      - Be familiar with the principles of treatment of major neurological disorders and be familiar with neuropsychiatric complications of such treatment.
      - The neuropsychiatrist should also be aware of the neurological manifestations and complications of psychiatric treatment and advise patients and professionals on evaluating the importance of these and in minimizing their occurrence and severity.

   (b) Be familiar with potential drug interactions between psychiatric and neurological medications and other treatments;

      - This requirement will include the awareness of the risks associated with prescribing psychotropic drugs to patients with neurological and neurosurgical diseases.

   (c) Be familiar with nonpharmacological treatments in neurological and neuropsychiatric disorders;

      - The trainee will have competence in the assessment for and the administration of ECT in its current form.
      - The trainee should have some understanding of the newer physical treatments such as transcranial magnetic stimulation (TMS), vagus nerve stimulation (VNS), deep brain stimulation (DBS), and other physical treatments.
      - The trainee should also acquire knowledge of the principles of neurorehabilitation and familiarity with the concepts of disability and handicap.

4. To diagnose and treat patients with medically unexplained symptoms that present as neurological and neuropsychiatric problems; this includes working with colleagues in other disciplines to determine which further tests and investigations are necessary or not as the case may be;

   (a) NP should involve competence in understanding the possible social, cultural, and family influences on unexplained neurological symptoms.
   (b) The trainee should be able to develop a grasp of the principles behind cognitive-behavioral treatments for such patients and be able to plan and oversee such treatments carried out by another professional such as a trained nurse or clinical psychologist.

(c) The trainee should be aware of the relationship between NP and allied psychiatric subspecialties such as old age, child and learning disability psychiatry, and which service patients might most appropriately be served by.

Critical Thinking in Neuropsychiatry: Research and Scholarship

A specialist training in NP will equip the trainee to think critically in the field. The trainee should be able to critically assess the empirical evidence in support of any clinical practice, including the ability to criticize published material. This skill can be developed by means of journal clubs, attendance at research meetings, research presentations, short-term courses, etc.

It is expected that in the second year of training, the trainee will undertake a research project. This work should ideally involve all the steps in an empirical project (background review, design of study, applying for ethics clearance, data gathering, analysis, and report preparation). However, it may take the form of a critical review of a current topic, or a case series. The trainee will produce a report of a publishable standard, as judged by the supervisors, and will be encouraged to publish in a peer-reviewed journal. The research report will be a mandatory component of the second year of training.

Specific Modules

Module 2.1: Cognitive Disorders

Specific Competencies

I. Dementias and predementia syndromes
   Be familiar with the diagnosis and investigation of dementias resulting from:

   1. Alzheimer's disease (AD)
   2. Vascular cognitive impairment (VCI)
   3. Dementia with Lewy bodies (DLB)
   4. Frontotemporal dementia (FTD), including semantic dementia, progressive aphasia, etc.
   5. Dementias related to Parkinsonism + syndromes (progressive supranuclear palsy, corticobasal degeneration, multiple system atrophy)
   6. Prion diseases, especially Creutzfeldt–Jakob disease and variant CJD
   7. Huntington's disease
   8. Dementia resulting from head injury, alcohol use, and medical conditions including human immunodeficiency virus (HIV), brain tumors, encephalitis, etc.

II. Other cognitive disorders
   1. Be familiar with the diagnosis and investigation of *specific memory disorders* (amnesic syndromes), in particular:

- Alcoholic Korsakoff's syndrome
- Other causes of thiamine deficiency
- Brain infection such as herpes encephalitis or other encephalopathies
- Brain dysfunction resulting from cerebral hypoxia, for example, carbon monoxide poisoning
- Vascular disorders, such as thalamic infarction or subarachnoid hemorrhage

2. Be familiar with the diagnosis and investigation of frontal/executive syndromes of disinhibitory and nonspontaneous types
3. Be familiar with the diagnosis and investigation of *other, more "posterior" cognitive disorders*:

   - Including language disorders (anomias, and disorders of comprehension or expression), reading disorders (surface and deep dyslexia), mental calculation (whether or not part of Gerstmann's syndrome), disorders of visuo-spatial awareness, perception, construction, and the agnosias.

III. Be familiar with the diagnosis and investigation of psychologically based cognitive impairments

- Hysterical conditions, including psychogenic amnesias
- Pseudo-dementias, as in depression
- Cognitive impairment as part of somatization, factitious or malingering syndromes

IV. Be familiar with the status and controversies regarding *mild cognitive impairment.*

Diagnostic Techniques

1. Understand clinical assessment including neurological and clinical cognitive examination.
2. Be familiar with the role, importance, and principles of neuropsychological testing.
3. Be familiar with the interpretation of occupational therapy and with speech and language therapy assessments and reports.
4. Be familiar with the relevant investigations in a clinical blood screen.
5. Be aware of when an EEG can be helpful or even crucial.
6. Be familiar with the purpose and interpretation of CT and MRI brain scans.
7. Be aware of the putative role of other forms of neuroimaging including SPECT, PET, diffusion tensor imaging (DTI), and functional MRI (fMRI).

Be familiar with the main principles involved in the management and treatment of cognitive disorders and of dementias

1. The work of a multidisciplinary team (MDT).
2. The contribution of cognitive behavior therapy and psychological counseling in specific conditions.

3. The use of cognitive-enhancing drugs including cholinesterase inhibitors and memantine.
4. The use of other medications in NP, including anticonvulsants and antidepressants.
5. The management of behavioral disturbances in dementia.
6. The use of outreach and community support services.

How Taught

1. Observation and modeling
2. Working as a team member
3. Supervised clinical practice
4. Review of suitable texts and papers in scientific publications, including review articles

How Assessed

1. Clinical supervision
2. Direct observation
3. Clinical logbook
4. Clinical audit
5. Case presentations, etc.

Module 2.2: Seizure Disorders

Specific Competencies

1. Undertake a clinical assessment of patients with suspected epilepsy:
    (a) Take a seizure history;
    (b) Take a neuropsychiatric history focusing on eliciting impact of seizure disorder on the patient;
    (c) Take a history from an informant;
    (d) Perform a neurological examination on patients with suspected epilepsy;
    (e) Construct a formulation with differential diagnoses for the seizure type and syndrome, along with discussion of etiology.
2. Assess patients suspected of having nonepileptic seizures (NEAD):
    (a) Be familiar with the main features differentiating epilepsy and NEAD;
    (b) Be familiar with the coexistence of epilepsy and NEAD;
    (c) Be familiar with the management of NEAD.
3. Undertake investigation of patients with suspected epilepsy:
    (a) Be familiar with EEG recording and interpretation (including the limitations) in people with epilepsy;

(b) Be familiar with the indications for and interpretation of structural and functional neuroimaging in people with epilepsy.

4. Prescribe treatment to patients with coexisting neurological disorder:

(a) Be familiar with social and psychological interventions for the treatment of epilepsy including relaxation techniques and other behavioral methods of controlling/inhibiting seizures;
(b) Be familiar with the principles of the medical treatment of the different seizure and syndrome types;
(c) Be familiar with potential drug interactions between psychiatric medications and anticonvulsants;
(d) Be aware of the risks associated with prescribing psychotropic agents to patients with epilepsy;
(e) Be familiar with the surgical treatment of epilepsy including vagal nerve stimulation.

5. Assess and manage special patient groups with epilepsy:

(a) Be familiar with the difficulties in assessing and managing seizure disorders in children and adolescents with epilepsy, including issues around puberty;
(b) Be familiar with the difficulties in assessing and managing seizure disorders in women with epilepsy, including catamenial epilepsy, contraception, pregnancy, teratogenicity, polycystic ovarian syndrome, and menopause;
(c) Be familiar with the difficulties in assessing and managing seizure disorders in older age patients, including cognition and issues regarding concomitant physical illnesses and medication;
(d) Be familiar with the difficulties in assessing and managing seizure disorders in patients with learning disability including etiology, difficulty eliciting a history, and cognitive and treatment issues.

6. Assess and manage psychiatric comorbidity in people with epilepsy: pre-ictal, ctal, post-ictal, inter-ictal, and iatrogenic:

(a) Be familiar with the diagnosis and management of depression in people with epilepsy, including the risk of suicide;
(b) Be familiar with the diagnosis and management of anxiety/panic attacks in people with epilepsy, including the difficulties in differentiating between panic attacks and ictal panic;
(c) Be familiar with the diagnosis and management of psychosis (post-ictal psychosis, chronic inter-ictal psychosis, and forced normalization) in people with epilepsy;
(d) Be familiar with the diagnosis and management of cognitive dysfunction in people with epilepsy, resulting from seizures and anticonvulsant medication, including the role of neuropsychological assessments;
(e) Be familiar with the diagnosis and management of sexual dysfunction in people with epilepsy;

(f) Be familiar with the diagnosis and management of disorders of impulse control (anger/irritability, drug/alcohol problems) in people with epilepsy;
(g) Be familiar with quality of life issues in people with epilepsy, such as stigma, locus of control, and employment/relationship difficulties.

7. Be aware of the issues involved in the medicolegal aspects of epilepsy:

(a) Be aware of the driving license implications of having epilepsy;
(b) Be familiar with the concept of automatisms when used as a defense in court.

8. Liaison with Epilepsy Surgery Program:

In centers affiliated with Epilepsy Surgery programs, the trainee should become familiar with the psychiatric issues involved in the assessment of candidates for epilepsy surgery and be able to provide preoperative consultations and postoperative follow-up to such patients.

Module 2.3: Movement Disorders

Specific Competencies

1. Clinical assessment

(a) Take a history of movement disorder
(b) Assess psychiatric history
(c) Assess neurological history
(d) Perform psychiatric examination
(e) Perform neurological examination
(f) Construct differential diagnosis of movement disorder

2. Investigation

(a) Review previous neurological examinations
(b) Review previous neurological treatment
(c) Review previous psychiatric treatment
(d) Order further relevant investigations

3. Treatment

(a) Review previous psychiatric treatment
(b) Review previous neurological treatment
(c) Recommend alterations to current treatment
(d) Prescribe new appropriate treatment
(e) Review effects of treatment

Suggested Learning Methods

1. Attend movement disorders clinic
2. Discuss neurological treatment of movement disorders with neurologist

Suggested Assessment Method: Clinic Logbook

1. Parkinson's disease
2. Tourette's syndrome: tics
3. Tremor
4. Dystonia
5. Catatonia
6. Neuroleptic-induced movement disorders: tardive dyskinesia, tardive dystonia, akathisia, NMS, drug-induced parkinsonism, etc.
7. Hysterical conversion/somatization disorders

Module 2.4: Traumatic Brain Injury

Clinical Settings

1. Emergency services, with patient presenting with psychiatric disturbance following head injury
2. Medical or surgical ward, involving patients with neuropsychiatric disturbance following head injury
3. Outpatient clinics
4. Neurorehabilitation settings
5. Medicolegal settings

Specific Competencies

1. To take a competent trauma history, including the assessment of posttraumatic amnesia (PTA), administration of Glasgow Coma Score (GCS), etc.
2. To assess psychiatric morbidity related to head injury.
3. To assess the relative contributions of brain injury, posttraumatic epilepsy, physical disability, personality, and psychosocial and medicolegal factors contributing to neuropsychiatric presentations.
4. To be able to assess cognitive disturbances following head injury, including the interpretation of neuropsychological assessments.
5. To be able to manage neuropsychiatric disturbances in head-injured patients using drug treatment, cognitive, and behavioral interventions.

Suggested Learning Methods

1. Participate in emergency, medical, and surgical consultations with supervisor.
2. Assess patients in outpatient clinics and follow up these patients.
3. Attend rehabilitation rounds and participate in consultations.

Module 2.5: Secondary Psychiatric Syndromes and Delirium

Clinical Settings

1. Psychiatric wards
2. Neuropsychiatric outpatient clinics
3. Medical and surgical wards

Specific Competencies

1. Familiarity with common presentations of delirium and secondary psychiatric syndromes, including secondary delusional disorder, secondary hallucinosis, secondary depression or mania, secondary anxiety disorder, secondary obsessive-compulsive disorder (OCD), and organic personality disorders.
2. Knowledge of the common causes of these syndromes.
3. Competency in the investigation of the etiology of secondary syndromes, and the interpretation of the results of the investigations.
4. Experience in the treatment of such syndromes, including the use of psychotropic and neurotherapeutic drugs.
5. Knowledge of the pathophysiological mechanisms underlying the development of secondary syndromes.

Suggested Learning Methods

1. Review of published material
2. Neuropsychiatric clinic attendance
3. Consultations on psychiatric, medical, and surgical wards
4. Case discussions

Module 2.6: Substance-Induced Neuropsychiatric Syndromes

Clinical Settings

1. Drug dependence clinic
2. Psychiatric wards
3. Neuropsychiatric outpatient clinics
4. Medical and surgical wards

Specific Competencies

1. Familiarity with common presentations of alcohol- and substance-related neuropsychiatric syndromes.

2. Competency in the investigation of these syndromes, including biological and psychosocial investigations.
3. Experience in the treatment of such syndromes, including the use of psychotropic drugs and psychosocial and rehabilitative interventions.
4. Knowledge of the pathophysiological mechanisms underlying the development of these syndromes.

Suggested Learning Methods

1. Review of published material
2. Clinic attendance
3. Consultations on psychiatric, medical, and surgical wards
4. Case discussions

Module 2.7: Attentional and Dysexecutive Syndromes (Including Adult ADHD)

Clinical Settings

1. Specialized adult ADHD clinic
2. Psychiatric wards
3. Neuropsychiatric outpatient clinics

Specific Competencies

1. Familiarity with common presentations of ADHD in adults.
2. Competency in the investigation of attentional and frontal dysexecutive syndromes, including biological and psychosocial investigations.
3. Experience in the treatment of such syndromes, including the use of psychotropic drugs and psychosocial and rehabilitative interventions.
4. Knowledge of the pathophysiological mechanisms underlying the development of these syndromes.

Suggested Learning Methods

1. Review of published material
2. Clinic attendance
3. Consultations on psychiatric, medical, and surgical wards
4. Case discussions

Module 2.8: General Hospital Liaison Neuropsychiatry

Key Competencies

Undertake assessment of patients with unexplained neurological symptoms:

1. Take an appropriate neuropsychiatric history.
2. Interpret previously performed investigations.
3. Perform examination of mental and physical status.
4. Assess the patients' function in the context of their disability.
5. Understand the concepts of conversion, somatization, and dissociation in a neurological context.
6. Formulate appropriate management plans.
7. Communicate information to the neurological team.

Learning and Assessment Methods

1. Take an appropriate neuropsychiatric history

   (a) Interpret previously performed investigations

Suggested learning methods	Suggested assessment methods
Observation/modeling	Validated self-assessment
Supervised clinical practice	Clinical supervision
Specific teaching from relevant health professionals (e.g., radiologist)	Case presentation

   Perform examination of physical and mental status (see other sections)

   (b) Assess patients' function in the context of their disability

Suggested learning methods	Suggested assessment methods
Observation/modeling	Validated self-assessment
Supervised clinical practice	Clinical supervision
Specific teaching from relevant health professionals (e.g., occupational therapist)	Clinical logbook
	Case presentation

   (c) Understand the concepts of conversion, somatization, and dissociation

Suggested learning methods	Suggested assessment methods
Supervised clinical practice	Clinical supervision
Reading relevant texts	Clinical logbook
Peer group discussion	Case presentation

   (d) Formulate appropriate management plans (see other sections)

(e) Communicate information to neurology team

Suggested learning methods	Suggested assessment methods
Obervation/modeling Supervised clinical practice	Clinical supervision Direct observation

2. Undertake assessment of patients with delirium

(a) Take a relevant clinical history from patient and informants
(b) Gather information from clinical staff

Suggested learning methods	Suggested assessment methods
Observation/modeling Supervised clinical practice Working as a team member	Clinical supervision Direct observation

Perform examination of physical and mental status

(c) Construct an appropriate differential diagnosis (delirium vs. depression vs. dementia)

Suggested learning methods	Suggested assessment methods
Supervised clinical practice Appropriate reading	Clinical supervision Case presentation Clinical logbook Validated self-assessment

(d) Perform investigation to ascertain etiology

Suggested learning methods	Suggested assessment methods
Supervised clinical practice Appropriate reading Specific teaching from other health professionals	Clinical supervision Case presentation Clinical logbook Validated self-assessment

(e) Initiate and monitor treatment where appropriate

Module 2.9: Developmental Neuropsychiatry

Preamble

Developmental NP is that branch of psychiatry concerned with the diagnosis and management of emotional, behavioral, and learning disorders that are associated with demonstrable or suspected organic brain dysfunction, and which manifest during childhood. Because these disorders are primarily disruptive to normal developmental attainments or adjustment, they are known as *neurodevelopmental* disorders. The practice of developmental NP requires skills and knowledge that encompass not only child psychiatry, in broad terms, but also pediatric neurology and learning disabilities.

Currently, there is no formal training program leading to a specific accreditation in developmental NP. In this respect, the subspecialty is in the same category as adult NP. Few child psychiatric training programs explicitly include training in developmental NP. However, it is arguable that within the clinical field of child psychiatry, neurodevelopmental disorders are now the predominant reason for specialist referral.

The competencies outlined below describe the minimum range of skills in developmental NP that should be acquired by consultant child psychiatrists in training. We recommend that all trainees have at least 1 year of experience in this specialty, but that those who intend to become specialists in this area may choose to spend additional time gaining particular skills.

Skills in Developmental Neuropsychiatry

Specific Competencies

1. Undertake clinical assessment of patients with apparent neurodevelopmental disorders

   (a) Take a developmental neuropsychiatric history

Suggested learning methods	Suggested assessment methods
Observation/modeling	Validated self-assessment
Working as a team member	In-training assessment
Supervised clinical practice	Clinical supervision
Focused training courses	Direct observation of clinical work
	Peer review
	Clinical logbook
	Clinical audit
	Case presentations
	Review of case notes and other records
	Chart-stimulated recall

   (b) Perform a neurobehavioral assessment;
   (c) Arrange for, and interpret, a neurocognitive examination;
   (d) Perform a neurological examination, and interpret signs;
   (e) Construct a neurodevelopmental differential diagnosis.

2. Undertake investigation of patients with apparent developmental neuropsychiatric disorders:

   (a) Be familiar with relevant hematological and metabolic investigations;
   (b) Be familiar with EEG recording and interpretation;
   (c) Be familiar with indications for and interpretation of structural neuroimaging.

3. Prescribe treatment to patients on basis of clinical assessment:

   (a) Be familiar with the evidence for the effectiveness of specific pharmacological treatments of common neurodevelopmental disorders;
   (b) Be familiar with the constraints on prescribing psychotropic medications to children, the indications, "approval status," and potential side effects;

(c) Be familiar with the need to undertake appropriate investigations before prescription, and the need for monitoring of treatments prescribed, to minimize side effects and complications;
(d) Be familiar with indications for nonmedical treatments including behavioral management techniques, educational interventions, skills, and training (e.g., motor, social, speech and language).

4. Work collaboratively with neuroscience colleagues:

(a) Obtain relevant information about patients' behavior from neuroscience staff;
(b) Advise neuroscience ward staff about interpretation and management of abnormal mental states and behaviors;
(c) Work collaboratively with neuroscience clinicians to establish correct diagnoses and treatment plans;
(d) Develop academic links within the neuroscience community.

Learning and Assessment Methods

1. Obtain relevant information about patients' behavior from neuroscience staff

Suggested learning methods	Suggested assessment methods
Observation/modeling	Clinical supervision
Supervised clinical practice	Direct observation

2. Advise staff about the interpretation and management of abnormal mental states and behaviors

Suggested learning methods	Suggested assessment methods
Observation/modeling	Clinical supervision
Supervised clinical practice	Direct observation

3. Work collaboratively with neuroscience colleagues to establish correct diagnosis and treatment plans

Suggested learning methods	Suggested assessment methods
Observation/modeling	Clinical supervision
Supervised clinical practice	Direct observation

4. Develop academic links with the neuroscience community

Suggested learning methods	Suggested assessment methods
Observation/modeling	Clinical supervision
Supervised clinical practice	Case presentation

5. Assess critically ill patients in a neuroscience setting

   (a) Assess the mental states of patients who are in the postoperative period or in a "neuro-critical care" setting

Suggested learning methods	Suggested assessment methods
Observation/modeling	Clinical supervision
Working as a team member	Direct observation
Supervised clinical practice	Clinical logbook
	Case presentation

   (b) Produce a differential diagnosis and formulation for patients with mental disorder in this setting

Suggested learning methods	Suggested assessment methods
Supervised clinical practice	Clinical supervision
Appropriate reading	Case presentation
	Clinical logbook

   (c) Make assessments of capacity in critically ill patients

Suggested learning methods	Suggested assessment methods
Supervised clinical practice	Clinical supervision
Observation/modeling	Case presentation

   (d) Advise on the management of disturbed behavior in critically ill patients

Suggested learning methods	Suggested assessment methods
Supervised clinical practice	Direct observation
Observation/modeling	Clinical supervision
Working as a team member	

Module 2.10: Sleep Disorders

Core competencies in assessment and management of patients with sleep disorders

Specific Competencies

Have knowledge of etiology, prevalence, diagnosis, categorization, and treatment of sleep disorders:

1. Primary insomnia
2. Secondary insomnia
3. Hypersomnias
4. Parasomnias
5. Neuropsychiatric consequences of sleep apnoea syndrome

Diagnostic Techniques

1. Take an appropriate history relevant to sleep problems.
2. Perform appropriate examination of mental, neurological, and physical status.
3. Be able to relate history and clinical findings to relevant medical, neurological, psychological, and social issues associated with etiology and treatment.
4. Have knowledge of use, reliability, and validity of generally accepted techniques and investigations for diagnostic assessment and the interpretation of results.
5. Have a basic understanding of the EEG, polysomnogram, oximetry, and actigraphy.
6. Understand the major theories of sleep mechanisms.
7. Have competence to form a differential diagnosis and to diagnose medical, neurological, and psychiatric sleep disorders and those sleep problems associated with medical, psychiatric, and neurological conditions.
8. Understand the biological, psychological, social, and economic factors that influence evaluation and management of sleep disorders.

Management

1. Formulate appropriate management plans.
2. Be familiar with therapies used [behavior therapy, psychotherapy, drug treatment, and physical treatments such as continuous positive airway pressure (CPAP)].
3. Have competence in being aware of when refer to a sleep disorders clinic.
4. Have basic knowledge relating to ethical and legal aspects of sleep medicine.

Suggested Learning Methods

1. Observation/modeling
2. Supervised clinical practice
3. Reading relevant texts
4. Peer group discussion
5. Multidisciplinary case conferences, journal clubs
6. Specific teaching from relevant health professionals (e.g., EEG, respiratory, neurology)
7. Primary responsibility for diagnosis and treatment of a reasonable number and adequate variety of patients with acute and chronic sleep disorders (e.g., at least five hypersomnia, five parasomnia, ten insomnia, of a range of ages)
8. Attendance at a respiratory sleep disorder clinic for the diagnosis of sleep apnea
9. Attendance at multidisciplinary national conferences

Suggested Assessment Methods

1. Validated self-assessment
2. Clinical supervision and feedback
3. Case presentation
4. Clinical logbook

Module 2.11: Rehabilitation Neuropsychiatry

Clinical Settings

1. Rehabilitation units providing neurophysical rehabilitation; District and/or Regional Rehabilitation Units.
2. Neuropsychiatric/Cognitive-Behavioral Rehabilitation Units for people with brain injury.
3. Neuropsychiatry/liaison psychiatry services to Clinical Neurosciences Centres, General District Hospitals, and nursing homes and other residential units.
4. Neuropsychiatry/liaison psychiatry outpatient clinics.

Knowledge

1. Of the pathophysiology of common causes of acquired brain injury.
2. Of brain–behavior relationships, in particular, following acquired focal lesions to the brain and diffuse brain injury.
3. Of the neuropsychiatric sequelae of acquired brain injury, including etiology and management of symptoms.
4. Of the principles of cognitive behavior therapy and behavior therapy for behavioral problems and other symptoms following brain injury.
5. Of the ICIDH (International Classification of Impairments, Disabilities, and Handicaps) model of impairment, disability, and handicap (impairment, activities, and participation).
6. Of outcome measures suitable for patients with acquired brain injury.
7. Of rehabilitation service provision, organization, and funding, including voluntary sector provision.

Skills

1. To undertake an assessment to understand the role of brain injury in neuropsychiatric symptom formation.
2. To assess the role of psychological processes and mental illness in symptom formation after acquired brain injury.
3. To use pharmacotherapy to manage neuropsychiatric symptoms after acquired brain injury.

4. To work with the MDT, including psychologists and other therapists, to produce an overall treatment strategy for symptoms.
5. To interpret neuropsychometric test results sufficiently to produce a neuropsychiatric formulation.
6. To set up, in collaboration with the MDT, a program of therapy based on goal planning.
7. To work alongside psychologists, behavioral nurse therapists, and others to implement cognitive-behavioral treatments and behavioral treatments.
8. To set up effective aftercare following inpatient rehabilitation, based on good communication across health services, social services, statutory services, and voluntary sector.
9. To undertake a risk assessment for all commonly occurring risks following acquired brain injury, and ensure that there are procedures in place to offer a reasonable risk management strategy.
10. To understand the symptoms and signs of the post-concussion syndrome and provide advice to patients following a brain injury to minimize the risk of problems on returning to work, and/or return to living in the community with family and/or carers.
11. To appreciate the psychodynamic processes that follow brain injury and other forms of disability and provide appropriate psychotherapeutic support.
12. To manage the common sequelae of brain injury, including disturbances of mood, psychotic disorders, personality change (especially associated with antisocial behavior), and reduced initiation and motivation.

Learning and Assessment Methods

1. Attending neuropsychiatric clinics, liaison assessments in rehabilitation units, general hospitals, etc.
2. Attachment to rehabilitation unit attending management rounds/ward rounds.
3. Attending postgraduate teaching programs/conferences on NP/brain injury.
4. Specific attachments to rehabilitation neuropsychologists and therapists.
5. Assessment methods: self-assessment, clinical supervision, and case presentation and clinical logbook.

Module 2.12: Forensic Neuropsychiatry

Key Competencies

1. Knowledge of organic basis of violence and of antisocial and criminal behavior.
2. Competence in the clinical assessment of individuals with violent or criminal behavior, from both biological and psychosocial perspectives.
3. Ability to intervene in the management of such behavior from a neuropsychiatric perspective, including drug management and psychosocial interventions.

4. Awareness of the ethical and medicolegal aspects of such disorders.
5. Ability to write an expert report for the court or other forensic settings.

Learning and Assessment Methods

1. Attending neuropsychiatric clinics in a forensic setting
2. Assessing patients referred for forensic reports
3. Preparation of reports under supervision
4. Attending court proceedings when medicolegal evidence presented

Acknowledgements We are grateful to the British Neuropsychiatric Association (H. Ring) and the American Neuropsychiatric Association (D. Arciniegas) for making their curricula available for use during the preparation of this document. Members of the Neuropsychiatric Section of the RANZCP made useful contributions (P. Hay, S. Starkstein, M. Hopwood, D. Velakoulis). Lauren Norton and Angie Russell assisted with manuscript preparation.

Recommended Reading

Neuropsychiatry Textbooks

1. Yudofsky SC, Hales RE (2008) Textbook of neuropsychiatry and clinical neurosciences, 5th edn. American Psychiatric Publishing, Arlington, VA
2. David A, Fleminger S, Kopelman M, Lovestone S (2009) Lishman's organic psychiatry: a textbook of neuropsychiatry. Wiley-Blackwell, London
3. Cummings JL, Mega MS (2003) Neuropsychiatry and behavioral neuroscience. Oxford University Press, New York
4. Schiffer RB, Rao SM, Fogel BS (2003) Neuropsychiatry: a comprehensive textbook, 2nd edn. Lippincott Williams & Wilkins, Baltimore
5. Coffey CE, Brumback RA (1998) Textbook of pediatric neuropsychiatry. American Psychiatric Publishing, Washington, DC
6. Coffey CE, Cummings JL (2000) Textbook of geriatric neuropsychiatry, 2nd edn. American Psychiatric Publishing, Washington, DC
7. Arciniegas DB, Beresford TP (2001) Neuropsychiatry: an introductory approach. Cambridge University Press, Cambridge
8. Sachdev P (with Keshavan M) (2010) Secondary schizophrenia. Cambridge University Press, Cambridge

Behavioral Neurology

9. M-Marsel M (2000) Principles of behavioral and cognitive neurology, 2nd edn. Oxford University Press, New York
10. Pincus JH, Tucker GJ (2003) Behavioral neurology, 4th edn. Oxford University Press, New York
11. Feinberg TE, Farah MJ (1997) Behavioral neurology and neuropsychology. McGraw-Hill, New York

12. Kirshner HS (2002) Behavioral neurology: practical science of mind and brain, 2nd edn. Butterworth-Heinemann, Boston
13. Leon-Carrion J, Giannini MJ (2001) Behavioral neurology in the elderly. CRC, Boca Raton
14. Strub RL, Black FW (1981) Neurobehavioral disorders: a clinical approach, 2nd edn. Davis, Philadelphia
15. Cummings JL, Trimble MR (2002) Concise guide to neuropsychiatry and behavioral neurology, 2nd edn. American Psychiatric Publishing, Arlington, VA
16. Trimble MR, Cummings JL (1997) Contemporary behavioral neurology (blue books of practical neurology), vol 16. Butterworth-Heinemann, Boston

Neuropsychology

17. Lezak MD, Howieson DB, Loring DW (with Hannay HJ, Fischer JS) (2004) Neuropsychological assessment, 4th edn. Oxford University Press, New York
18. Walsh K, Darby D (1999) Neuropsychology: a clinical approach, 4th edn. Churchill Livingstone, Edinburgh

Neuroscience

19. Kandel ER, Schwartz JH, Jessell TM (2000) Principles of neural sciences, 4th edn. McGraw-Hill, New York
20. Squire LR, Bloom FE, Spitzer NC, du Lac S, Ghosh A, Berg D (2008) Fundamental neuroscience, 3rd edn. Academic, Burlington

General Neuropsychiatric Education

21. Sachdev P (2002) Neuropsychiatry: a discipline for the future. J Psychosom Res 53:625–627 (Editorial)
22. Sachdev P (2005) Whither neuropsychiatry? J Neuropsychiatry Clin Neurosci 17:140–144
23. Price BH, Adams RD, Coyle JT (2000) Neurology and psychiatry: closing the great divide. Neurology 54:8–14
24. ANPA Standards for Fellowship Training in Neuropsychiatry (2001) I. Definition of neuropsychiatry. http://www.neuropsychiatry.com/ANPA
25. Accreditation Council on Graduate Medical Education (2001) Program requirements for training in psychiatry. http://www.acgme.org/RRC/Psy_Req2.asp
26. Accreditation Council on Graduate Medical Education (2002) Program requirements for training in neurology. http://www.acgme.org/RRC/Psy_Req2.asp
27. American Board of Psychiatry and Neurology, Inc (2003) Information for applicants for certification in the subspecialties of addiction psychiatry, clinical neurophysiology, forensic psychiatry, geriatric psychiatry, and neurodevelopmental disabilities. http://www.abpn.com/Downloads/2003subspec_ifa.pdf
28. Academy of Psychosomatic Medicine (1998) Standards for fellowship training in consultation-liaison psychiatry. http://www.apm.org/fellow.html

Index

V

W